Skills for **Midwifery Practice**

For Elsevier

Commissioning Editor: Mairi McCubbin
Development Editor: Carole McMurray
Project Manager: Frances Affleck
Senior Designer: Charles Gray

Skills for Midwifery Practice

THIRD EDITION

Ruth Johnson (now Bowen) BA (Hons) RGN RM
Clinical Midwife; Formerly Senior
Lecturer Midwifery, University of
Hertfordshire, Hatfield, UK

Wendy Taylor BSc (Hons) MSc RN RM
Clinical Midwife, Whangarei,
New Zealand; Formerly Senior Lecturer
Midwifery, University of Hertfordshire,
Hatfield, UK

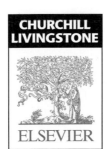

CHURCHILL LIVINGSTONE

ELSEVIER

Edinburgh   London   New York   Oxford   Philadelphia   St Louis   Sydney   Toronto   2010

CHURCHILL
LIVINGSTONE
ELSEVIER

First published 2000
Second edition 2006
Third edition 2010
  Reprinted 2010

1006312092

ISBN 9780702031465

British Library Cataloguing in Publication Data
A catalogue record for this book is available from the British Library.

Library of Congress Cataloging in Publication Data
A catalog record for this book is available from the Library of Congress.

ELSEVIER your source for books, journals and multimedia in the health sciences
www.elsevierhealth.com

Working together to grow
libraries in developing countries
www.elsevier.com | www.bookaid.org | www.sabre.org

ELSEVIER   BOOK AID International   Sabre Foundation

The Publisher's policy is to use paper manufactured from sustainable forests

Printed in China

Contents

Contents

Preface

Welcome to the third edition of this text. On each occasion when we rewrite the book we are surprised at just how much new material has been published and, on this occasion, how much is still ongoing. We have several times encouraged you to seek out findings that will be published in the near future. All of this, we hope, will contribute to the best available care for women, babies and their families. As midwives and educators, it is also our personal hope that midwives, too, will find enjoyment and satisfaction in their roles, knowing that their contribution is to individuals and society. We trust that this text contributes to this, both in the UK and in other parts of the world.

As in previous editions, we acknowledge the contribution of all midwives, whatever their gender. However, purely for the purposes of clarity, this text considers midwives to be female and babies to be male. We are also aware that there are many more skills that midwives utilise than are featured here. Some of them are implied, e.g. communication, rather than featured. There are frequent encouragements to 'gain informed consent', this is a standardised way of noting the significance of good communication that allows the woman/parents to make decisions following a full, open and honest conveying of the facts for their consideration.

Student midwives will be able to undertake many of the skills detailed in this text, but with overseeing and guidance from qualified midwives. This is particularly the case for the countersigning of records and for actions such as 'Document the findings and act accordingly'. In taking action with regard to a particular response it is the midwife who carries the responsibility and so acts according to knowledge, experience, local and national protocols.

It's our hope that you'll enjoy reading and using this text as much as we have enjoyed writing it, will be challenged by it and will find that your practice is developed yet further!

Todmorden &
Whangarei, 2009

Ruth Johnson
(now Bowen)
Wendy Taylor

Acknowledgements

The authors gratefully acknowledge the unstinting support of family and friends, namely, for Ruth Bowen: Robbie, Hannah, Daniel, Jean and Harold, and for Wendy Taylor: Ian, Helen, Ann, John and Jade.

We are also grateful for the professional and technical support from the library staff at the Calderdale and Huddersfield NHS Trust (both hospital sites); Stephen Rowley & Patricia Fernandes at ANTT, University College London Hospitals NHS Foundation Trust; Dr Suzanne Colson, Canterbury Christ Church University; Carole McMurray & Mairi McCubbin at Elsevier; and for the photographic skills of Ian Taylor in providing photographs on which some of the illustrations are based.

Principles of abdominal examination: during pregnancy and labour

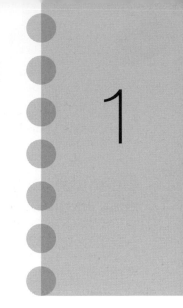

1

Maternity care is changing. According to the National Institute for Health and Clinical Excellence (NICE 2008), the emphasis is moving from the woman having 'lots done to her' to a much more holistic approach in which psychological and social issues are prioritized with physical care. This means that skills such as palpating the abdomen in the antenatal period are perhaps undertaken less often, but that they nevertheless remain skills that midwives need to maintain. This chapter considers the skill of abdominal examination, what is learned from it and how it is undertaken both antenatally and during labour.

Routine antenatal auscultation of the fetal heart is no longer recommended, but it is a much needed skill when caring for a labouring woman and it *is* needed for aspects of non-routine antenatal care. This chapter discusses the use of a Pinard stethoscope, fetal Doppler and cardiotocograph (CTG). Some of what is described overlaps with labour care and so should be read in conjunction with Chapters 30, 31 and the glossary. The final part of the chapter considers the other aspect of abdominal examination in labour, that of palpating uterine activity.

LEARNING OUTCOMES

Having read this chapter the reader should be able to:

- discuss the indications for abdominal examination in pregnancy and labour
- discuss the different components of an abdominal examination, indicating the nature of the information sought and the rationale for it
- describe the ways in which the fetal heart can be auscultated
- explain the indications for using a CTG, how it is applied and how to interpret the tracing

- describe the criteria used to identify normal, suspicious and pathological CTG tracings
- describe how uterine contractions are palpated in labour, why this is undertaken and the significance of the findings
- explain the midwife's role and responsibilities in relation to each of these aspects of care.

Antenatal abdominal examination

Undertaking an abdominal examination antenatally has historically sought to:

- assess fetal growth, size, wellbeing, position and presentation
- detect deviations from the norm.

However, in the climate of evidence-based best practice, NICE (2008) considers some of these aims to be questionable. Fetal wellbeing is more likely to be assessed by discussions about the fetal movements than it is by listening to the fetal heart for 1 minute. Equally, the position and presentation of the fetus have little bearing on care until the end of pregnancy, when labour is approaching. Consequently, the recommended components (NICE 2008) for abdominal examination are:

- the measuring and recording of symphysis fundal height on each occasion from 24 weeks gestation
- assessment for fetal presentation at and after 36 weeks.

It is likely that multiparous women in particular, having had prior experience, will expect to have a thorough abdominal examination at much earlier gestations than 36 weeks. Women are often reassured to hear the fetal heart and to know which way the 'baby' (fetus) is lying. The skill of abdominal palpation increases with both knowledge and experience and, whereas the current requirements in pregnancy are limited, the authors recognise the need to maintain the skill (for the times when it is much needed) or lose it! As with all guidelines, the midwife will exercise her clinical judgement and might, at times, need to deviate from them.

Indications

- At antenatal assessments after 24 weeks of pregnancy, adapted according to gestation.
- Prior to auscultation of the fetal heart and use of CTG equipment.

- Before a vaginal examination.
- Throughout labour.

Contraindications

As the uterus can be stimulated when this examination is performed, it should be undertaken cautiously when there is:

- placental abruption
- preterm labour.

Abdominal examination: principles

The assessment begins by appreciating the woman – how she is looking, feeling, coping and what she reveals in conversation. A woman who describes lots of indigestion, some breathlessness and 'the baby right under her ribs' might cause the midwife to begin wondering whether the fetus is a breech presentation, for example.

Informed consent should be obtained for palpation. Olsen (1999) discovered that women didn't like palpation and thereafter made efforts to explain the procedure, to seek permission before doing anything and to ensure greater comfort. Explanations should be given during and after the examination, there should be full discussion of the findings, contemporaneous documentation and explanations as to what has been written. These are some of the ways in which women can experience greater empowerment.

Although the midwife should have clean hands, other standard precautions are unlikely to be necessary as contact with body fluids does not occur. Care should be taken to ensure that aortocaval occlusion is avoided and the woman should be encouraged to empty her bladder. She should be comfortable, in a private location and her dignity should be maintained throughout. A woman might choose to have others present or absent and she needs to know that she has the option to cease the examination if she so desires.

Visual appearance of the abdomen

The visual appearance of the abdomen can influence the midwife's findings and add to the holistic care offered:

- Size: may be affected by obesity, lax abdominal muscles, multiple pregnancy, poly- and oligohydramnios, fetal size and lie, uterine fibroids and the gestation period.
- Shape: may give an indication of the fetal position or presentation, e.g. a dip at the umbilicus can be indicative of an occipitoposterior position.
- Skin changes: linea nigra, striae gravidarum, signs of previous abdominal surgery, presence of rash or itching.
- Fetal movements may be seen.
- Signs of potential domestic violence may be observed.

Assessing the uterine fundus

Using the hands on the abdomen, the uterine fundus can be located. Using the hand nearest to the woman, the pads of the fingers are placed on the abdomen below the xiphisternum and moved gently downwards until the firmness of the fundus is felt. As the fetus grows, so does the uterus, making the fundal height a possible indicator as to fetal growth. The presence of a fetal pole in the fundus (e.g. buttocks) is confirmatory of what is suspected as the presenting part.

The height of the fundus can be affected by several maternal factors, including size, parity and a full bladder. Fundal height can be assessed in two ways,

although neither is considered to have absolute reliability (Rosser 2000):

1. using a traditional set of indicators that consider landmarks on the abdomen (Fig. 1.1)
2. measuring with a tape measure.

Neilson (1998) undertook a Cochrane review of the value of measuring the symphysis fundal height. He concluded that there was not enough evidence to evaluate its use. Other studies consider that when plotted on customized growth charts it has some (but still limited) predictive value (Gardosi & Francis 1999, Wright et al 2006). NICE (2008) recommends that each woman has the fundal height measurement recorded and plotted at each consultation from 24 weeks gestation.

Measuring the symphysis fundal height

A disposable tape measure is used to measure in centimetres (cm): 0 cm is placed scale down on the upper border of the symphysis pubis, the tape measure is placed smoothly straight along the midline of the abdomen, to the top of the fundus. Once the top of the fundus is confirmed the tape measure is held securely, turned over and the number of centimetres read. The fundal height in centimetres generally equates with the weeks of gestation; a margin of error of ± 2 cm is generally permitted, but this

Figure 1.1 • Fundal height at different stages of pregnancy

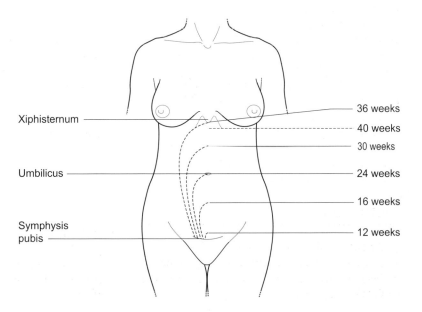

Xiphisternum

Umbilicus

Symphysis pubis

36 weeks
40 weeks
30 weeks
24 weeks
16 weeks
12 weeks

will depend on local protocols. A fundal height inconsistent with gestation may indicate:

- unreliable landmarks, e.g. long abdomen
- inaccurate dates
- that the fetus is larger or smaller than expected
- that the amount of amniotic fluid might be greater or lesser than expected
- multiple pregnancy
- abnormal lie, e.g. transverse
- uterine mass, e.g. fibroid, cyst or tumour
- poor technique
- intrauterine death.

NICE (2008) recommends that, until 36 weeks gestation, it is not necessary to offer routine abdominal palpation, considering that it is only from this gestation that the information is of clinical value.

Presentation of the fetus

Assessing the presentation

The fundus is located as described above. The palmar surfaces of both hands are used to palpate and identify the fetal pole (Fig. 1.2):

- buttocks: feel softer, less ballotable, bulkier, less clearly defined
- head: feels firmer, more rounded and ballotable, i.e. can be moved gently from side to side.

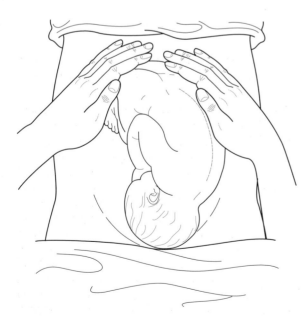

Figure 1.2 • Fundal palpation

If a pole is not located in the fundus, the lie is not longitudinal (see Fig. 1.3); the lateral palpation (below) will then identify the position.

Pelvic palpation (Fig. 1.4) assesses the presentation, i.e. the part of the fetus lying in the lower segment of the uterus or at the pelvic brim, and then determines:

- if the fetus is flexed
- if any of the presenting part has engaged in the pelvis
- how 'mobile', or moveable, the presenting part is if it has not engaged.

There are five main presentations (Fig. 1.5) and two methods of undertaking pelvic palpation:

1. Using both hands, one either side of the presentation (fingers facing towards the woman's feet), press in gently. The presentation can be felt beneath the hands, as described for fundal palpation and identified according to its features (Fig. 1.4A). It is helpful if the woman can take a deep breath and hold it for a moment while the hands are able to feel deeply around the presentation.
2. Pawlik's manoeuvre can be considered. Using one hand with fingers facing the woman's head, the presenting pole is held between the fingers and thumb (Fig. 1.4B). This should be done very gently, as it is uncomfortable for the woman. Ideally it is avoided.

Engagement into the pelvis is assessed according to the passage of the widest transverse diameter through the pelvic brim. In a cephalic presentation this is the biparietal diameter (9.5 cm). Engagement is generally measured in fifths; for example, a cephalic presentation that is 3/5 palpable has 3/5 of the head palpable out of the pelvis, indicating that 2/5 of the head has passed through the pelvic brim into the pelvis; 1/5 palpable would mean 4/5 has engaged, and so on. When 3/5 of the head has passed through the pelvic brim the presentation is 'engaged'. A non-engaged presentation may be referred to as 'free' or 'at the brim' and may necessitate referral at term, particularly for the primigravid woman.

Position of the fetus

An abdominal examination is often undertaken as one seamless procedure for which the midwife may alter the 'order' accordingly. Many midwives

Figure 1.3 • The lie of the fetus

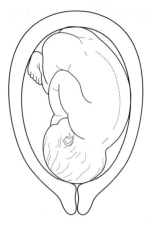

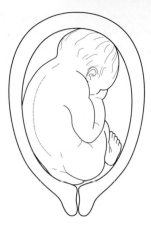

Longitudinal

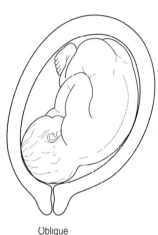

Oblique

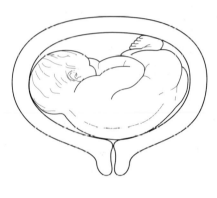

Transverse

will begin at the fundus, undertake the lateral palpation and end with the pelvic palpation.

Lateral palpation assesses the main body of the uterus to identify the fetal position. It combines with the fundal and pelvic palpations to confirm the lie. It also gives information about the fetal size, volume of amniotic fluid, uterine tone and fetal movements.

The fetal spine is usually firmer and smoother; the limbs on the opposing side are less regularly defined, with that side of the uterus being softer. There are two methods of undertaking lateral palpation:

1. The hands are placed one on either side of the uterus at about umbilical level: support one side of the uterus while the other hand progresses down the length of the uterus (Fig. 1.6); palpate the other side of the uterus in the same way.

2. 'Walk' both hands across the uterus from side to side, from the fundus to the symphysis pubis (Fig. 1.7).

The lie of the fetus is determined by the relationship of the long axis of the fetal spine to the long axis of the maternal uterus. The lie is normally longitudinal, but can be oblique or transverse (Fig. 1.3).

With a longitudinal lie, the position of the fetal spine indicates the position of the fetal head. The position is defined according to the approximation of the fetal denominator (occiput for cephalic presentation) to a pelvic landmark. Figure 1.8 indicates the relevant landmarks on the pelvic brim. For example, if the occiput is in apposition with the iliopectineal eminence of the pelvis, it is described as occipitoanterior (Fig. 1.9). It is further defined according to whether it is on the maternal left or right. If the occiput is in apposition with the sacroiliac joint, it is described as

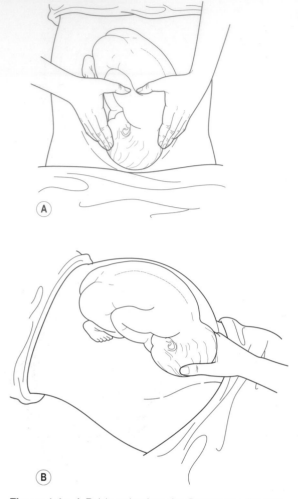

Figure 1.4 • A Pelvic palpation: the fingers are directed inwards and downwards. B Pawlik's manoeuvre

occipitoposterior. For occipitolateral the occiput is found midway on the iliopectineal line (Fig. 1.9). If the denominator were the sacrum (breech presentation) the same pelvic landmarks apply, and the terminology would be right or left sacroanterior, etc.

Abdominal examination in labour

This may be more uncomfortable for the woman and harder to do when the uterus is contracting regularly, but is an aspect of care that supports and informs other aspects of care, for example, vaginal assessments, indicators of maternal and fetal wellbeing. The midwife should ensure that the procedure is not undertaken unnecessarily and is completed promptly. The examination should be undertaken between contractions, to minimise discomfort and make it easier to palpate the fetus.

This procedure requires the woman to be in an almost recumbent position, which is not ideal for labour. Thus the midwife should ensure that the woman is encouraged to adopt a more upright position following the examination, whenever possible. It is indicated:

- To gain a baseline on which care is provided and subsequent progress assessed, by determining the gestation, lie, position, presentation, engagement and auscultation of the fetal heart.
- To monitor progress by assessing descent and rotation of the presenting part.
- Prior to auscultation of the fetal heart or commencing monitoring using CTG.
- Prior to undertaking an examination *per vaginam*.
- Multiple births, following delivery of each baby, to determine the lie, position and presentation of the remaining fetuses.

Documentation

The findings from the abdominal palpation should be recorded in the relevant documentation, which should include the antenatal/labour obstetric/midwifery notes, the partogram and CTG [Nursing and Midwifery Council (NMC) 2005]; the NMC (2005) states that abbreviations should not be used. Observations and actions undertaken should include:

- the woman's comments and observations
- fundal height (cm)
- if undertaken: the fetal lie, position, presentation and degree of engagement
- presence of fetal movements
- if undertaken: the fetal heart rate and equipment used
- any additional information, e.g. contractions, amniotic fluid volume, observations on inspection.

Any deviations from the norm should be reported to the appropriate personnel (NMC 2004).

PROCEDURE: abdominal examination

- Establish the woman's health and wellbeing, discuss her thoughts e.g. fetal movements, growth, possible position.
- Gain informed consent and ensure privacy.

Figure 1.5 • Five presentations of the fetus

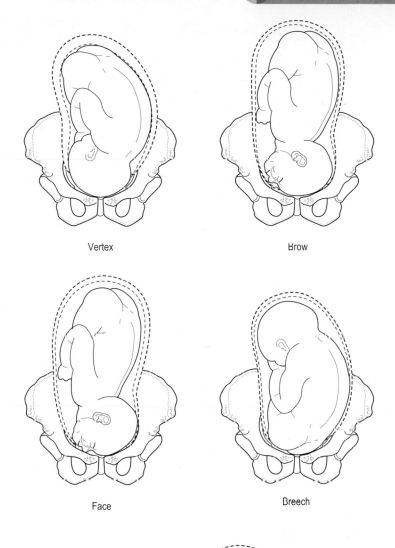

Vertex

Brow

Face

Breech

Shoulder

- Gather equipment:
  - single-use tape measure
  - if needed, Pinard stethoscope, watch with a second hand, sonicaid, gel and tissues
  - sheet
  - antenatal/labour record.

- Encourage the woman to empty her bladder.
- Ask the woman to adopt an almost recumbent position (use a wedge to avoid aortocaval occlusion if necessary), with her knees slightly bent and her arms by her side. Cover her legs with the sheet.
- Wash hands.

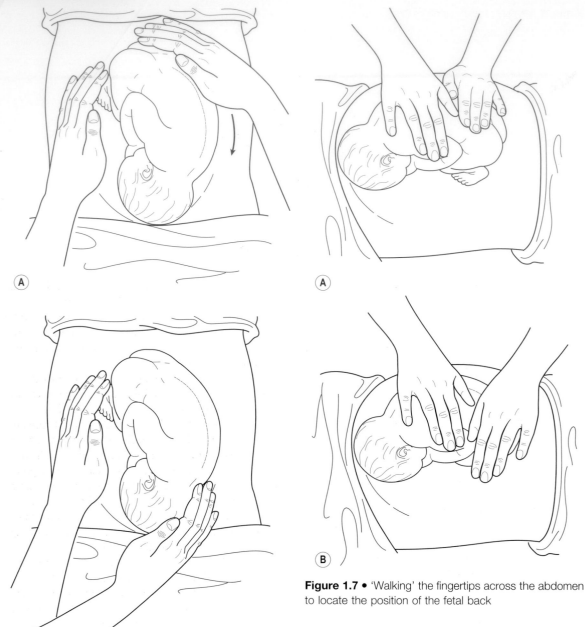

Figure 1.6 • Lateral palpation. One side of the uterus is supported as the other hand progresses down the uterus. Both sides are palpated in this way

Figure 1.7 • 'Walking' the fingertips across the abdomen to locate the position of the fetal back

- Expose and inspect the abdomen, ensuring that her legs and upper torso remain covered.
- Undertake fundal palpation and use the tape measure to assess symphysis fundal height, undertake lateral and pelvic palpations (if gestation >36 weeks) (all described above).
- If requested or indicated, auscultate the fetal heart (described below) using watch and Pinard stethoscope while simultaneously palpating the maternal radial pulse; use the Doppler to allow the woman to hear also/apply CTG monitor.
- Replace the clothing, assist the woman into a comfortable position and discuss the findings.
- Document the findings and act accordingly.

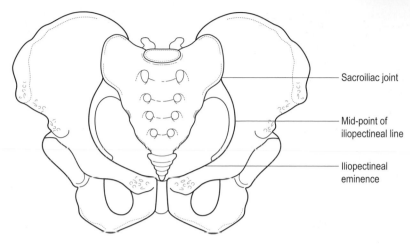

Sacroiliac joint

Mid-point of
iliopectineal line

Iliopectineal
eminence

Figure 1.8 • Relevant landmarks on the pelvic brim

Auscultation of the fetal heart

As suggested earlier, if the fetal movements are present, then there is limited value that can be gained from auscultating the fetal heart on a routine antenatal visit. However, auscultation:

* should be undertaken prior to the application of a CTG monitor
* is necessary throughout labour to monitor fetal reaction and wellbeing: this may be undertaken intermittently (Pinard stethoscope or Doppler) or continuously using electronic fetal monitoring. If using intermittent monitoring NICE (2007) recommend that the fetal heart is auscultated for at least 1 minute (after a contraction) every 15 minutes in the first stage of labour, every 5 minutes in the second stage of labour. The average is recorded and maternal pulse is assessed simultaneously
* can determine fetal life in the event of absence of fetal movements
* is often reassuring to the mother and can anecdotally aid parent/child bonding.

It is easier to auscultate the fetal heart by first having undertaken an abdominal palpation (described above). Locating the fetal presentation and position indicates where the equipment should be placed on the woman's abdomen to hear the fetal heart. Blindly placing the equipment on the abdomen can raise anxieties in the midwife and mother if the fetal heart is not immediately located.

The clearest fetal heart sounds are heard through the fetal shoulder (scapula). They can sometimes be heard through the chest wall, depending on the fetal position. The sound is a rapid double beating (often rather like a tapping sound) between 110 and 160 beats per minute (bpm). Changes in the rate occur with fetal movements and both regularity and variability can be heard too.

Using a Pinard stethoscope allows the midwife to confirm that it is the fetal heart that has been heard: electrical equipment can confuse the fetal and maternal heart rates. The midwife should palpate the maternal radial pulse while listening to the fetal heart to ensure that the fetal heart has been heard. Using the Pinard stethoscope is a learned and practised skill; Wickham (2002a) agrees and encourages lots of practice. It can be used from 24 weeks gestation but many midwives would not use one until 28 weeks gestation. A smaller fetus that is moving significantly can be hard to 'stabilize' and therefore listen to. This is true for any auscultatory equipment.

Wickham (2002b) suggests that variability is assessed using a Pinard stethoscope by counting the beats over a series of 5-second intervals. A difference for each 5-second observation indicates changing variability; no change may indicate fetal sleep and so auscultation should be repeated later. Up to 40 minutes of decreased variability is acceptable, longer than this constitutes a deviation from the norm.

There are some maternal positions that make Pinard use difficult or impossible (on all fours or very upright, particularly as the fetus descends in the second stage of labour). A Doppler ultrasound may be used instead on these occasions, or the woman may be prepared to adjust her position for a short while.

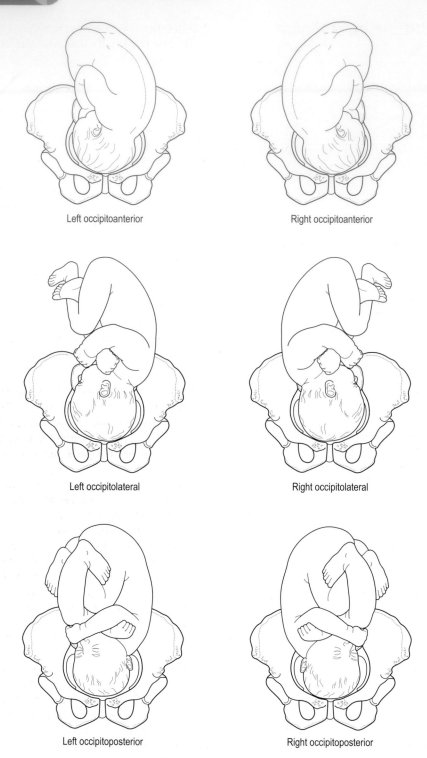

Left occipitoanterior

Right occipitoanterior

Left occipitolateral

Right occipitolateral

Left occipitoposterior

Right occipitoposterior

Figure 1.9 • Six positions in a vertex presentation

PROCEDURE: using a Pinard stethoscope

- Undertake abdominal examination.
- Place the Pinard stethoscope over the area where heart sounds are expected (Fig. 1.10).
- Place the ear over the hole and remove the hand so that the ear, stethoscope and abdomen are in direct contact (this increases the sound variance); gentle pressure is needed.
- Listen and count the fetal heart for 1 minute; simultaneously palpate the woman's radial pulse (see Chapter 4).
- Discuss the results with the woman.
- Document the findings and act accordingly.

Use of the sonicaid

A fetal Doppler (sometimes called a sonicaid) can also be used to auscultate the fetal heart. One advantage of using a Doppler is that the woman can hear the sounds too and be reassured. It can detect the fetal heart at earlier gestations than a Pinard stethoscope. The midwife should always be alert to the possibility of an absent fetal heart and therefore may choose to confirm its presence with a Pinard stethoscope first. The sonicaid often needs to be placed directly over the fetal shoulder in order to hear the fetal heart. Sometimes less pressure is needed on the abdomen than with a Pinard and it is possible to use one whatever the woman's position, including in water. Other sounds (swooshing of uterine vessels, fetal hiccoughs, fetal movements, etc.) all need explaining to listening parents.

PROCEDURE: using a fetal Doppler

- Undertake abdominal examination and auscultate fetal heart using a Pinard stethoscope.
- Lubricate the Doppler probe with a suitable conductive gel.
- Place the sonicaid over the area where heart sounds are expected.
- Count the heart beat for 1 minute (some sonicaids give a digital reading) while simultaneously counting the maternal pulse.
- Reassure the woman about the other sounds that can be heard.

- Wipe the gel off with a tissue.
- Discuss the results with the woman.
- Document the findings and act accordingly.

Cardiotocography

CTG – also known as electronic fetal monitoring (EFM) – has increased the maternal intervention rates, but with no reduction in perinatal mortality or cerebral palsy (NICE 2007). Low-risk women should not be offered CTG antenatally or in labour; it is unproven, and is offered to women only with potential or existing risk factors (NICE 2007). These include (not an exhaustive list):

- a reduction in fetal movements
- preterm labour, significant meconium-stained liquor, ante- or intrapartum bleeding, use of oxytocin
- on maternal request
- abnormalities found on intermittent auscultation (bradycardia, tachycardia or decelerations)
- maternal pyrexia
- other fetuses at risk: small for gestational age, multiple pregnancy, diabetes and pre-eclampsia.

CTG should be used twice weekly for gestations >42 weeks and for 30 minutes after the establishment of epidural analgesia and after each bolus top up.

CTG monitors vary, but the principles are that the fetal heart and uterine pressure can be monitored abdominally or within the uterus (Fig. 1.11); commonly, both are monitored abdominally. Electrical interference can occur, the most likely source for this being the use of a transcutaneous electrical nerve stimulation (TENS) machine. The heart rate and uterine activity are printed on graph paper, the monitor should run according to local protocol, often 1 cm per minute. The actual pressure changes in the uterus do not equate exactly with the printed strength of contractions, and so electronic monitoring should not replace the regular assessment of uterine activity by the midwife. As the fetus moves, there can be loss of contact, which might be accompanied by an increase in the heart rate. The length of time that the monitor is left *in situ* will depend on the condition of the woman and fetus, allowing sufficient time to make an assessment of normality.

Mandatory updating is often undertaken for the use and interpretation of CTG. The midwife should

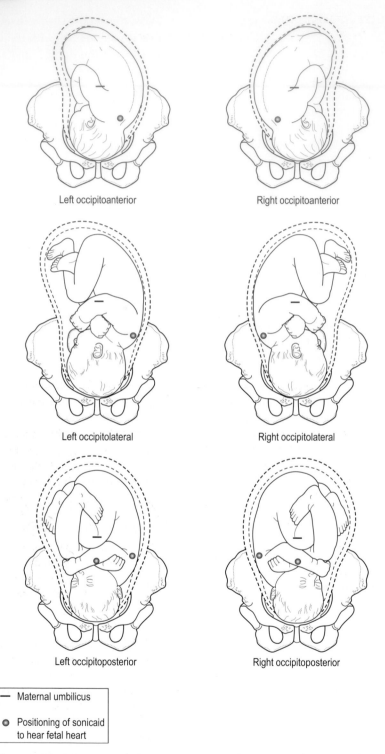

Left occipitoanterior

Right occipitoanterior

Left occipitolateral

Right occipitolateral

Left occipitoposterior

Right occipitoposterior

— Maternal umbilicus

● Positioning of sonicaid to hear fetal heart

Figure 1.10 • The approximate points of the fetal heart sounds with a vertex presentation

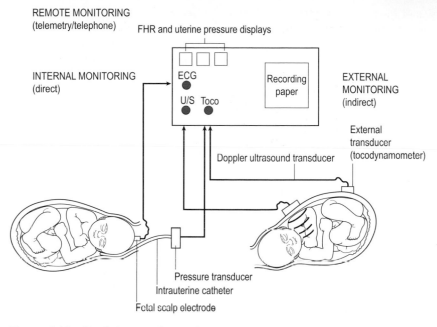

REMOTE MONITORING
(telemetry/telephone)

FHR and uterine pressure displays

INTERNAL MONITORING
(direct)

ECG

Recording
paper

U/S   Toco

EXTERNAL
MONITORING
(indirect)

External
transducer
(tocodynamometer)

Doppler ultrasound transducer

Pressure transducer
Intrauterine catheter
Fetal scalp electrode

Figure 1.11 • Cardiotocography monitor

ensure that the equipment is used, stored, cleaned and maintained correctly. The Medicines and Healthcare Products Regulatory Agency (MHRA 2002) indicates that errors have occurred in which the fetus was stillborn, despite the monitor providing a tracing of wellbeing. The maternal pulse should always be assessed alongside the fetal heart rate to ensure that they are different.

According to NICE (2007), fetal blood sampling should be available when CTG is in use to assist with any decisions about early delivery. However, this is questionable; Alfirevic et al (2006) found that the presence of fetal blood sampling made no difference to neonatal outcome.

PROCEDURE: application of the CTG monitor

- Gain and record informed consent; invite the woman to empty her bladder.
- Undertake maternal observations: temperature, blood pressure and pulse.
- Undertake an abdominal examination and auscultation of the fetal heart using a Pinard stethoscope (pp 6 & 11).
- Position the woman in a sitting or semi-recumbent position; her position may be changed

once the monitor has been applied. Ensure the two belts are in position and that the woman is sufficiently covered.
- Apply gel to the ultrasound transducer.
- Place the transducer over the area where heart sounds are expected; the signal should indicate that the positioning is good.
- Secure the transducer in position using an abdominal belt. Reassess the maternal pulse to ensure that the two are different.
- Place the tocodynamometer on the fundus of the uterus; secure it with an abdominal belt.
- Adjust the toco setting on the machine (with the uterus relaxed) to 0 mmHg, unless set automatically or local protocol suggests a different figure.
- Start the paper printing (1 cm per minute); document the date, woman's name and ID number, time commenced, indication for monitoring, all of the maternal observations and any other relevant details on the trace, e.g. epidural analgesia, oxytocin, etc. Sign and print name.
- Establish that any automatic printing of data (e.g. time, date) is correct.
- Encourage the woman to record fetal movements. Ensure that she understands the

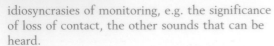

idiosyncrasies of monitoring, e.g. the significance of loss of contact, the other sounds that can be heard.

- Record the indication and commencement of the monitoring in the records with date, time and signature.
- Ensure that anyone else who reviews the trace should sign with the date, time and findings both on the trace and in the records.
- Remove the monitor when satisfied that the tracing is within normal limits. Wipe the gel off the abdomen.
- Sign and store correctly the tracing, record completion of the monitoring and the indications for care. If birth has occurred, the date, time and mode of delivery should also be recorded on the tracing.
- Discuss the results with the woman.
- Clean, restock and store the equipment correctly.

Cardiotocograph interpretation

CTG interpretation begins with knowledge of the woman's history and current clinical profile and that the monitor has been correctly applied. Changes of maternal position, vomiting, vaginal examination, epidural analgesia and other such variables should be noted and considered. The absence/presence of uterine contractions should be noted for their frequency, strength and length. The fetal heart tracing is assessed (in conjunction with uterine activity) by the:

- Baseline rate: this should be between 110 and 160 bpm and is the rate to which the fetal heart returns after accelerations or decelerations. It is determined over a period of 5–10 minutes (between contractions if in labour).
- Baseline variability: a variation in heart rate of between 5 and 15 bpm over a 10- to 20-second period of time, assessed by subtracting the lowest number of beats from the highest number. Variability can be reduced when the fetus is asleep. This is acceptable for up to 40 minutes; reduced variability for longer than this is suspicious. Variability is an important part of assessing the fetus. If variability is unclear using the abdominal transducer, a fetal scalp electrode can be considered.
- Accelerations: a rise in the heart rate of 15 bpm from the baseline over a 15-second period at

least; a reactive trace should include two or more accelerations over a 20-minute period.

- Decelerations: the heart rate decelerates from the baseline, often 15 bpm and lasting for 10 seconds or more; the depth and time of recovery are observed in conjunction with the timing of the contractions. Often obvious but sometimes very subtle.

A CTG is described as being 'reassuring' when the baseline and variability are within normal limits, there are accelerations and no decelerations (NICE 2007). A reassuring CTG is also a normal one (Fig. 1.12).

In labour, decelerations are currently defined as:

- Early: decelerations occur with the contraction, often associated with head compression during the second stage of labour, with the peak of the contraction mirroring the nadir of the deceleration.
- Variable: the timing and shape are variable; the fetal heart usually accelerates before and after the deceleration before returning to the baseline – referred to as 'shouldering' – distinguished by a rapid fall and return to the baseline, often a result of cord compression.
- Late: decelerations occur after the onset of the contraction, and recovery takes place after the end of the contraction, often a result of reduced uteroplacental blood flow. Some decelerations are subtle, particularly if they are shallow with reduced variability.
- Prolonged: occurring at any time, there is a significant decrease in heart rate for more than 2 minutes; the fetus might be compromised and delivery is generally indicated.

A CTG is classified as 'non-reassuring' when:

- the baseline is 100–109 or 161–180 bpm
- the variability is <5 for 40–90 minutes
- there are typical variable decelerations with more than half of the contractions over 1½ hours *or*
- there is a single prolonged deceleration for up to 2 minutes.

The presence of one feature from the above non-reassuring list, with all other features being reassuring, would make the tracing suspicious.

A pathological CTG has two or more non-reassuring features (above) and one or more abnormal features. 'Abnormal features' are:

- a baseline rate of <100 bpm, >180 bpm or a sinusoidal rhythm for >10 minutes

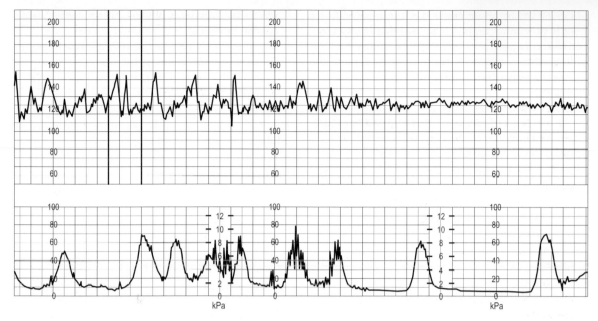

Figure 1.12 • A reassuring cardiotocography (CTG): baseline and variability are within normal limits, there are accelerations and no decelerations. This CTG shows a period of fetal activity, followed by sleep

- variability <5 bpm for 1½ hours
- atypical variable or late decelerations with more than half of the contractions for ½ hour *or*
- single prolonged deceleration for more than 3 minutes.

(adapted from NICE 2007)

CTG interpretation is a skill for which even experienced practitioners vary in their opinions. Categories such as the ones described above aim to give a working guide that encourages referral should any suspicions occur.

Palpation of uterine contractions

The second aspect of abdominal assessment during ante/intrapartum care is that of assessing uterine activity. Antenatally, many women experience the painless tightenings known as Braxton Hicks contractions. These may occasionally be palpated while undertaking an abdominal assessment; the midwife should be able to distinguish between these and the contractions of labour, both to reassure the woman and to inform clinical care. Women who present in preterm labour might not always appreciate that the uterus is contracting, commonly experiencing

the discomfort as backache or constipation. The midwife should always be alert to the signs of uterine contraction whatever the gestation.

When beginning or established in labour, the midwife uses the information gained from the palpation of contractions to assess progress and to inform care, e.g. to aid the appropriate use of Entonox (see Chapter 24). Contraction of the fibres of the myometrium causes the uterus to become firm. These contractions begin and end in the fundus, sweeping down over and back up the uterus. This makes the fundus the best place to detect the contraction occurring and fading away. Contractions can be palpated through the abdominal wall; their length and frequency can be determined with relative accuracy (this is a learned skill), although the strength is somewhat more subjective. The resting tone of the uterus is also observed by assessing the tone of the uterus between the contractions. The abdomen should be soft when the uterus is at rest.

As the labour progresses, it would be expected that the length, strength and frequency of contractions would increase. The midwife assesses this by palpation of the uterine fundus along with all the other signs of progress seen in the reactions and observations of the woman. As with other examinations, the findings are not taken in isolation, but form part of an overall assessment. Cardiotocography may aid some of the observations, i.e. the frequency and length of contractions if the tocodynamometer is set to record appropriately, but the midwife should still be sure of what is happening by palpation. This is particularly true when assessing contraction strength (the monitor may not detect this accurately), if the woman has epidural analgesia and if using oxytocics to induce or augment labour. Excessive contraction (>5 in 10 minutes) requires the administration of oxytocics to be reduced.

Indications

- To assess progress of labour in relation to the length, strength and frequency of the uterine contractions.
- Correct administration of Entonox (see Chapter 24).
- During the second stage of labour: if the woman is being guided when to push, e.g. with epidural analgesia.
- During active management of the third stage of labour: to determine if the uterus is contracted prior to undertaking controlled cord traction to deliver the placenta and membranes (see Chapter 32).

Contraindications

- An incorrect technique can lead to stimulating the uterus unnecessarily. Palpation should be done with care when trying to stop a preterm labour or if there is uterine irritability for any other reason, e.g. antepartum haemorrhage, fever.
- Excessive interference with the uterine fundus can cause it to have uncoordinated activity as opposed to its usual coordination across the uterus. This would result in poor cervical dilatation.

PROCEDURE: assessing uterine contractions

- A watch/clock with a second hand is required to time the contraction.
- Gain informed consent.
- Wash and warm hands.
- Ensure the woman is in a comfortable position, with access to the area of the abdomen beneath

which the fundus is located; the abdomen can remain covered.
- Place one hand on the top part of the abdomen, over the fundal region of the uterus.
- Keeping the hand still, feel for the contraction along the length of the fingers (not just the fingertips).
- Note the time when the abdomen (and uterus) first contracts.
- Observe the length of time the contraction lasts and the extent to which the uterus hardens.
- Keeping the hand on the abdomen to await the next contraction, observe the time between contractions to assess frequency and note the relaxed, resting tone of the uterus.
- If the contractions are irregular, palpate the contractions for 10 minutes to calculate the number occurring in a 10-minute period. (This is more intrusive; it might be preferable to ask the woman to note the number of contractions in a 10-minute period, provided she is aware of them.)
- Discuss the findings with the woman.
- Document the findings and act accordingly.

ROLE AND RESPONSIBILITIES OF THE MIDWIFE

These are summarised as:
- knowledge and application of current evidence-based practice
- undertaking all procedures correctly
- appropriate CTG trace interpretation and regular update of such skills
- education, advice and support of the woman
- accurate contemporaneous record keeping
- referral for deviations from the norm.

Summary

- Abdominal examination antenatally and in labour is a skill from which significant information can be gained.
- The midwife has a responsibility to undertake it competently, record the findings and make a referral if necessary. It is more uncomfortable for women when in labour.
- The fetal heart can be auscultated using a Pinard stethoscope, fetal Doppler or CTG monitor. It is always preceded by an abdominal examination.

- CTG monitors should be correctly applied and the trace interpreted accordingly.
- The palpation of uterine contractions in labour assess the frequency, strength, length and resting tone of the uterus. It is a significant aspect of labour care.

SELF-ASSESSMENT EXERCISES

The answers to the following questions may be found in the text:

1. Describe the different components of an abdominal examination, discussing the rationale for each aspect.
2. Describe how to measure the symphysis fundal height.
3. Discuss the means by which the fetal heart rate is auscultated.
4. Describe the procedure when applying a CTG monitor.
5. Discuss which factors the midwife needs to consider when interpreting a CTG tracing.
6. If a CTG tracing was described as 'non-reassuring' what would this mean?
7. Describe how to successfully palpate uterine contractions in labour.
8. Summarise the role and responsibilities of the midwife in relation to abdominal examination and use of electronic fetal monitoring.

References

Alfirevic Z, Devane D, Gyte G. Continuous cardiotocography (CTG) as a form of electronic fetal monitoring (EFM) for fetal assessment during labour, *Cochrane Database Syst Rev* 3: CD006066, 2006. DOI:10.1002/14651858. CD006066.

Gardosi J, Francis A: Controlled trial of fundal height measurement plotted on customized antenatal growth charts, *Br J Obstet Gynaecol* 106(4):309–317, 1999.

MHRA (Medicines and Healthcare Products Regulatory Agency): 2002 SN2002(23) *Cardiotocograph (CTG) monitoring of fetus during labour – update*. Online. Available: http://www.mhra.gov.uk 2009.

Neilson JP: Symphysis-fundal height measurement in pregnancy, *Cochrane Database Syst Rev* (1): CD000944, 1998. DOI: 10.1002/14651858.CD000944.

NICE (National Institute for Clinical Excellence): *Intrapartum care. Care of healthy women and their babies during childbirth*, London, 2007, NICE.

NICE (National Institute for Clinical Excellence). *Antenatal care. Routine care for the healthy pregnant woman*, London, 2008, NICE.

NMC (Nursing and Midwifery Council): *Midwives rules and standards*, London, 2004, NMC.

NMC (The Nursing and Midwifery Council): *Guidelines for records and record keeping*, London, 2005, NMC.

Olsen K: 'Now just pop up here, dear...'. Revisiting the art of antenatal abdominal palpation, *Pract Midwife* 2(9):13–15, 1999.

Rosser J: Symphysis-fundal height measurement, *Pract Midwife* 3(1):10, 2000.

Wickham S: Pinard wisdom tips and tricks from midwives, part 1, *Pract Midwife* 5(9):21, 2002a.

Wickham S: Pinard wisdom tips and tricks from midwives, part 2, *Pract Midwife* 5(10):35, 2002b.

Wright J, Morse K, Kady S, Francis A: Audit of fundal height measurement plotted on customized growth charts, *MIDIRS Midwifery Digest* 16(3): 341–345, 2006.

Principles of abdominal examination: during the postnatal period

2

CHAPTER CONTENTS

Gale (2008: 281) believes that postnatal care is '...vital because it prepares parents for a lifetime of parenting'. Postnatal morbidity is something for which many women are unprepared; without adequate care, it is also something for which mortality is a possibility. Depending on other indicators, assessment of the uterus postnatally is one aspect of care that the midwife can undertake as part of holistic and individualised postnatal care. This chapter includes a description of the physiology of uterine involution and discussion of the ways in which normality is assessed.

LEARNING OUTCOMES

Having read this chapter the reader should be able to:

- briefly outline the physiology of involution
- discuss the possible deviations from the norm that can be identified when palpating the uterus postnatally
- describe the procedures (verbal and physical) necessary to assess involution of the uterus
- discuss the role and responsibilities of the midwife when undertaking abdominal examination during the postnatal period.

Physiology of involution

Involution is the process by which the uterus returns approximately to its pre-pregnant size, position and tone. This involves a reduction in weight from 1000 to 60 g and reduction in size from $15 \times 11 \times 7.5$ cm to $7.5 \times 5 \times 2.5$ cm. The term 'autolysis' refers to the digestion of excess muscle fibres by proteolytic enzymes, a process that is assisted by the continuing contraction and retraction of the uterus that began during labour. As the uterus reduces in size, the decidua is shed within the lochia (the discharges from the vagina following childbirth) and new endometrium begins to grow from the basal layer of the endometrium. New endometrial growth is evident from about the tenth day after delivery; by 6 weeks the endometrium has reformed. Strong contraction of the muscle fibres occurs in the first 12–24 hours, decreasing in strength and frequency over the next few days. They are often stronger and persist for longer in multiparous women (Blackburn 2007). Women recognise these contractions as 'after pains'. The rate at which the uterus involutes is considered to be approximately 1 cm per day. Therefore, after 6 days, the fundus is usually about halfway between the umbilicus and the symphysis pubis and should be just palpable by the end of 10 days. For many women, the fundus may not be palpable at this time, and is usually no longer palpable after the twelfth postnatal day (Fig. 2.1).

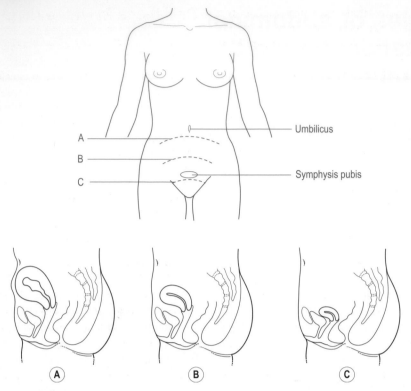

A — Umbilicus

B

C — Symphysis pubis

(A)   (B)   (C)

Figure 2.1 • The position of the uterus during involution. **A** Following delivery.
B 1 week after delivery – the fundal height is palpable approximately 5 cm above
the symphysis pubis. **C** 2 weeks after delivery – the fundal height is not usually
palpable above the symphysis pubis

Whereas most textbooks report the changes described here as standard postpartum physiology, Cluett et al (1997) noted several variations in their assessment of 28 women, including several days without uterine involution and uteri palpable at 23 days, both without signs of abnormality. Subinvolution of the uterus is considered to be less likely if the mother is breastfeeding (due to the increased action of oxytocin on uterine fibres) but more likely if there has been surgery or trauma. Pathological subinvolution usually relates to endometritis (infection within the uterus), often stemming from retained products. This creates the potential risk of a secondary postpartum haemorrhage (PPH).

Changes in the colour and amount of the lochia reflect the changes occurring within the endometrium and may vary with individual women. During the first 2–4 days after the birth of the baby, the lochia contain blood cells, necrotic deciduas, fragments of the amnion and chorion (lochia rubra),

and are usually red in colour (initially bright, changing to dark red then brown as the proportion of blood cells within the lochia decreases). From around the third to fourth day, the lochia change to a pinkish-red colour (lochia serosa) and also contain leucocytes and organisms. The lochia then change to a pink or whitish-yellow discharge, usually from the tenth to fourteenth postnatal day (lochia alba) and lasting until approximately 6 weeks (Blackburn 2007, NCT 2008).

Rationale for the procedure

The evidence to support the action of uterine palpation (both method and frequency) remains inadequate. The National Institute for Health and Clinical Excellence (NICE 2006) concluded that, as a routine assessment, abdominal palpation or measurement of the uterus was unnecessary.

However, it also noted that in the presence of other symptoms (fever, excessive or offensive vaginal lochia, abdominal pain) abdominal assessment of the uterus is indicated. If no uterine abnormality is found, other causes for the symptoms should be sought.

What is assessed?

As suggested above, the active 'descent' of the uterus back to a pelvic organ forms the largest part of the assessment. In conjunction, the position and tone of the uterus, colour, amount and odour of the lochia (discussed above) are all assessed. Bick et al (2009) suggest that an initial 'baseline' palpation of the uterus should be undertaken after delivery, thereafter the assessment begins with a detailed conversation with the woman. If this conversation reveals the need to palpate, then it is undertaken. It is clear, however, that this will work only if the woman has received guidance on what to expect realistically (and can therefore suggest when there is potentially a deviation from the norm) and if the midwife utilises good communication skills with open questioning (discussed further below).

The uterus should be positioned centrally within the abdomen. A full bladder can displace the uterus, causing it to deviate to one side. This can interfere with myometrial contraction, predisposing to postpartum haemorrhage. Thus, when the uterus is deviated, the lochia should be assessed to ensure the woman is not haemorrhaging and she should be encouraged to empty her bladder. The tone of the uterus should be firm, indicating a well contracted uterus. If the tone is poor, the uterus will feel soft, which again is associated with postpartum haemorrhage. A full rectum, retained products of conception or blood clots can cause the uterus to feel bulky. Additionally, the uterus should not feel tender when palpated, and discomfort could be indicative of infection.

Palpating after caesarean section

The uterus is often very tender for several days and is slower to involute. Although there is less likelihood of retained products, there is a risk of endometritis. In the event of needing to palpate the uterus, the hand should be placed gently over the uterus. The action of feeling the tone of the fundus described below is likely to be too painful.

Deviations from the norm

If a deviation from the norm is identified, the midwife's decision making should include the severity of the deviation in order to inform the action taken. Any clinical signs that suggest actual or pending haemorrhage should prompt a swift referral to hospital. Signs of infection also need referral, the severity may determine whether this is to hospital or the general practitioner. A minor deviation, for example the uterus being slow to involute with no other concerning signs, should prompt the midwife to reassess soon, advising the woman what to be aware of in the meantime.

Verbal assessment

Initially, Bick et al (2009) suggest that the following should be considered after delivery:

- Antenatal and delivery records, including antenatal haemoglobin and third-stage management.
- When palpating the uterus, explanations should be given to the woman as to what is being felt and why; she is then invited to palpate her own uterus.
- Discuss the pattern of her vaginal loss, expected pattern, factors affecting it (e.g. feeding, signs of infection or clots), hygiene and pad changes.
- Visually assess the lochia.

At subsequent assessments it is necessary to discuss:

- Is she feeling well? Are there any signs of pyrexia or pain?
- How much lochial loss is there? Has it changed particularly? What colour is it? Any offensive smell? Any accompanying abdominal discomfort?

If the conversation gives the midwife any cause for concern then the uterus should be palpated.

PROCEDURE: postnatal abdominal palpation of the uterus

- Confirm that palpation is necessary (see above), gain informed consent.
- Ask the woman to empty her bladder if she has not done so recently.
- Wash and warm hands.

- Ask the woman to lie in a recumbent position with her arms by her side, ensure she is comfortable and that privacy is maintained.
- Expose the woman's abdomen, note any features that might affect the palpation, e.g. obesity, degree of healing for caesarean section wound.
- Using the outer aspect of one hand, gently depress the abdomen to feel for the fundus. If the fundus is not found, remove the hand and reposition higher or lower and gently press down again.
- When the fundus is felt, use the outer aspect of the hand to estimate the height and position of the uterus. Depress slightly further down into the abdomen to feel over the top of the fundus, assess the uterine tone. A well-contracted uterus is often described as feeling like a cricket ball.
- Note whether the woman displays any non-verbal discomfort or expresses any pain on palpation.
- If it has not already been done, the lochial loss should be assessed by examining the pad. Check when the pad was last changed to obtain an idea of the extent of the loss. This can be done with the woman in the same position or in left lateral; she may prefer to stand up and remove the pad. Gloves should be worn if contact with body fluids is anticipated. If the lochial loss is heavy the uterus should be palpated at the same time as examining the pad to see if on palpation any clots are expelled from the uterus.
- Re-cover the woman, assisting the woman to a comfortable position. Wash hands.
- Discuss the findings with the woman.
- Document the findings and act accordingly.

ROLE AND RESPONSIBILITIES OF THE MIDWIFE

These can be summarised as:

- careful communication, undertaking a physical examination correctly if indicated
- recognising deviations from the norm and instigating referral
- education, explanations and support of the woman
- appropriate record keeping.

Summary

- It is unnecessary to palpate the uterus routinely postnatally. If a suspected deviation from the norm is revealed on discussion or there are any other clinical signs observed (pyrexia, abdominal pain or offensive lochia) uterine palpation and assessment of lochial loss are then indicated.
- Uterine palpation includes the height, position and tone of the uterus.
- A deviation from the norm may suggest current or pending haemorrhage or infection. Urgent attention is needed to reduce the morbidity and mortality risks.

SELF-ASSESSMENT EXERCISES

The answers to the following questions may be found in the text:

1. Describe how involution occurs.
2. Based on what information should the midwife palpate the uterus during the postnatal period?
3. What is being assessed for when palpating the uterus during the postnatal period?
4. The lochia may be examined following abdominal palpation. What information may be gained from this in relation to involution?
5. What factors may influence the rate of involution?

References

Bick D, MacArthur C, Winter H: *Postnatal care: evidence and guidelines for management*, ed 2, Edinburgh, 2009, Elsevier.

Blackburn ST: *Maternal, fetal and neonatal physiology: a clinical perspective*, ed 3, St. Louis, 2007, Saunders.

Cluett ER, Alexander J, Pickering RM: What is the normal pattern of uterine involution? An investigation of postpartum uterine involution measured by the distance between the symphysis pubis and the uterine fundus using a paper tape measure, *Midwifery* 13(1):9–16, 1997.

Gale E: Throwing the baby out with the bathwater? *MIDIRS Midwifery Digest* 18(2):277–281, 2008.

NCT (National Childbirth Trust): *Blood loss after birth. NCT information sheet*, London, 2008, NCT.

NICE (National Institute Health and Clinical Excellence): *Routine postnatal care of women and their babies*, London, 2006, NICE.

Assessment of maternal and neonatal vital signs: temperature measurement

3

This chapter considers the means and significance of obtaining an as-accurate-as-possible temperature measurement. There is discussion about the different sites for temperature assessment, followed by the equipment available.

LEARNING OUTCOMES

Having read this chapter the reader should be able to:

- discuss the midwife's role and responsibilities in relation to temperature measurement, identifying when it should be undertaken
- define normal body temperature for the childbearing woman and baby
- describe the factors that influence body temperature and the changes relating to child bearing
- discuss the suitable sites for temperature measurement, highlighting their rationale for use, accuracy, normal temperature ranges and the equipment that can be used
- describe the types of thermometer and how each one is used correctly and safely
- demonstrate taking a baby's temperature.

Body temperature

Body temperature is the balance between heat gain and heat loss. Humans are homeothermic, that is, their core temperature is maintained at 37°Celsius (°C) ± 1°C whatever the external environmental temperature. The hypothalamus acts as the body's thermostat. Humans cannot tolerate extreme changes at either end of the temperature range; should the temperature rise to 40.5°C, cellular damage will begin; temperatures above 42°C can result in brain dysfunction, coma, cardiovascular collapse and death. Conversely, a body temperature less than 28°C can result in uncoordinated muscle activity and fatigue, unconsciousness, cardiac arrhythmias and death.

The core temperature refers to the temperature within the brain, the abdominal and the chest organs, reflecting the warmest parts of the body. Core temperatures are usually reached about 2 cm below the body surface (Hinchliff et al 1996), with two-thirds of body mass maintained at core temperature. The most accurate measurement of the core temperature, the 'gold standard', is found in the pulmonary artery (Board 1995). Maintenance of the body temperature at a constant level is essential to ensure optimal functioning of all cells. Rises in body temperature increase the demands for oxygen and therefore increase the heart rate. This is of significance for the pregnant woman; the nature of oxygen transfer to the fetus means that it is more likely to be compromised if the mother is pyrexial.

Peripheral temperature

The peripheral temperature generated by skin and skeletal muscle is often lower than the core temperature, and so helps to regulate the core temperature by assisting with heat loss and gain. Peripheral temperatures reduce proportionally as distances increase from the core.

Normal values

Different body sites have different normal values. These are usually determined according to the nearness of the site to a major blood vessel and the route that it is taking to/from the heart. According to

Dubois (1948), the normal oral temperature is set within a range of 35.8–37.3°C; however, everyone has their own 'normal' oral temperature setting within this range. Thus, a rise in core temperature of 1°C may be difficult to detect if a person's normal oral temperature is 36.0°C.

Factors influencing body temperature

The hypothalamus regulates body temperature by both instigating and responding to the body's chemistry. The factors listed below are known to influence the body temperature. The midwife should be aware of these factors so that inappropriate treatments are not commenced or pathologies overlooked if a false temperature reading is obtained.

Diurnal variations

Circadian rhythms influence both the core and the peripheral temperature. Body temperature is lowest during the night and peaks in the evening.

Menstrual cycle

Body temperature is lower during the postmenstrual period of the menstrual cycle, increasing by 0.3–0.5°C after ovulation. This rise in body temperature is maintained until progesterone levels decrease prior to the onset of menstruation (Hinchliff et al 1996, Houdas & Ring 1982).

Digestion

A slight increase in temperature of 0.1–0.2°C has been noted to occur with normal digestion.

Basal metabolic rate

Heat is produced as a result of chemical reactions within the body. When the body is at rest, this is referred to as the basal metabolic rate (BMR). The amount of heat produced can be altered by various regulatory mechanisms to ensure the body temperature is maintained within the normal range: the higher the BMR, the more heat is produced, the higher the temperature (Houdas & Ring 1982). BMR decreases with age, thus babies have a higher BMR than adults; also, women have a slightly lower BMR than men (Chinyanga 1991). Certain diseases/disorders will increase the BMR (e.g. hyperthyroidism). Exercise can also cause a rise in temperature; Closs (1987) suggests that strenuous exercise might increase the core temperature to 40°C.

Hot baths

These can raise the body temperature by 0.5–1.0°C for up to 45 minutes.

Fever

Leucocytes release endogenous pyrogens in response to stimulation by pyrogenic substances such as bacterial, viral and protozoal infection and necrotic tissue. This causes the thermostat within the hypothalamus to be 'reset' at a higher level. The affected person feels cold and the body attempts to raise the temperature to maintain it within its higher 'normal' range. When the level of endogenous pyrogens decreases, the thermostat returns to its original setting. The person then feels hot, with the body attempting to lower the temperature to its normal setting.

General anaesthesia

The drugs used during general anaesthesia can interfere with the normal homeothermic mechanisms that assist with heat loss and gain, predisposing to heat loss (Schönbaum & Lomax 1991). Chinyanga (1991) proposes that the greatest decrease in body temperature will occur during the first hour of anaesthesia and that this can induce postanaesthetic shivering.

Alcohol

Kalant and Lé (1991) conclude from their review of the literature that large amounts of alcohol will lower the body temperature.

Child bearing

This is discussed in detail below.

Temperature changes related to childbirth

Pregnancy: maternal

During pregnancy, progesterone and a raised metabolic rate increase the amount of heat generated by 30–35%. Although the body attempts to compensate for this by increasing heat loss mechanisms, the maternal temperature can increase by 0.5°C (Blackburn 2007).

Pregnancy: fetal

Intrauterine temperature is determined partly by maternal temperature and partly by the maternal–fetal gradient, as the fetus is unable to regulate its own temperature. Generally, the fetal temperature is approximately 0.8°C higher than the maternal oral temperature (Banerjee et al 2004). Therefore, a raised maternal body temperature will result in a higher fetal temperature and is associated with intrauterine hypoxia, fetal tachycardia, teratogenesis and preterm labour (Blackburn 2007).

Labour

During labour, a rise in temperature can be indicative of infection, dehydration or the result of increased muscular activity from uterine contractions. It is often associated with the use of epidural analgesia.

Postnatal period: maternal

A transient rise in maternal temperature can occur within the first 24 hours after delivery; it might result from the stress of labour and be related to dehydration. Blackburn (2007) suggests that up to 6.5% of women have a rise in temperature to 38°C in the 24 hours following a vaginal birth. In the majority of cases, this is physiological and resolves spontaneously. However, for a small number of women, the temperature rise could be due to an infection, such as a puerperal infection, mastitis or a urinary tract infection, or might result from an inflammatory process, such as the development of a deep venous thrombosis. The temperature may also rise in breastfeeding women around the second to third day as milk production occurs. This will resolve spontaneously once lactation is established although it can take several days.

Postnatal period: baby

Babies emerge from the warmth of the uterus (i.e. a temperature of 37°C+) into an environment of approximately 21°C. They are wet and need to establish several adaptations to extrauterine life simultaneously. Thermoregulation is difficult for the immature systems, and is further affected by:

- The large ratio of surface area to body mass with thin layers of insulating subcutaneous fat. This creates an increased opportunity to lose body heat, especially from the head.
- The changeable nature of the environment, especially open doors or windows, fans, cold mattresses, etc.

Consequently, babies lose heat by evaporation, especially before thorough drying, by convection when draughts blow over them, by radiation and conduction to nearby items and surfaces. A decrease in temperature of between 1 and 2°C might occur during the first hour after birth. If action is not taken to remedy this, a normal body temperature may not be achieved for 4–8 hours afterwards (Black 1972). Various measures can be taken at birth to protect the baby's temperature. The World Health Organization (WHO 1997) calls this 'the warm chain' (consideration to room temperature, immediate drying, postponing weighing and bathing, etc.), and skin-to-skin contact has value for both temperature regulation and breastfeeding success.

Heat production comes mainly from metabolic processes, moving and shivering both being limited activities. External clothing helps, while the stores of brown fat are utilised, along with calories from milk. Metabolism requires both glucose and oxygen; a cold baby rapidly becomes hypoxic and hypoglycaemic and can have a serious metabolic acidosis. The problems are compounded significantly if the baby is preterm or small for gestational age.

Attention to careful management of the baby's temperature immediately following birth and in the first weeks of postnatal life is essential, including education of the parents. Danger exists for hyperthermia as well as hypothermia. An infected baby may display a changeable or cool temperature rather than the expected high temperature.

Temperature assessment

A literature search reveals that there is only one point on which there is consensus: the pulmonary artery is the 'gold standard' site for temperature measurement. This is highly impractical in day-to-day midwifery, but all other sites and types of equipment used are suspect in their reliability. The published studies are often small, criticize each other for their methodologies and are contradictory in their conclusions (cited throughout this chapter). Consequently, it falls to the midwife to:

- keep up to date with evaluated current research
- work with the protocols of their employment, influencing these for the better if possible
- maintain consistency with temperature measurement, using the same equipment in the same site (documented) for that woman/baby
- undertake temperature measurement as part of a complete assessment, and not in isolation.

The taking of a temperature, as for any clinical investigation, might lead to other actions, for example, further screening with swabs, blood tests or urine specimens, use of antibiotics or other drugs, augmentation of labour if ruptured membranes. Consequently, the result needs to be as accurate as possible; this is achieved by completing the procedure correctly with approved equipment.

Indications

As stated above, temperature may be recorded if other observations suggest a deviation from the norm. What the woman looks like (e.g. hot, pale, flushed, sweaty) and how she is feeling or behaving also add to the observation. Although midwives offer individualised care to women and babies based on their needs, there are circumstances when routine temperature measurement is required, for example, 4-hourly in labour (NICE 2007). The value of a baseline recording (particularly prior to surgery) is a means of ensuring that deviations from the norm for that woman are quickly noticed and acted upon. Other likely indications are:

- after delivery (by whichever mode) initially for both the woman and baby, then as required [National Collaborating Centre for Women's and Children's Health (NCCWCH) 2004, NICE 2007]
- as clinical condition requires for woman and baby

- preterm labour
- prelabour rupture of the membranes, especially if prolonged
- loin or abdominal pain (i.e. possible urinary tract infection)
- known infection, e.g. group B streptococcus
- blood transfusion.

Sites for temperature recording

Choosing a site

Although the presence or absence of certain equipment can automatically reduce the choice of site, the following should be considered when making a choice:

- known reliability of the site
- accessibility
- ability of the woman to comply
- safety
- local protocol
- equipment available.

As suggested above, no one site is deemed totally reliable in adults or children. These sites are generally readily accessible and therefore are commonly used:

- oral (mouth or buccal cavity)
- tympanic (ear)
- axilla
- forehead.

These four sites will be discussed in detail below. Other less common sites can also be used:

- Rectum: this has a good blood supply, is well insulated and correlates closely with core temperature (approximately 0.5°C higher than the oral normal value); however, it is slower to react to changes than other sites. It is less frequently used, being inaccessible and embarrassing for adults. Vagal stimulation can be a danger in children and babies (Bailey & Rose 2000). If necessary, a lubricated catheter is used to check anal patency at birth, rather than a thermometer.
- Oesophagus and pulmonary artery: only accessible in high-dependency care (e.g. intensive therapy unit), when such accuracy is essential and the readings can be safely obtained.
- Skin probes are used in environments such as the neonatal intensive care unit.

Oral site

Rationale for use and normal values

The thermometer is placed in one of the sublingual pockets, located on either side of the tongue (Fig. 3.1). A branch of the carotid artery, the sublingual artery, runs beneath the sublingual pocket (Closs 1987). The blood within this vessel is travelling to the hypothalamus, therefore it responds rapidly to changes in body temperature. It is a readily accessible site, with little inconvenience to the woman and minimal contact with body fluids. An acceptable adult oral temperature reading is between 35.8 and 37.3°C (Dubois 1948). The temperature in other parts of the mouth is lower than in the sublingual pocket. The temperature within the mouth can be affected by environmental factors. Drinking hot fluids and smoking can create an artificially high reading, whereas mouth breathing, tachypnoea, drinking iced fluids and not placing the thermometer far enough into the mouth can all create a falsely low reading.

Safety and compliance

The woman will be required to hold the apparatus in her mouth with her mouth closed. The oral site should be avoided due to lack of compliance and/or potential danger for:

- babies and young children
- labouring women

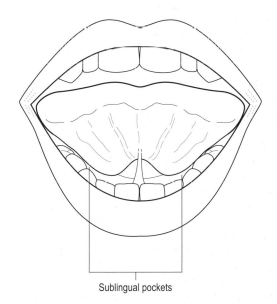

Sublingual pockets

Figure 3.1 • Sublingual pockets of the mouth

- anaesthetised, semi-conscious or unconscious women
- women likely to experience seizure, e.g. fulminating pre-eclampsia
- facial or oral impairment/injury
- known oral infection
- nausea or vomiting
- failure to gain consent.

It is therefore only a safe temperature measurement route for a coherent adult or an understanding older child.

Suitable equipment

Electronic and disposable thermometers (pp 29–32) are suitable for oral use, each with a disposable protective cover.

Tympanic membrane

Rationale for use and normal values

The tympanic membrane of the ear shares the same blood supply as the hypothalamus and is positioned close to it. It is considered to be an accurate approximation of core temperature. The auditory canal is insulated (maintaining the temperature of the site) and easily accessible. A direct normal value is not quoted but calibration of the equipment by the manufacturer may be according to oral or core body temperature, the user needs to know which this is prior to using the equipment.

Suitable equipment

Temperature recordings from the tympanic membrane can only be taken with a specific tympanic thermometer (p 30). Disposable covers reduce the cross-infection risk.

Accuracy

This is dependent upon an ambient temperature in the ear and the correct positioning of the equipment (p 31). Any of the following factors in the ear can affect the validity of the recording:

- presence of moisture, e.g. vernix caseosa, amniotic fluid
- presence of hearing aid within the last 20 minutes (Pullen 2003)
- excessive wax
- infection
- recent surgery
- raised air temperature, e.g. an incubator.

The Medical and Healthcare Products Regulation Agency (MHRA 2003) has received several alerts as to the problems of incorrect use of tympanic thermometers, particularly in the home. It points out that the probe must be clean and that the ear canal must be straightened for the scan to be of the ear drum and not just the canal wall (see pp 30, 31 for correct use of this thermometer).

Several studies or reviews (adult and neonatal) now suggest that tympanic thermometers (partly for their ease of use) are the most reliable (Bailey & Rose 2001, Dowding et al 2002, Woodrow et al 2006), but this is not by any means a consistent recommendation (Fawcett 2001, Fountain et al 2008, Scanga et al 2000). Fountain et al (2008) reviewed four studies and considered tympanic thermometers to be unreliable with poor performance.

Safety

The technique uses single-use covers, eliminating the danger of cross-infection. The manufacturers suggest that it is safe for all age groups.

Axilla site

Rationale for use and normal values

Actual evidence on the reliability of this site is scarce. Fulbrook (1993) believes that axilla temperatures are closely correlated with core temperature and therefore concludes that normal values for an adult axilla temperature equate with those of the oral route: 35.8–37.3°C. Bailey et al (2008) disagree, pointing out that skin temperatures vary with the environment, and that the axilla is also not in close proximity to any major vessels and so therefore not a reliable site. Nicol et al (2008) have stated that the axilla temperature is 0.5°C less than the oral site. It is, however, the site generally recommended for temperature measurement in babies. An inaccurate reading will be gained if the thermometer is left *in situ* for insufficient time or if the skin folds of the armpit are not in good contact with the thermometer. The thermometer should be placed centrally in the axilla. The effects of sweat, deodorant and vernix on temperature measurement have not been evaluated within the literature.

Safety and compliance

The axilla is usually accessible by moving clothes slightly and so compliance is good. The woman needs to be mindful of the fact that the thermometer is in the armpit and that mobility is restricted at that time. A baby's arm needs to be supported.

Suitable equipment

Disposable and covered electronic thermometers are all suitable for use in the axilla.

Forehead

Rationale for use and normal values

The superficial temporal artery (containing blood from the heart) also stems from the external carotid artery (see oral site, p 27). It runs up in front of the ear, then bifurcates so that one branch runs along the forehead and the other horizontally above the ear. It is considered to be about 1 mm beneath the skin of the forehead and it is its 'accessibility' and its nearness to the core body temperature that have caused its proponents to recommend it as an appropriate site. The literature does not suggest any normal values. Woodrow et al (2006) calibrated their forehead scanner to equate with oral ones, one manufacturer (Exergen 2005) suggests that with its equipment a temperature 0.4°C higher than oral values (at 36.3–37.8°C) is the expected norm.

Suitable equipment

Disposable liquid crystal thermometers and temporal artery thermometers may both be used on the forehead. Temporal artery (TA) thermometers are infrared heat scanners and can only be used to scan the temporal artery.

Accuracy

Anything insulating the forehead (hair, hats, wigs or bandages) would create a falsely high reading when using a TA thermometer. Perspiration also affects the accuracy of TA thermometers, and users need to be aware of the manufacturer's instructions with regard to this (Exergen 2005, Woodrow et al 2006). They appear to be unaffected by skin colour (Roy et al 2003) but Woodrow et al (2006) speculate that it may be affected by forehead skin thickness. As a relatively new piece of equipment, there are few reliable studies on its accuracy and this technology is likely to improve over the next few years. Fountain et al (2008) consider that whereas some researchers (Frommelt et al 2008, Greenes & Fleisher 2001, Lawson et al 2007, Roy et al 2003) have concluded that the accuracy of the TA

thermometer is acceptable, they are often critical of the study design and so caution against application. Their own findings declared these thermometers to be inadequate (Fountain et al 2008).

Morley et al (1998) suggested that chemical dot thermometers (pp 31, 32) had greater reliability than liquid crystal forehead thermometers, whereas Manandhar et al (1998) found that liquid crystal forehead results were comparable with axilla readings. Both were paediatric studies and care should be taken as to the application of these findings with adults.

Safety and compliance

The disruption to the woman or baby by using the forehead is minimal. Liquid crystal thermometers are disposable, some TA thermometers don't need to touch the skin, others have individual covers. The infection risk is therefore small with both.

Types of thermometer

Choosing the equipment for temperature measurement will depend on the site chosen and the availability of suitable apparatus. There is again no consensus as to the most accurate piece of equipment to use; Latman et al (2001) have doubts about the whole range of clinical thermometers in use.

Training should be given and the equipment must always be used according to the manufacturer's instructions. It should also be maintained and cleaned properly. The availability of some of the equipment discussed below may depend upon finance, local protocol, safety and suitability.

Electronic thermometers

These will vary in appearance but are generally available in two designs (Fig. 3.2):

1. a digital reading at the end of the thermometer
2. a digital reading on the hand-held box attached to the temperature probe.

The reading usually occurs within 1 minute and an alarm sounds to indicate that this has happened. Oral, axilla or rectal sites may be used for the adult; the axilla is used for the baby. There is a danger of cross-infection, as the thermometer is often used for more than one woman. Disposable covers must be used and the thermometer must be cleaned and maintained according to the manufacturer's guidelines.

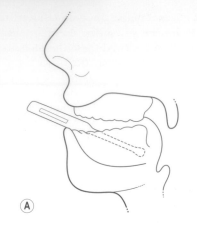

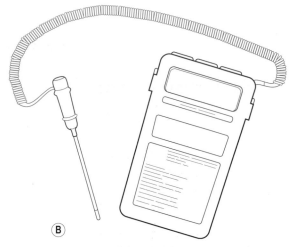

Figure 3.2 • A Electrical thermometer with digital reading. B Electrical thermometer with temperature probe (Adapted with kind permission from Jamieson et al 1997)

Some electronic thermometers have a separate probe for rectal use. Fountain et al (2008) suggest that electronic oral thermometers have a good level of agreement with core body temperature.

PROCEDURE: electronic thermometer use in oral and axilla sites

- Gain informed consent.
- Wash hands.
- Take the thermometer and cover to the woman.

- Clarify if any environmental factors exist that may affect the reading, e.g. a recent hot drink.
- Apply a disposable cover, switch on the thermometer, allow it to self-calibrate and when ready insert correctly into the chosen site (sublingual pocket or centrally against chest wall).
- Remove and read when the alarm sounds.
- Dispose of the cover correctly.
- Clean the thermometer if indicated.
- Discuss the findings with the woman.
- Wash hands.
- Document findings and act accordingly.

Summary

- Use a rapid, easy-to-use and easy-to-read thermometer.
- Pay attention to the prevention of cross-infection and proper maintenance.

Tympanic thermometers

Tympanic membrane thermometers scan the tympanic membrane using an infrared scanner to take temperature measurements. Readings are made in less than 30 seconds and are displayed digitally. Clearly, the thermometer is only ever placed in the ear, but can be used with both adults and babies. As discussed earlier, some environmental conditions can affect the accuracy of the result (p 28). It can be expensive initially and will require regular servicing and calibration. The user should be properly instructed in its use, various parts of the auditory canal will be scanned unless the probe is correctly directed to the tympanic membrane and the canal sealed with the probe.

PROCEDURE: tympanic thermometer use

Due to differences in manufacturers' designs, the reader is encouraged to read the specific instructions with their thermometer. These are general guidelines:

- Gain informed consent.
- Cover the thermometer tip with the supplied sheath.
- Switch the thermometer on.

- Aim to use the same ear for each assessment.
- When it is ready to scan, insert into the ear, ensuring that the auditory canal is sealed. To do this, for adults and children over 1 year of age, the pinna is pulled gently but firmly upwards and backwards, prior to inserting the thermometer (Fig. 3.3A,B). For babies of less than 1 year of age, the pinna is pulled straight back and the tip inserted into the ear opening (Fig. 3.3C) (MHRA 2003). Mains et al (2008) suggest that the tip should then be horizontal (pointing towards the opposite ear).
- Press the scan button, remove and read the thermometer when the alarm sounds.
- Remove and dispose of the sheath.
- Switch off the thermometer.
- Discuss the findings with the woman.
- Document the findings and act accordingly.

A baby cared for laterally in an incubator should have the ear nearest to the sheet used (downwards ear) rather than the upper ear, which will have been exposed to the environmental heat.

Summary

A rapid technique causing minimal disruption to the woman, but with a high margin of error if technique is poor.

Disposable (chemical dot) thermometers

Disposable thermometers are widely available. Research into their accuracy is limited; however, Fountain et al (2008) noted only non-significant differences between it and an electronic thermometer.

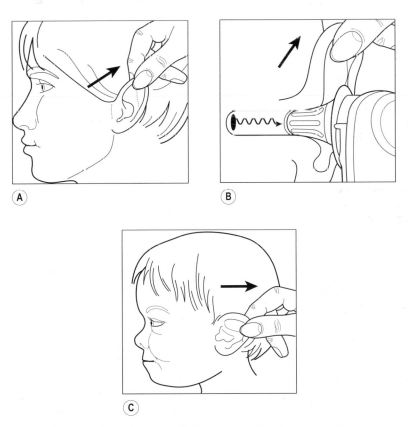

Figure 3.3 • A,B Use of a tympanic thermometer in adults and children >1 year: the pinna is pulled up and back to straighten the auditory canal. C Use of a tympanic thermometer in babies <1 year: the pinna is pulled straight back and the tip of the thermometer inserted into the ear opening (Adapted with kind permission from HMSO (MHRA))

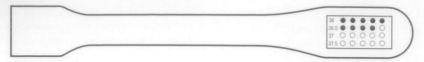

Figure 3.4 • Disposable thermometer indicating a reading of 36.8°C (Adapted with kind permission from Jamieson et al 2002)

They are considered to be cheap, safe and comfortable to use (Board 1995). They are made of flexible plastic with a series of chemical dots at one end. As the temperature rises the dots undergo a chemical reaction and colour change (each one is 0.1°C higher than the previous one (Macqueen 2001). The level to which the colour change occurs is the point at which the temperature is read (Fig. 3.4). They are suitable for oral, axilla and rectal use for the adult, axilla only for the baby. Reliability is impaired if the thermometers are stored in too hot an environment. The manufacturer's instructions should be read before the thermometer is used.

PROCEDURE: disposable thermometer use

The thermometer is used in the same way as an electronic thermometer (p 30) except that:

- Oral recordings can be made after 1 minute, axilla and rectal after 3 minutes (Blumenthal 1992); an accurate time source is needed.
- In the axilla, the chemical pads should be placed against the chest wall in a vertical position (Nicol et al 2008).
- The thermometer is given 10 seconds to stabilize before being read (may vary according to manufacturer).
- When reading the thermometer the first dot on the line is the same as the number next to it. The number is then counted along according to the number of dots that have changed colour (Fig. 3.4 indicates 36.8°C).
- The thermometer should be disposed of correctly.

Summary

- Disposable thermometers are easy to use and eliminate the dangers of cross-infection.
- Accuracy can be impaired under certain environmental conditions.

Conclusion

When choosing a site for temperature recording, consideration should be given to its accessibility, acceptability, known reliability and safety. The midwife needs to recognise the strengths and limitations of each site and piece of equipment available in order to make accurate recordings of a temperature. Temperature assessment can provide evidence of the clinical condition and may lead to further investigations and treatment.

Taking a baby's temperature

Taking a baby's temperature is different from taking that of an adult. The site used is generally the axilla with a disposable or electronic thermometer (Fig. 3.5). Tympanic thermometers can also be used, some of which will be a specific paediatric size and need to be inserted correctly (as described on p 31). The normal values for an axilla recording are between 36.5 and 37.0°C.

Indications

- Following birth.
- Repeat later (at 1 hour of age) if active resuscitation was needed.
- At any time postnatally when the baby looks or feels cool, hot, red, pale, sweaty, unwell, is not feeding or is behaving strangely (the abdomen is the best guide when assessing the skin temperature).
- If mother was pyrexial in labour or had a known infection (e.g. group B streptococcus) or if the baby is receiving antibiotics for a suspected or confirmed infection.
- If receiving phototherapy treatment.
- If preterm or low birth weight, this might be alongside regular feeding, or it may be a part of the care given in the high-dependency unit.

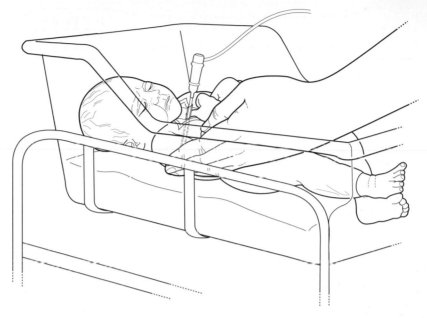

Figure 3.5 • Taking a baby's temperature: axilla site using electronic thermometer

PROCEDURE: taking a baby's temperature (axilla site)

- Parents should accompany the baby, their informed consent having been gained.
- Observe the baby generally, particularly noting its colour, behaviour and known clinical indicators.
- The baby is placed in a safe and warm environment, e.g. in the cot or in the mother's arms.
- Clothing is loosened so that the axilla is accessible; the baby is not allowed to chill, but if respiration is being counted at the same time then the chest may be exposed (see Chapter 6).
- The covered or disposable thermometer is placed into the axilla and the arm held gently across the chest to keep the thermometer secure.
- After the required length of time the thermometer is removed and read. The clothing is replaced and the baby returned to his parents.
- Records are made and action taken according to the findings.

ROLE AND RESPONSIBILITIES OF THE MIDWIFE

These can be summarised as:

- recognising the need to undertake temperature measurement
- use of appropriate equipment in the correct sites
- referral if indicated
- contemporaneous record keeping.

SELF-ASSESSMENT EXERCISES

The answers to the following questions may be found in the text:

1. Discuss the factors that influence body temperature.
2. List the occasions when temperature assessment is undertaken for a childbearing woman and a newborn baby.
3. What is the normal temperature range for the woman and how does this alter during the ante-, intra- and postpartum periods?
4. What is an accepted normal temperature range for a newborn baby?
5. Discuss the advantages and disadvantages of each of the sites for temperature assessment.
6. What would you say to someone who did not know what a temporal artery thermometer was?
7. Demonstrate taking a woman's temperature using a tympanic thermometer.
8. Demonstrate taking a baby's temperature using the axilla site.
9. Summarise the role and responsibilities of the midwife when undertaking temperature assessment.

References

Bailey J, Rose P: Temperature measurement in the preterm infant: a literature review, *J Neonatal Nurs* 6(1):28–32, 2000.

Bailey J, Rose P: Axillary and tympanic membrane temperature recording in the preterm neonate: a comparative study, *J Adv Nurs* 34(4):465–474, 2001.

Bailey M, Crossen S, Hofland J, et al: Observations. In Doughty L, Lister S, editors: *The Royal Marsden Hospital Manual of Clinical Nursing Procedures Student Edition*, ed 7, Oxford, 2008, Wiley Blackwell, pp 656–666.

Banerjee S, Cashman P, Yentis SM, et al: Maternal temperature monitoring during labor: concordance and variability among monitoring sites, *Obstet Gynecol* 103(2):287–293, 2004.

Black L: *Neonatal emergencies and other problems*, Oxford, 1972, Butterworth Heinemann.

Blackburn ST: *Maternal, fetal and neonatal physiology: a clinical perspective*, ed 3, St. Louis, 2007, W B Saunders.

Blumenthal I: Should we ban the mercury thermometer?*J R Soc Med* 85(9):533–555, 1992.

Board M: Comparison of disposable and mercury in glass thermometers, *Nurs Times* 91(33):36–37, 1995.

Chinyanga HM: Temperature regulation and anaesthesia. In Schönbaum E, Lomax P, editors: *Thermoregulation: pathology, pharmacology and therapy*, New York, 1991, Pergamon Press, ch 9.

Closs J: Oral temperature measurement, *Nurs Times* 7:36–39, 1987.

Dowding D, Freeman S, Nimmo S, et al: An investigation into the accuracy of different types of thermometers, *Prof Nurse* 18(3):166–168, 2002.

Dubois EF: *Fever and the regulation of body temperature*, Springfield, 1948, C C Thomas.

Exergen: Temporal artery thermometer instructions for use, http://www. exergen.com/medical/TAT/tatfaq. html Online. Available: (educational video also available) 24 March 2009.

Fawcett J: The accuracy and reliability of the tympanic membrane thermometer: a literature review, *Emergency Nurse* 8(9):13–17, 2001.

Fountain C, Goins L, Hartman M, et al: Evaluating the accuracy of four temperature instruments on an adult oncology unit, *Clin J Oncol Nurs* 12(6):983–987, 2008.

Frommelt T, Ott C, Hays V: Accuracy of different devices to measure temperature, *MEDSURG Nursing* 17(3):171–182, 2008.

Fulbrook P: Core temperature measurement in adults: a literature review, *J Adv Nurs* 18:1451–1460, 1993.

Greenes D, Fleisher G: Accuracy of a Noninvasive temporal artery thermometer for use in infants, *Archives of Pediatric Medicine* 155:376–381, 2001.

Hinchliff SM, Montague SE, Watson R: *Physiology for nursing practice*, ed 2, London, 1996, Baillière Tindall.

Houdas Y, Ring EFJ: *Human body temperature*, New York, 1982, Plenum Press.

Jamieson EM, McCall J, Whyte L: *Clinical nursing practices*, ed 4, Edinburgh, 2002, Churchill Livingstone.

Jamieson EM, McCall JM, Blythe R, et al: *Clinical nursing practices*, ed 3, Edinburgh, 1997, Churchill Livingstone.

Kalant H, Lé AD: Effects of ethanol on thermoregulation. In Schönbaum E, Lomax P, editors: *Thermoregulation: pathology, pharmacology and therapy*, New York, 1991, Pergamon Press, ch 15.

Latman N, Hans P, Nicholson L, et al: Evaluation of clinical thermometers for accuracy and reliability, *Biomed Instrum Technol* (3594):259–265, 2001.

Lawson L, Bridges E, Ballou I, et al: Accuracy and precision of noninvasive temperature measurement in adult intensive care patients, *Am J Crit Care* 16(5): 485–496, 2007.

Macqueen S: Clinical benefits of 3M Tempa·DOT thermometer in paediatric settings, *Br J Nurs* 10 (1):55–57, 2001.

Mains JA, Coxall K, Lloyd H: Measuring temperature, *Nurs Stand* 22(39): 44–47, 2008.

Manandhar N, Ellis M, Manandhar D, et al: Liquid crystal thermometry for the detection of neonatal hypothermia in Nepal, *J Trop Pediatr* 44(1):15–17, 1998.

Medicines and Healthcare products Regulatory Agency: http://www. mhra.gov.uk/ MDA/2003/010 Infrared ear thermometer home use, *MHRA.* Online. Available: 24 March 2009.

Morley C, Murray M, Whybrew K: The relative accuracy of mercury, Tempa-DOT and FeverScan thermometers, *Early Hum Dev* 53(2):171–178, 1998.

NCCWCH (National Collaborating Centre for Women's and Children's Health): *Caesarean Section*, London, 2004, RCOG Press.

NICE (National Institute for Health and Clinical Excellence): *Intrapartum care: care of healthy women and their babies during childbirth*, London, 2007, NICE.

Nicol M, Bavin C, Cronin P, Rawlings-Anderson K: *Essential Nursing Skills*, ed 3, Edinburgh, 2008, Mosby.

Pullen R: Using an ear thermometer, *Nursing* 33(5):24, 2003.

Roy S, Powell K, Gerson L: Temporal artery temperature measurements in healthy infants, children and adolescents, *Clin Pediatr (Phila)* 42(5):433–437, 2003.

Scanga A, Wallace R, Kiehl E, et al: A comparison of four methods of normal newborn temperature measurement, *MCN* 25(2):76–79, 2000.

Schönbaum E, Lomax P: Temperature regulation and drugs: an introduction. In *Thermoregulation: pathology, pharmacology and therapy*, New York, 1991, Pergamon Press, ch 1.

WHO (World Health Organization): Thermal protection of the newborn: a practical guide, 1997: http://www. who.int/reproductive-health/ publications. Online. Available: Accessed 24 March 2009.

Woodrow P, May V, Buras-Rees S, et al: Comparing no-touch and tympanic thermometer temperature recordings, *Br J Nurs* 15(18): 1012–1016, 2006.

Assessment of maternal and neonatal vital signs: pulse measurement

4

The pulse is a direct indicator of the action of the heart; the midwife should recognise the significance of it as an assessor of wellbeing. From such a straightforward observation much information can be gained, and using the correct technique each time increases the reliability of the results. This chapter examines pulse assessment: what it is, how, when and why it is completed. Factors affecting heart rate are also discussed; other means of pulse assessment are discussed briefly. Assessment of the fetal heart is discussed in Chapter 1.

LEARNING OUTCOMES

Having read this chapter, the reader should be able to:

- discuss the midwife's role and responsibilities in relation to pulse assessment, identifying when, where and how it is undertaken
- identify the normal range for the childbearing woman and baby
- discuss factors that influence the heart rate.

Definition

A pulse is a rhythmic expansion and recoil of the elastic arteries as the left ventricle ejects blood into the circulation (Jamieson et al 2002). The sinoatrial (SA) node is the heart's pacemaker and ensures that the heart meets the body's needs. The autonomic nervous system relays the cues which cause the heart to beat faster or slower to the SA node. The effects both extend to and come from the inter-relation of other body systems (e.g. the lungs). If, for example, running for a bus causes shortness of breath, one of the effects will be that the heart beats faster to supply more oxygen to the body tissues. Other factors affecting the heart rate are discussed below. These changes mean that it is necessary to assess a person's pulse for its rate, rhythm and amplitude.

Factors influencing the heart rate

The following factors increase the rate:

- pregnancy and labour (discussed below)
- emotions: stress, anxiety, nervousness and excitement
- pain
- infection: almost any infection (with or without changes to other vital signs)
- elevated body temperature
- haemorrhage
- shortage of red blood cells, e.g. iron-deficiency anaemia
- changes in position, e.g. from sitting to standing
- fluid and/or electrolyte imbalances, including dehydration
- exercise
- allergic reactions: anaphylaxis causes the pulse to be weak, tachycardic and irregular
- medications: drugs can cause tachycardia or bradycardia, e.g. salbutamol causes tachycardia and digoxin bradycardia
- disease: may affect heart rate, e.g. hyperthyroidism causes tachycardia.

The following factors reduce the rate:

- rest and relaxation: calm, controlled breathing can reduce the heart rate
- insult or injury: myocardial infarction or other injury might cause the heart to slow or stop
- hypothermia
- good exercise tolerance: in athletes
- age: heart rate decreases with age.

Normal values

A healthy, non-pregnant female adult has a regular heart rate of approximately 65–85 beats per minute (bpm) (Docherty & Coote 2006), with the normal range between 60 and 100 bpm. Tachycardia refers to an abnormally fast pulse rate above 100 bpm and bradycardia is a slow heart rate, generally considered to be below 60 bpm, although Higgins (2008) suggests it should be considered bradycardic when the pulse rate is below 50 bpm.

The pulse rhythm should be regular; an irregular pulse reflects an irregular pumping action of the heart. The amplitude indicates changes in the amount of blood being pumped around the body, the pulse strength and elasticity of the arterial wall. It is subjectively described as 'normal', 'weak' or 'thready' (may be due to hypovolaemia), 'rapid', 'full' or 'bounding' (may be due to infection) (Trim 2005).

A newborn baby has a heart rate of 110–160 bpm, with the average being approximately 130 bpm. Heart rate varies noticeably with respiration in the newborn, hence it is important to count for 1 minute.

Changes related to childbirth

Pregnancy

During pregnancy the maternal heart rate increases from 7 weeks gestation by approximately 10–20 bpm, peaking by 32 weeks, due to changes in cardiac output and stroke volume, corresponding with an increase in total blood volume. The rate declines slightly during the third trimester, and positional changes are particularly obvious throughout pregnancy. The rate is higher in the sitting or supine position than the lateral recumbent position (Blackburn 2007).

Mild cardiac arrhythmias (e.g. extra beats) may occur as a result of these changes and are harmless, usually resolving without treatment. However, the presence of cardiac disease places additional stress on the cardiovascular system of a pregnant woman. Nelson-Piercy (2007) reports 48 deaths from cardiac disease in childbirth in the period 2003–2005. It was the most common cause of death overall, and the highest number since reporting began. Women with existing cardiac problems or any presenting symptoms need careful combined cardiac and obstetric care.

Labour

During labour each contraction returns 300–500 mL of blood to the circulation. The heart rate rises accordingly, but this might also be due to other factors, for example pain, anxiety or exercise (Blackburn 2007).

Postnatal period: maternal

Blackburn (2007) suggests there is cardiac instability in the immediate postpartum period due to the changes in circulation (loss of placenta), blood loss and the body's compensatory mechanisms; there is an increased cardiac output followed by a bradycardia after 15 minutes. By 1 hour after delivery, cardiac output has returned to its prelabour values. As diuresis occurs and hormones change the majority of the cardiovascular system begins to return to its prepregnant state. Most changes are complete by 6–8 weeks postpartum; cardiac output generally takes up to 12 weeks although for some women this can be up to 24 weeks (Blackburn 2007).

Sites for pulse measurement

A pulse can be felt anywhere in the body where an artery near to the surface can be palpated against something firm, usually bone. The heart rate can also be heard (e.g. using a stethoscope).

The most commonly used site in the adult is the radial artery, being readily accessible; other sites are indicated in Figure 4.1. The radial pulse of the right wrist is best palpated by the midwife's left hand, and vice versa. The right radial pulse is less accurate in assessing amplitude due to its distance from the heart compared to the left radial pulse, but can be used for assessing the rate and rhythm (Docherty & Coote 2006). To find the radial pulse, place the index and middle finger gently in the groove of the woman's wrist that lies beneath the thumb. If a pulsation cannot be felt, the fingers should be moved gently along the groove until the pulse is located. The amount of pressure applied may need to be increased or decreased as well.

The brachial artery is used in the measurement of blood pressure and is located in the antecubital fossa. The woman should have her arm slightly bent with the palm uppermost and the midwife places her index and middle finger on the inner side of the crease of the elbow. Apply firm pressure for 5 seconds, if no pulsation is felt, begin again in the centre of the crease moving the fingers towards the woman's body.

The carotid or femoral arteries may be palpated in the case of collapse, where cardiac output cannot be detected in the peripheral circulation or with the critically ill person as they assess the quality of the left ventricular function better than the radial or brachial pulse (Docherty & Coote 2006). The carotid pulse is found by placing 3–4 fingertips against the larynx (at the top of the neck just under the jaw, mid-point between the chin and earlobe), using gentle pressure on one side only. If both sides are compressed the arterial circulation to the brain can be cut off. To locate the femoral pulse, the woman needs to be lying flat with the groin exposed. Three fingers are placed over the superior pubic ramus (near the crease of the groin) and direct downward pressure is applied (this may be quite deep) to feel the pulsation. It may take several attempts to locate and is difficult to find in obese, agitated or confused people (Docherty & Coote 2006).

Where there is an inconsistency between the heart beating and the pulse felt at the periphery, the two can be counted together (apical and radial) by two midwives. The midwife counting the apical assessment uses the diaphragm side of the stethoscope, placing it in the midline on the left side of the chest between the fifth and sixth ribs. Both midwives should have access to the watch, and agree when to begin and finish the minute's recording so they both record for the same period of time (Jevon 2007). Both readings are recorded using different coloured inks.

In the baby, the most usual site of pulse measurement is either apical (which can be heard or felt) or if this is not accessible, the brachial (Fig. 4.2). The radial pulse is not a site of choice in any child under 2 years of age, the palpable area being so small and the rapidity of the pulse being hard to count (Bailey et al 2008). Listening to the apical beat has greater reliability and is recommended.

Indications

While care should be individual and according to need, indications for pulse assessment are:

Maternal

- On admission, as a baseline recording.
- Any deviation from the norm or signs of illness or accident.
- When using a Pinard stethoscope to auscultate the fetal heart.

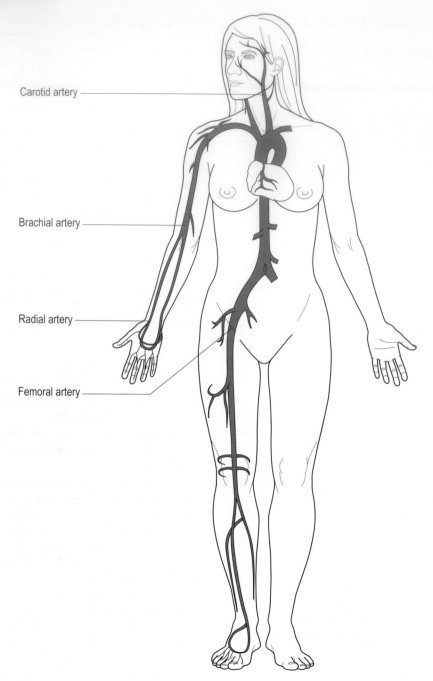

Carotid artery

Brachial artery

Radial artery

Femoral artery

Figure 4.1 • Main sites for adult pulse assessment (Adapted with kind permission from Thibodeau & Patton 1999)

- During labour (the pulse should not be taken during a contraction) and prior to transfer of care following labour.
- During and following surgery. NICE (NCCWCH 2004) recommends 5-minute recordings for the first 30 minutes after surgery, 30-minute recordings for the next 2 hours, then hourly recordings until the pulse rate is stable.
- Postnatal assessment, if indicated.
- Prelabour spontaneous rupture of membranes.

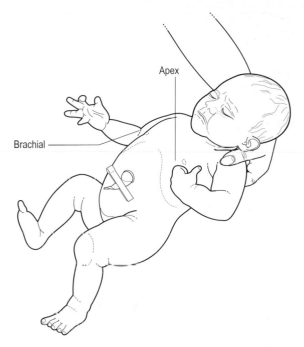

Apex

Brachial

Figure 4.2 • Main sites for neonatal pulse assessment

- During blood transfusion.
- Treatment for preterm labour using tocolytic drugs.

Baby

The heart rate is only generally monitored if the baby is ill or preterm, requiring intensive care. Other occasions include:

- at delivery as part of Apgar scoring and resuscitation
- any signs of cyanosis, irritability or illness
- as part of vital sign observations for suspected or potential infection, e.g. if prolonged spontaneous rupture of membranes or known maternal group B streptococcus or meconium aspiration.

Documentation

Pulse assessment can be written in the woman's/baby's records as prose. However, if repeated observations are undertaken, an overall picture is obtained if the findings are recorded pictorially on an observations chart or partogram. This will show at a glance if there is a pattern emerging or if the condition is changing.

PROCEDURE: adult radial pulse

- Obtain informed consent, ensure the woman is comfortable and if possible in the same position as the last assessment.
- Locate the radial artery, placing the index and middle fingers over it, supporting the woman's wrist and arm across her chest (if the wrist is held too firmly the pulse may be occluded, if held too lightly it is difficult to count).
- Count the pulse, for 30 seconds if it is completely regular, then double it, or 60 seconds if irregular or slow, noting also the rhythm and amplitude.
- Undertake respiration assessment (see Chapter 6) if necessary.
- Discuss the results with the woman, explaining whether it will be necessary to assess the pulse again.
- Document the findings and act accordingly.

PROCEDURE: baby

The baby should be peaceful and not crying when undertaking pulse assessment:

- Obtain informed consent from the parents, expecting at least one parent to be present throughout.
- Loosen the clothing and access the chosen site.
- Place the index and middle fingers over the brachial artery; *or* place a warmed stethoscope over the apex of the heart (midline, left side of the chest); *or* place index and middle fingers over the apex. Count the pulse for 60 seconds, noting amplitude and rhythm.
- Observe the colour, behaviour and general condition of the baby at the same time. Other vital sign observations may also be undertaken, e.g. temperature or respiratory assessment.
- Replace the clothing and ensure comfort.
- Discuss the results with his parents.
- Document the findings and act accordingly.

Other means of pulse measurement

- ECG (electrocardiogram) monitors give a continuous or single reading, or printout of the heart rate and pattern.

- Pulse oximeters (see Chapter 6) also give a heart rate reading, as do cardiotocograph machines for fetal heart assessment (see Chapter 1).

- Assessment of the general condition of the woman or baby is made simultaneously.

ROLE AND RESPONSIBILITIES OF THE MIDWIFE

These can be summarised as:

- recognising when pulse assessment is indicated
- undertaking the assessment correctly
- referral if indicated
- contemporaneous record keeping.

Summary

- Pulse assessment is a straightforward, non-invasive skill of considerable importance.
- An accurate assessment includes the rate, rhythm and amplitude of the pulse.

SELF-ASSESSMENT EXERCISES

The answers to the following questions may be found in the text:

1. Discuss the significance of pulse assessment and when it should be undertaken for the childbearing woman.
2. What changes occur to the heart rate during pregnancy and labour and why do they occur?
3. List the normal ranges for the antenatal woman, labouring woman, postnatal woman and newborn baby.
4. Discuss the factors that affect the heart rate.
5. Describe how a baby's heart rate can be measured immediately after birth.
6. Summarise the role and responsibilities of the midwife when undertaking pulse assessment.

References

Bailey M, Crossen S, Hofland J, et al: Observations. In Dougherty L, Lister S, editors: *The Royal Marsden Hospital manual of clinical nursing procedures*, ed 7, Oxford, 2008, Blackwell Science, pp 504–511.

Blackburn ST: *Maternal, fetal and neonatal physiology: a clinical perspective*, ed 3, St. Louis, 2007, Saunders.

Docherty B, Coote S: Monitoring the pulse as part of track and trigger, *Nurs Times* 102(43):28–29, 2006.

Higgins D: Patient Assessment: part 5 – Measuring Pulse, *Nurs Times* 104(11):24–25, 2008.

Jamieson E, McCall J, Whyte L: *Clinical nursing practices*, ed 4, Edinburgh, 2002, Churchill Livingstone.

Jevon P: Cardiac Monitoring part 4: Monitoring the apex beat, *Nurs Times* 103(4):28–29, 2007.

NCCWCH (National Collaborating Centre for Women's and Children's Health: *Caesarean Section*, London, 2004, RCOG Press.

Nelson-Piercy C: Cardiac Disease. In Lewis G, editor: *The Confidential Enquiry into Maternal and Child health (CEMACH). Saving Mothers Lives: reviewing maternal deaths to make motherhood safer – 2003–2005.*

The seventh report on confidential enquiries into maternal deaths in the United Kingdom, London, 2007, CEMACH, pp 117–130.

Thibodeau GA, Patton K: *Anatomy and physiology*, ed 4, St Louis, 1999, Mosby.

Trim J: Monitoring pulse, *Nurs Times* 101(21):30–31, 2005.

Assessment of maternal and neonatal vital signs: blood pressure measurement

5

CHAPTER CONTENTS

Maternal deaths from pre-eclampsia and eclampsia are the second highest direct cause of maternal deaths in the UK (Lewis 2007). The midwife is ideally placed to measure blood pressure in the childbearing woman, confirming normality and detecting deviations from the norm. It is essential that the midwife is able to undertake this procedure as accurately as possible as changes in blood pressure can have serious consequences for both the woman and the fetus/baby.

This chapter considers the issues surrounding the accurate measurement of arterial blood pressure, physiology, influencing factors and changes that occur during childbirth. The equipment available, technique of blood pressure measurement and factors influencing the accuracy of the recording are discussed, concluding with a discussion of venous blood pressure measurement.

LEARNING OUTCOMES

Having read this chapter the reader should be able to:

- discuss the midwife's role and responsibilities in relation to the measurement of blood pressure, identifying when and how it is undertaken

- define blood pressure, identifying the difference between systolic and diastolic pressure and the normal range for the childbearing woman and baby
- discuss the factors that influence blood pressure and the changes relating to child bearing
- discuss factors that influence the accuracy of blood pressure measurement and consider how the midwife can minimise these
- describe how central venous pressure is measured using a manual manometer.

Definition

Blood pressure is the force exerted by the blood on the blood vessel walls. It varies within the different blood vessels, being highest in the large arteries closest to the heart and decreasing gradually within the smaller arteries, arterioles and capillaries. Blood pressure continues to reduce as blood returns to the heart via the venules and veins. Blood pressure measurement (measured in millimetres of mercury – mmHg) usually reflects the arterial blood pressure although venous pressure may also be measured.

Arterial blood pressure

This is the pressure exerted on the arterial walls. Arterial blood pressure facilitates blood flow around the body to ensure adequate oxygenation of the tissues and vital organs. It is not constant, increasing during ventricular contraction (systole) and decreasing when the ventricles relax (diastole). When recording blood pressure it is important to assess both the highest and lowest levels of pressure as these reflect differing physiological responses of the cardiac cycle.

Mean arterial pressure

The mean arterial pressure (MAP) is the average pressure needed to push the blood through the circulatory system and provides a sensitive indicator of acute changes in perfusion pressure making it a valuable tool in caring for the critically ill woman (Roberts 2006). The MAP helps to interpret the changes that occur in blood pressure measurements when the systolic and diastolic pressures alter at different rates. It can be estimated electronically or mathematically, using the formula:

$$\text{Mean arterial pressure} = 1/3 \text{ systolic pressure} + 2/3 \text{ diastolic pressure}$$

Alternatively, it can be calculated quickly by doubling the diastolic pressure reading, adding it to the systolic reading and dividing the total by 3. Thus a blood pressure of 100/70 mmHg has a MAP of 80 mmHg and a blood pressure of 140/80 mmHg has a MAP of 100 mmHg.

Systolic pressure

This is the pressure exerted on the blood vessel walls following ventricular systole, when the arteries contain the most blood and is the time of maximal pressure. Systolic pressure is determined by the:

- amount of blood ejected into the arteries (stroke volume)
- force of the contraction
- distensibility of the arterial wall.

An increase in the first two factors, or a decrease in the third factor, raises systolic pressure and vice versa.

Diastolic pressure

This is the pressure exerted on the blood vessel wall during ventricular diastole, when the arteries contain the least amount of blood, resulting in the least pressure being exerted on the blood vessel walls. Diastolic pressure is influenced by the:

- degree of peripheral resistance
- systolic pressure
- cardiac output.

Diastolic pressure is lower when these are reduced, particularly when the heart rate is slower as there is less blood remaining in the arteries.

Pulse pressure

This is the difference between the systolic and diastolic pressure and reflects the stroke volume. The normal pulse pressure is 20 mmHg (Roberts 2006). A rise in pulse pressure is associated with pyrexia, infection, bradycardia and exercise whereas a decrease in pulse pressure can be the result of hypovolaemia, for example shock, haemorrhage and increased systemic vascular resistance.

Venous blood pressure

This is the pressure exerted on the walls of the veins, reflecting venous flow to the heart (particularly circulating blood volume) and cardiac function.

Central venous pressure measures the pressure within the right atrium and is determined by:

- the volume of blood entering the right atrium (venous return)
- right ventricular function
- venous tone
- intrathoracic pressure.

Normal maternal arterial values

The normal range for a healthy adult is 100–140/60–90 mmHg (Bailey et al 2008), but varies according to age and other variables. Both the National Institute for Health and Clinical Excellence (NICE 2006) and the World Health Organization (WHO 2003) define hypertension (raised blood pressure) as a systolic blood pressure of 140 mmHg or above and a diastolic blood pressure of 90 mmHg or above. Bailey et al (2008) define hypotension (low blood pressure) as occurring when the systolic pressure is below 100 mmHg. Blood pressure may vary between the right and left arm. Consequently Beevers et al (2001a), the British Hypertension Society (2009a), NICE (2006) and Poon et al (2008) recommend that blood pressure should be measured in both arms initially to determine if significant differences are present (20 mmHg systolic pressure, 10 mmHg diastolic pressure). Thereafter, the same arm should be used to measure blood pressure to ensure consistency.

Blood pressure changes related to childbirth

Pregnancy

Haemodynamic changes occur during pregnancy primarily as a result of hormonal and anatomical changes, resulting in an increased blood volume, increased cardiac output and heart rate. In the non-pregnant individual this would result in an increase in blood pressure; however, during pregnancy these changes are counterbalanced by the effect of progesterone on the blood vessel walls, resulting in decreased peripheral resistance. Pregnancy is not normally associated with significant changes in arterial blood pressure. Blood pressure usually begins to decrease during the first trimester, as the effects of progesterone are evident before blood volume has increased to its maximum point in the third trimester. Blood pressure begins to rise gradually from the middle of pregnancy, returning to prepregnancy levels by term. The early decrease in blood pressure is much less for systolic pressure than for diastolic pressure (Blackburn 2007). Murray & Hassell (2009) suggest the systolic blood pressure decreases by an average of 5–10 mmHg, whereas the diastolic blood pressure can decrease by up to 10–15 mmHg below the baseline by 24 weeks' gestation. Venous pressures do not alter significantly during pregnancy, although venous pressure below the uterus does increase with gestation. This may impede venous return to the heart but does not usually create problems. However, some women may experience a transient hypotensive episode (supine hypotensive syndrome) due to the weight of the gravid uterus compressing the inferior vena cava, impeding venous return. This occurs more commonly when in a supine position and is quickly rectified by changing to a lateral or recumbent position and it is advisable that women are not laid flat on their back during the second half of pregnancy.

Labour

Increased anxiety and pain levels can result in a rise in blood pressure. Additionally, both systolic and diastolic blood pressures increase during uterine contractions; the greater increase is seen in the systolic values. Both these increases return to the baseline level once the contraction is over (Blackburn 2007). It is therefore important to estimate the blood pressure between contractions.

Postnatal period: maternal

Increased venous return following delivery results in higher venous pressures. As the blood volume and physiological effects of pregnancy decrease, the blood pressure will return to its prepregnant level.

Postnatal period: baby

Blood pressure increases with gestational age; blood pressure is lower in the preterm baby than the term baby. A rapid rise in arterial blood pressure occurs during the first week of life, with blood pressure increasing gradually with age (Swinford et al 2006).

Factors influencing arterial blood pressure

A variety of factors influence arterial blood pressure, including:

- Blood volume: a reduction in circulating blood volume (e.g. haemorrhage, shock), resulting in a decrease in both systolic and diastolic blood pressure.
- Heart rate: blood pressure increases with an increasing heart rate providing the circulating blood volume is unaltered.
- Age: blood pressure increases with age due to loss of elasticity of the arterial walls.
- Diurnal variations: systolic pressure is highest in the evening, lowest in the morning and changes during rest and sleep periods.
- Weight: overweight people tend to have higher blood pressure.
- Alcohol: a consistently high alcohol intake is associated with higher blood pressure, although alcohol may also lower blood pressure by inhibiting the effects of antidiuretic hormone, resulting in vasodilatation.
- Smoking: smoking increases blood pressure, with effects lasting up to 30–60 minutes.
- Eating: blood pressure increases for 30–60 minutes following ingestion of food.
- Stress, fear, anxiety: these can all raise blood pressure by stimulating the sympathetic nervous system; 'white coat' syndrome refers to anxiety-related hypertension resulting from attending a healthcare setting.
- Exercise: exercise increases blood pressure, with effects lasting 30–60 minutes.
- Distended bladder: this can increase blood pressure, with effects lasting 30–60 minutes.
- Hereditary factors: some people have an inherited predisposition to raised blood pressure; where one parent is hypertensive there is a 10–20% risk of the offspring developing hypertension with the risk increasing to 25–45% where both parents are hypertensive (Dungan et al 2008).
- Disease: any disease process affecting stroke volume, blood vessel diameter, peripheral resistance or respiration will alter blood pressure.
- Renin: high renin levels cause vasoconstriction and an increase in blood volume (due to increased salt and fluid retention within the kidneys), resulting in a rise in blood pressure.

Indications

Blood pressure is often recorded as a matter of routine throughout pregnancy and labour, less so during the postnatal period. While the circumstances in which the estimation of blood pressure is undertaken can vary, they include:

- the initial booking history to establish a baseline, ideally by 10 weeks gestation (NICE 2008)
- at each antenatal visit (NICE 2008)
- during labour, initially and then 4 hourly (NICE 2007)
- following each epidural bolus/top-up (see Chapter 25)
- as the clinical condition dictates, e.g. shock and haemorrhage, symptoms such as headaches, visual disturbances, proteinuria
- pregnancy-induced hypertension
- preterm or sick babies
- blood transfusion (see Chapter 49)
- before, during and after surgery: with other vital sign observations, it should be taken at 5-minute intervals for 30 minutes, every 30 minutes for 2 hours and then hourly until stable after caesarean section (NICE 2004).

Equipment

Sphygmomanometer

The basis of measuring blood pressure is to exert a measured pressure on an artery (commonly brachial), usually with a sphygmomanometer, which comprises a manometer (pressure gauge) and an inflatable cuff. The blood flow is occluded and as the pressure is released and blood begins to flow through the artery, different sounds can be heard through a stethoscope (auscultatory). Oscillatory sphygmomanometers detect the pulsation of blood flow via a pressure sensor in the cuff, avoiding the need to listen for sounds.

Different types of sphygmomanometer are available and can be divided into two categories: (1) auscultatory (manual) and (2) oscillatory (automated, electronic). Aneroid and mercury column manometers are the two forms of auscultatory sphygmomanometer available and are seen more commonly in the community setting. Auscultatory sphygmomanometers are considered to be the gold standard for blood pressure measurement [Medicines and Healthcare Products Regulatory Agency (MHRA) 2006] and Beevers et al (2001a) consider mercury manometers to be more accurate than aneroid devices. Oscillatory systolic values tend to be higher than auscultatory values, but oscillatory diastolic values tend to be lower than auscultatory values. To ensure accurate blood pressure comparisons between different recordings, measurements should be undertaken on similar equipment. It is important to record the type of sphygmomanometer used. The use of oscillatory manometers is increasing, particularly within hospitals.

All sphygmomanometers should be maintained properly, with manometers being recalibrated every 6–12 months to maintain accuracy. Turner et al (2006) suggest that lack of sphygmomanometer calibration can result in both over- and underdetection of hypertension, proposing that systolic hypertension is not detected in 20% adults but might be falsely detected in 15% of adults. Diastolic hypertension may be undiagnosed in 28% of adults and falsely diagnosed in 31% adults, indicating that some women will be wrongly treated for hypertension and some who should be treated will be missed. The date of the last calibration should be marked on the machine. The tubing should also be checked regularly for signs of deterioration and replaced accordingly. The control valves should be able to hold a pressure of 200 mmHg for 10 seconds, allowing for a rate of fall of 1 mmHg per second (Jolly 1991); it is important for the control valves to be checked regularly to ensure the free passage of air without undue force.

Aneroid manometers

This type of manometer has a circular gauge encased in glass, with a needle that points to numbers. Pressure variations within the inflated cuff cause metal bellows within the gauge to expand and collapse, moving the needle up and down the gauge. Prior to use, the needle should be set at zero.

These are lightweight, compact and portable but less accurate than mercury column manometers as the metal parts are liable to expand and contract with temperature changes. Aneroid manometers should undergo biomedical calibration on a regular basis to increase accuracy. Beevers et al (2001a) suggest these devices lose accuracy with time, resulting in falsely low readings.

Mercury column manometers

This type of manometer has mercury contained within a glass column, with ascending numbers on either side of the column. The mercury should be clearly visible, have no gaps and rest at the zero level. If the mercury is below zero, the reservoir can be topped up. The column of mercury usually needs to be upright; some mercury manometers are read at an inclined angle but these are not commonly used in midwifery. The mercury should be read at eye level as looking up or down at the mercury can result in distorted readings. When examining the manometer, ensure the air vent or filter at the top of the column is clear and clean (oxidation of mercury can make it appear dirty and difficult to read, columns should be cleaned every year). If it becomes blocked, the mercury response is sluggish, leading to false results (Jolly 1991).

Mercury manometers underestimate systolic pressure by up to 10 mmHg and overestimate the diastolic (based on phase V sounds) pressure by up to 8 mmHg (Jolly 1991).

Mercury is a substance hazardous to health and should a spillage occur, appropriate steps should be taken to remove the mercury and minimise the risks of contamination. Each NHS Trust should have a policy to deal with this situation. The use of mercury-based equipment is decreasing due to the associated environmental risks.

Oscillatory manometers

These are electronic machines that measure blood pressure automatically. A cuff is placed around the arm, as with a manual manometer, and is attached to the machine. The machine can be set to record blood pressure on a regular basis, inflating and deflating the cuff at the desired time. A stethoscope is not required. The systolic and diastolic pressures are displayed visibly. The pulse is often counted and recorded at the same time.

Oscillatory manometers can reduce the errors associated with auscultatory sphygmomanometers (e.g. sampling error) and observer bias, such as terminal digit preference, threshold avoidance (Gupta et al 1997). However, talking with the woman while blood pressure is being recorded may increase the measurement by 10–40% (Fetzer 1999). Ma et al (2008) measured blood pressure using an automated machine on both bare and sleeved arms and found no significant differences in blood pressure. Thus using an automated machine may be appropriate for women who are unwilling or unable to have a bare arm.

Heinemann et al (2008) found that automated machines consistently recorded lower blood pressure for both systolic and diastolic measurements and conclude that whilst they can be used with some degree of confidence for recording the systolic pressure, caution should be used with recording the diastolic pressure. Thus it would be sensible to estimate the blood pressure manually on any woman thought to have or be at risk of raised blood pressure.

Summary

Various sphygmomanometers are available for use:

- Aneroid manometers are lightweight and portable; however, there is a tendency to error due to expansion and contraction of the metal parts with temperature changes.
- The mercury column manometer is considered the gold standard for non-invasive blood pressure measurement.
- Automated manometers reduce errors such as terminal digit preference and threshold avoidance.
- All manometers should be properly maintained and serviced.

The cuff

The sphygmomanometer has a cuff that is placed around the upper part of the arm (Fig. 5.1), or occasionally around the forearm or lower thigh. The cuff is an inelastic cloth that encircles the arm and contains a bladder. Inside the bladder is an inflatable balloon that, when inflated to a pressure higher than the pressure within the artery, occludes the artery. At this point, blood flow ceases and the pulse is no longer palpable. The cuff is held in place either by Velcro fastenings or, if a long tapering cuff is used, by wrapping it around the arm several times and securely tucking the end into the cuff. A loose cuff can distort the reading. The bladder is attached to tubing with a bulbous end that is squeezed to inflate the bladder. For cuffs attached to manual sphygmomanometers, a valve on the bulb controls the pressure within the bladder.

If the upper arm cannot be used, the lower arm can be used by placing the cuff centrally above the radial artery, or the lower third of the thigh with the cuff placed above the posterior popliteal artery. Systolic pressure is 20–30 mmHg higher in the leg

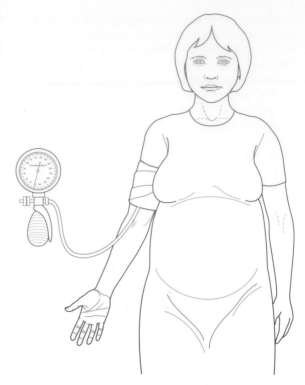

Figure 5.1 • The position of the cuff on the upper arm

than in the arm. The lower arm and leg are rarely used in midwifery.

It is important to use the correct cuff size; a cuff that is too small in length or depth can give falsely high readings (cuff hypertension). Conversely, a cuff that is too large can give falsely low readings (Oliveira et al 2002). The British Hypertension Society (2009b) recommends the length of the inside bladder of the cuff should be at least 80% of the arm circumference and the depth should be at least 40%. The correct cuff width is 20% greater than the arm diameter (Jolly 1991, Oliveira et al 2002). Thus, standard cuff sizes (12 cm wide) are not appropriate for all adults as this is too small for large arms (use the wider 15–16 cuff) and too large for lean arms. Cuff lengths vary from 22 to 36 cm. Lean arms require a cuff length of 35 cm, larger arms 42 cm (Bardwell 1995).

Stethoscope

By placing a stethoscope over the artery, the sounds of the blood flow and vibrations in the surrounding tissues can be heard. The level at which the artery is occluded and no sounds heard is equal to the systolic pressure. As the cuff is deflated, the pulse reappears and pulsating sounds are heard with each beat of the heart.

The stethoscope head may be in two parts, with a bell-shaped end and a flat diaphragm side, or it might have just the diaphragm shape. Either side of the stethoscope head can be used for auscultation as similar results are obtained with each (Kantola et al 2005). However, the British Hypertension Society (2009b) recommends the use of the diaphragm and it is often easier to hold in this position.

Care should be taken not to press too hard on the stethoscope head as this compresses the brachial artery, resulting in a misleading murmur and possibly lowering the diastolic pressure reading. Bardwell (1995) suggests a pressure of 10 mmHg on the stethoscope significantly reduces the diastolic blood pressure and, of more concern, a pressure of 100 mmHg maintains the Korotkoff sounds until zero, making a recording impossible. It is also important to ensure the stethoscope is not tucked under the cuff edge as this can have the same effect.

The stethoscope should be in good condition, particularly the earpiece, which should be clean and well fitting.

Ultrasound (Doppler) stethoscopes can be used if the arterial pulse is too weak to be heard on auscultation.

Korotkoff sounds

The different sounds heard are named after the man who defined them in 1905. Korotkoff defined the sounds according to five phases, reflecting different stages in the measurement of blood pressure (Table 5.1)

Individual variations can occur in the sequencing of these sounds. In around 5% of hypertensive people, the phase II sounds may be absent, replaced by a short period of silence: the 'auscultatory gap'. This can last through a change of 40 mmHg. Audible Korotkoff sounds may be absent in 20–30% of obese people (Bardwell 1995).

The muffling sounds of phase IV are heard when the pressure gauge is 7–10 mmHg higher than the intra-arterial diastolic pressure. This is due to a loss of transmission of pressure from the cuff to the artery. The absence of sounds associated with phase V is considered to be more closely related to the intra-arterial diastolic pressure. However, phase V sounds may be very low or absent in some adults, particularly during pregnancy.

Whether to use phase IV or phase V sounds to record blood pressure has been the subject of debate, particularly when measuring blood pressure in pregnancy. From their analysis of the evidence, Beevers et al (2001b) recommend phase V, as this is 'the most accurate measurement of diastolic pressure'. If, however, phase V continues to zero, phase IV should be used and it should be documented that this is the Korotkoff phase used.

PROCEDURE: blood pressure estimation using a manual manometer

- Obtain informed consent.
- Encourage the woman to empty her bladder.
- Take the sphygmomanometer and stethoscope to the woman.
- Wash and dry hands.
- If the woman has been active, allow her to rest for at least 5 minutes.
- Position the sphygmomanometer so that the base of the manometer is level with the woman's heart, whenever possible.
- Assist the woman into a suitable position, legs uncrossed and expose her upper arm, ensuring no constriction from tight clothing.
- Support her arm, and ask the woman to turn the palm of her hand upwards.
- Palpate the brachial artery and position the cuff 2–3 cm above the site of brachial pulsation in the antecubital fossa, with the bladder of the cuff placed centrally above the artery to ensure even distribution of pressure during cuff inflation, and ensure the valve is closed.

Phase	Sound
I	Faint tapping sounds that increase in intensity
II	Softening, swishing sounds
III	Crisper sounds with an intense pitch, not as intense as phase I
IV	Abrupt, muffled sounds, which become soft and blowing
V	Silence – no sounds heard

Table 5.1 Blood-pressure phases and Korotkoff sounds

- Palpate the brachial or radial artery with the fingertips of one hand and, with the other hand, inflate the cuff rapidly by pumping the bulb until the pulse disappears; continue to inflate the cuff 30 mmHg above this.
- Slowly deflate the cuff by opening the valve slightly, taking note of when the pulse reappears; this gives an approximate reading of the systolic pressure and prevents confusion arising from the presence of an auscultatory gap.
- Quickly deflate the cuff by opening the valve fully and wait for 30 seconds then close the valve.
- Place the stethoscope earpieces in your ears (allowing the angle of the earpieces to follow the angle of the external auditory canal) and position the head of the stethoscope over the brachial artery.
- Inflate the cuff to a pressure 30 mmHg higher than the palpated systolic pressure.
- Slowly deflate the cuff at 2–3 mmHg per second, listening for the appearance of the first clear sound (Korotkoff I).
- Read the needle position or mercury level (systole) (at eye level).
- Continue to deflate the cuff slowly until the sounds become absent.
- When the sounds are no longer audible (Korotkoff V), read the needle position or mercury level (diastole) to the nearest 2 mmHg, deflate the cuff rapidly.
- Assist the woman into a comfortable position, removing the cuff and readjusting her clothing.
- Discuss the findings with the woman.
- Document the findings and act accordingly.

Factors affecting accuracy

The whole procedure of recording blood pressure can take up to 5 minutes (Nolan & Nolan 1993). Care should be taken throughout to minimise the risk of inaccuracies occurring. Accuracy can be considered under three main headings: technique, equipment and operator bias.

Technique

Position

The arm should be at the level of the heart (midsternum). If above this level, the blood pressure may give a falsely low reading, whereas placing the arm below this level can give a falsely high reading, with differences of up to 10 mmHg (Beevers et al 2001b, British Hypertension Society 2009c, Petrie et al 1986). Blood pressure is altered by 0.49 mmHg (systolic pressure) and 0.47 mmHg (diastolic pressure) for each centimetre the arm is above or below the heart (Adiyaman et al 2006). The arm should be horizontal and supported; if left dangling at the hip, blood pressure may increase by 11–12 mmHg (Bailey et al 2008). An unsupported, extended arm may result in the diastolic pressure rising by up to 10% (Beevers et al 2001b).

The woman can adopt any position that is comfortable, although her legs should not be crossed at the knees as this can result in a falsely high recording (Adiyaman et al 2007). If the woman changes her position immediately prior to this procedure, it is better to wait for a few minutes before recording the blood pressure to avoid erroneous results. Beevers et al (2001b) suggest waiting 3 minutes if a supine or sitting position is used, and 1 minute for a standing position. It is better to measure the blood pressure using the same position each time as blood pressure is lower when standing compared to sitting and supine positions and is highest in the supine position (particularly the systolic pressure) Eser et al 2007).

Cuff position

The bladder needs to be over the brachial artery and fitted properly, as discussed earlier.

Deflation of the cuff

Rapid deflation can result in an inaccurate measurement (Reinders et al 2006) with the systolic pressure being underestimated and the diastolic being overestimated. The measurement should be recorded to the nearest 2 mmHg.

Never stop deflating the cuff between systolic and diastolic readings or reinflate the cuff to recheck the systolic reading. Blood will begin to flow into the lower arm, increasing the blood volume below the cuff, reducing the intensity and loudness of sounds (Hill 1980).

Rechecking the measurement

If the reading is abnormal, it should be repeated twice more and the mean value calculated (Cook 1996). However, if multiple recordings are taken, at least 2 minutes should elapse between recordings

(Hill 1980). Cook (1996) further recommends that if an abnormal blood pressure is found on the initial assessment, it should be estimated in both arms.

Equipment

- Auscultatory and oscillatory manometers can yield different results.
- Inappropriate cuff size.
- Equipment not properly maintained.

Operator bias

Operators might have an unconscious bias about what they expect to hear, influenced by knowledge of earlier recordings. If checking a woman's blood pressure that has already been recorded, accuracy is increased if previous findings are not known.

Monitoring blood pressure in the baby

Blood pressure estimation in the baby is of particular significance as babies, especially preterm babies, are unable to tolerate fluctuations in blood pressure, predisposing them to intracranial haemorrhage.

Blood pressure can be read intermittently with a manometer system, using either auscultatory or oscillatory manometers, or continuously, using a transducer attached to an arterial line, connected to an oscilloscope. However O'Shea & Dempsey (2009) found that non-invasive methods of blood pressure measurement overestimated the mean blood pressure compared with invasive methods. If the manometer system is used, minimal handling is required; oscillatory manometers are preferred. If the cuff is left on between measurements, it should be repositioned every 4–6 hours to reduce the risk of skin damage, nerve palsy or limb ischaemia. Blood pressure is recorded as for the adult; however, it may be difficult to auscultate the brachial artery with a stethoscope, and thus Doppler stethoscopes are often used. It is important to use the correct cuff size to obtain an accurate measurement, and neonatal cuff sizes are available. The cuff can be placed around either the arm or the leg as values are similar (O'Shea & Dempsey 2009).

Normal range

Blood pressure in the baby varies according to postnatal age, birth weight, body weight, cuff size and state of arousal. It is lowest in babies who are sleeping, increasing during periods of wakefulness, agitation, crying and suckling. While systolic and diastolic pressures can be recorded, it is more usual to record the mean arterial pressure. Normal values have been developed by body weight and postnatal age. Blood pressure begins low but increases by 1–2 mmHg a day for the first 3–8 days then by 1 mmHg per week for the next 5–7 weeks (Swinford et al 2006).

Central venous pressure

Central venous pressure (CVP) is the pressure within the superior vena cava or right atrium, measured in centimetres of water (cmH_2O) when using a manual manometer and mmHg when monitoring with a pressure transducer. The central venous catheter is inserted via the femoral, brachial, subclavian or internal jugular vein and the catheter tip positioned in the right atrium or upper portion of the superior vena cava (or inferior vena cava if access is via the femoral artery). It is a direct measurement of blood pressure and is considered an important determinant of venous return measuring the pressure of blood filling the right atrium and cardiac output. It provides a more accurate reading of blood pressure and informs fluid management in the critically ill woman (Holloway 1993).

There is a difference in normal values depending on whether a water manometer or pressure transducer is used. Normal CVP measurements are 5–8 cmH_2O (water manometer) and 0–6 mmHg (pressure transducer) (Morton et al 2005). To convert from cmH_2O to mmHg, divide by 1.36; to convert from mmHg to cmH_2O, the number should be multiplied by 1.36.

The position of the woman should always be recorded and ideally the same position used for each measurement; however, this will depend on the woman's condition, for example, if she becomes breathless she might need to alter position from supine to semi-recumbent/upright. The zero point of the manometer should be in line with the base of the woman's right atrium; this is the phlebostatic axis and is located at the fourth intercostal space where it joins the sternum. An imaginary line is extended from here to the side of the chest to

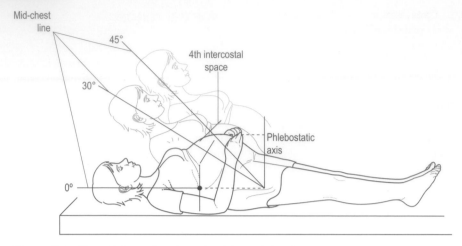

Figure 5.2 • The phlebostatic axis and phlebostatic level

intersect with a second imaginary line between the front and back of the chest (Fig. 5.2). This is known as the phlebostatic level and the site of intersection is marked on the side of the woman's chest to highlight the place used to obtain the reading.

CVP readings are affected by the amount of blood in the right ventricle prior to systole, the contractility of the right ventricle and the amount of resistance to blood being ejected from the right ventricle. A low CVP reading is associated with haemorrhage, dehydration, hypovolaemia, drug-induced vasodilatation and vigorous diuresis. A high CVP reading is associated with ventricular failure, fluid overload, fluid retention in cardiac and renal disease, pulmonary obstruction, congestion and/or embolism.

Equipment

CVP readings can be obtained via a water manometer, suitable for low pressures (<40 cmH$_2$O) or a pressure transducer and oscilloscope. The transducer converts the pressure waves to electrical energy, displayed on the oscilloscope. It is useful when pressures are high or where waveform depiction is required. Water manometers provide intermittent readings, whereas pressure transducers provide continuous readings of a CVP trace with a clear waveform that moves up and down in line with the respiratory pattern.

The CVP line is attached to a three-way tap, allowing for movement of fluid between the central venous line, intravenous infusion (saline, dextrose or dextrose saline) and manometer (Fig 5.3). This

allows for fluid infusion directly into the larger veins, and the tap is usually open to facilitate this. By moving the tap, the fluid can be redirected to an alternative site (e.g. the manometer) or prevented from flowing altogether. It is important to note the position of the tap prior to, during and following CVP measurement.

PROCEDURE: measuring central venous pressure using a manual manometer

- Gain informed consent, gather equipment and ascertain site to be used.
- Wash and dry hands.
- Assist the woman in a supine or semi-recumbent position to allow the baseline of the manometer to be level with the woman's right atrium.
- Place the manometer so that the baseline is level with the woman's right atrium (in line with the mark on the side of the woman's chest).
- Slide the scale up or down by loosening the securing screw until the baseline figure is next to the arm of the spirit level – this should correspond to zero.
- Extend the arm of the spirit level to ensure the baseline and right atrium are level.
- Move the manometer to position the bubble between the parallel lines of the spirit level.
- Turn off all intravenous infusions running through the same site as the CVP line.

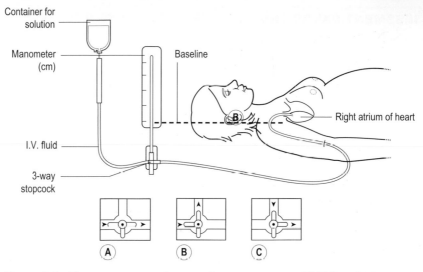

Figure 5.3 • Three-way tap on the central venous pressure (CVP) line. **A** The position prior to reading or between readings, with fluid running from the fluid solution to the woman. **B** The position at the beginning of the procedure, as the manometer fills with fluid. **C** The position during the recording (Adapted with kind permission from Jamieson et al 1997)

- Turn the three-way tap to open the access from the intravenous infusion to the manometer, allowing the fluid to run slowly into the manometer.
- Allow the manometer to fill several centimetres above the expected reading, without the upper end of the manometer becoming contaminated with fluid, then switch off the infusion line.
- Remove any bubbles in the manometer as this can distort the reading.
- Turn the three-way tap to direct the fluid from the manometer to the central venous line, allowing the fluid from the manometer to enter the woman's right atrium.
- The column of fluid will fall rapidly and begin to oscillate with respiration between two numbers (usually 1 cmH_2O). The pressure in the column of fluid in the manometer is now equal to the pressure in the right atrium.
- Note where the fluid is and read off the higher number.
- Turn off the three-way tap to the manometer, and recommence the intravenous infusion, adjusting the infusion rate accordingly.

- Assist the woman into a comfortable position, readjusting her clothing.
- Wash and dry hands.
- Document the findings and act accordingly.

ROLE AND RESPONSIBILITIES OF THE MIDWIFE

These can be summarised as:

- recognising the need to undertake blood pressure measurement
- completing the procedure correctly
- documenting the findings and acting on them accordingly
- ensuring that any equipment used is properly serviced and maintained.

Summary

- CVP measurement provides an accurate reading of blood pressure in the critically ill woman.
- The zero point of the manometer should be sited using the mark on the side of the woman's chest indicating the phlebostatic axis.

SELF-ASSESSMENT EXERCISES

The answers to the following questions may be found in the text:

1. What is the difference between systolic and diastolic blood pressure?
2. What is the normal blood pressure and how is this altered during childbirth?
3. Discuss the factors that may influence blood pressure.
4. Discuss the factors that influence the accuracy of the measurement and how the midwife can minimise this.
5. What is the central venous pressure and how can it be measured?

References

Adiyaman A, Tosun N, Elving LD, et al: The effects of crossing legs on blood pressure, *Blood Press Monit* 12(3): 189–193, 2007.

Adiyaman A, Verhoeff R, Lenders JWM, et al: The position of the arm during blood pressure measurement in sitting position, *Blood Press Monit* 11(6):309–313, 2006.

Bailey M, Crossen S, Hofland J, et al: Observations. In Dougherty L, Lister S, editors: *The Royal Marsden Hospital manual of clinical nursing procedures*, ed 7, Oxford, 2008, Blackwell Science, pp 504–511.

Bardwell J: For good measure... blood pressure measurement, *Nurs Times* 91(27):40–41, 1995.

Beevers G, Lip GYH, O'Brien E: ABC of hypertension. Blood pressure measurement Part 2 – conventional sphygmomanometry: technique of auscultatory blood pressure measurement, *Br Med J* 322:1043–1047, 2001a.

Beevers G, Lip GYH, O'Brien E: ABC of hypertension. Blood pressure measurement Part 1 – sphygmomanometry: factors common to all techniques, *Br Med J* 322:981–985, 2001b.

Blackburn ST: *Maternal, fetal and neonatal physiology: a clinical perspective*, ed 3, St. Louis, 2007, Saunders.

British Hypertension Society: Factfiles for health professionals blood pressure measurement. Online, 2009a: Available: http:www.bhsoc. org.publications_leaflets.stm 15 March 2009.

British Hypertension Society: How to measure blood pressure. Online, 2009b: Available: http:www.bhsoc. org/bp_monitors_BLOOD_ PRESSURE_17846.pdf 15 March 2009.

British Hypertension Society: Factfiles for health professionals blood pressure measurement. Online, 2009c: Available: http:www.abdn.ac. uk/medical/bhs/booklets.proced. htm 15 March 2009.

Cook R: Measuring and recording blood pressure (continuing education credit), *Nurs Stand* 11(7):51–53, 1996.

Dungan J, Yucha CB, Artinian NT: Hypertension as a risk factor. In Moser DK, Riegel BR, editors: *Cardiac Nursing A Companion to Braunwald's Heart Disease*, St. Louis, 2008, Saunders, pp 431–445.

Eser I, Khorshid L, Yapucu Gunes U, et al: The effect of different body positions on blood pressure, *J Clin Nurs* 16(1):137–140, 2007.

Fetzer SJ: Vital signs. In Potter PA, Perry AG, editors: *Basic nursing: a critical thinking approach*, ed 4, St Louis, 1999, Mosby, pp 434–477.

Gupta M, Shennan AH, Halligan A, et al: Accuracy of oscillometric blood pressure monitoring in pregnancy and pre-eclampsia, *Br J Obstet Gynaecol* 104:350–355, 1997.

Heinemann M, Sellick K, Rickard C, et al: Automated versus manual blood pressure measurement: a randomised cross over trial, *Int J Nurs Pract* 14(4):296–302, 2008.

Hill MN: What can go wrong when you measure blood pressure? *Am J Nurs* 80(5):942–946, 1980.

Holloway NM: *Nursing the critically ill adult*, ed 4, California, 1993, Addison Wesley.

Jamieson EM, McCall JM, Blythe R, et al: *Clinical nursing practices*, ed 3, Edinburgh, 1997, Churchill Livingstone.

Jolly A: Taking blood pressure, *Nurs Times* 87(15):40–43, 1991.

Kantola I, Vesalainen R, Kangassalo K, et al: Bell or diaphragm in the measurement of blood pressure, *J Hypertens* 23(3):499–503, 2005.

Lewis G editor: The Confidential Enquiry into Maternal and Child Health (CEMACH) Saving Mothers' Lives: reviewing maternal deaths to make motherhood safer – 2003–2005, The Seventh Report on Confidential Enquiries into Maternal Deaths in the UK, London, 2007, CEMACH.

Ma G, Sabin N, Dawes M: A comparison of blood pressure measurement over a sleeved arm versus a bare arm, *Can Med Assoc J* 178(5):585–589, 2008.

MHRA (Medicines and Healthcare Products Regulatory Agency): Device bulletin blood pressure measurement devices DB2006(03), 2006: Online. Available: http://www.mhra.gov.uk/ Publications/Safetyguidance/ DeviceBulletins/CON2024245 16 March 2009.

Morton PG, Tucker T, Van Rueden K: Patient assessment: Cardiovascular system. In Morton PG, Fontaine DK, Hudak CM, et al, editors: *Critical Care Nursing A Holistic Approach*, ed 8, Philadelphia, 2005, Lippincott, Williams & Wilkins, pp 211–291.

Murray I, Hassell J: Change and adaptation in pregnancy. In Fraser DM, Cooper MA, editors: *Myles textbook for midwives*, ed 15, Edinburgh, 2009, Churchill Livingstone, pp 189–225.

NICE (National Institute for Health and Clinical Excellence): *Caesarean Section*, London, 2004, NICE.

NICE (National Institute for Health and Clinical Excellence): *Hypertension: management of hypertension in adults in primary care*, London, 2006, NICE.

NICE (National Institute for Health and Clinical Excellence): *Intrapartum Care care of healthy women and their babies during childbirth*, London, 2007, NICE.

NICE (National Institute for Health and Clinical Excellence): *Antenatal care routine care for the healthy pregnant woman*, London, 2008, NICE.

Nolan J, Nolan M: Can nurses take an accurate blood pressure? *Br J Nurs* 2(14):724–729, 1993.

Oliveira SMJV, Arcuri EAM, Santos JLF: Cuff width influence on blood pressure measurement during the pregnant-puerperal cycle, *J Adv Nurs* 38(2):180–189, 2002.

O'Shea J, Dempsey EM: A comparison of blood pressure measurements in newborns, *Am J Perinatol* 26(2): 113–116, 2009.

Petrie JC, O'Brien ET, Littler WA, et al: Recommendations on blood pressure measurement: British Hypertension Society, *Br Med J* 293:611–615, 1986.

Poon L, Kametas N, Strobl I, et al: Inter-arm blood pressure differences in pregnant women, *Br J Obstet Gynaecol* 115:1122–1130, 2008.

Reinders LW, Mos CN, Thornton E, et al: Time poor: rushing decreases accuracy and reliability of blood pressure measurement technique in pregnancy, *Hypertens Pregnancy* 25:81–91, 2006.

Roberts M: Blood pressure monitoring: Invasive and Noninvasive. In Schell HM, Puntillo KA, editors: *Critical Care Nursing SECRETS*, ed 2, St. Louis, 2006, Mosby, pp 36–46.

Swinford RD, Bonilla-Felix M, Cerda RD, et al: Neonatal Nephrology. In Merenstein GB, Gardner SL, editors: *Handbook of Neonatal Intensive Care*, ed 6, St. Louis, 2006, Mosby, pp 736–772.

Turner MJ, Irwig L, Bune AJ: Lack of sphygmomanometer calibration causes over- and under-detection of hypertension: a computer simulation, *J Hypertens* 24(10):1931–1938, 2006.

World Health Organization: World Health Organization (WHO)/International Society of Hypertension (ISH) statement on management of hypertension, *J Hypertens* 21(11):1983–1992, 2003.

Assessment of maternal and neonatal vital signs: respiration assessment

6

Changes in the respiratory and heart rate have been identified as being the earliest and most sensitive indicator of deterioration of wellbeing (Hogan 2006). Thus although respiration assessment is rarely undertaken for the healthy woman and baby, it is of significance in the event of ill health. This chapter considers the effects of pregnancy upon the respiratory system, other factors affecting respiration and the midwife's role and responsibilities in completing the observation correctly. Pulse oximetry is also discussed.

LEARNING OUTCOMES

Having read this chapter the reader should be able to:

- define external respiration, identifying the normal ranges, factors that influence it and the principles for correct assessment
- discuss the safe and accurate use of pulse oximetry.

Definition

External respiration is the means by which the body gains oxygen (inspiration) and excretes carbon dioxide (expiration). Assessment of respiration includes observation of the rate (number per minute), depth and regularity of breaths and any associated signs (e.g. skin colour). Breath sounds may also be heard, or the chest felt to rise and fall, as well as being visually observed.

Normal values

There is some debate as to the normal respiratory rate for a healthy adult at rest. Mooney (2007) suggests this is 12–18 times per minute; Docherty & Coote (2006) state the rate is 10–20 breaths per minute whereas Bailey et al (2008) propose the respiratory rate to be 14–18 per minute.

Respiration can be consciously controlled (e.g. for swimming, singing, etc.) but is unconsciously determined by definite and precise mechanisms.

Tachypnoea is an increased respiratory rate, above 20 breaths per minute. It can be due to pain or fever (Bailey et al 2008, Nelson & Schell 2006), although Docherty & Coote (2006) suggest that tachypnoea occurs with respiratory rates above 30 breaths per minute.

Bradypnoea refers to a decreased but regular respiratory rate of below 8 (Docherty & Coote 2006) or, more commonly, 10 breaths per minute (Nelson & Schell 2006). Dyspnoea refers to difficulty with breathing and the woman may be seen to use some accessory muscles of respiration, e.g. shoulder or neck, have nasal flaring and/or pursed lips.

The newborn baby may breathe irregularly with a respiration rate of 40–60 breaths per minute (Michaelides 2004). Due to the weakness of the intercostal muscles, the baby may appear to be breathing abdominally, as the diaphragm is extensively used (Blackburn 2007). Tachypnoea in the newborn (above 60 breaths per minute) is often an early sign of illness, particularly cardiac, respiratory, metabolic or infection (Gardner & Johnson 2006). The baby may show other signs of respiratory difficulty when tachypnoeic, such as nasal flaring (where the nares increase in size to decrease the airway resistance up to 40%), grunting (from forced expiration through a partially closed glottis) and using accessory muscles of respiration (the thin chest walls are pulled inwards on inspiration – recession/retraction, usually seen around the sternum, intercostal, subcostal and supracostal muscles).

Changes related to childbirth

Pregnancy

When supporting both the fetus and the woman, the body's oxygen demands are high. The function and anatomy of the respiratory tract changes. Breathing is largely diaphragmatic, with the diaphragm being displaced upwards as the lower ribs flare. Progesterone relaxes the smooth muscle of the alveoli and despite the gravid uterus splinting the diaphragm from below, each breath is deeper. The rate of respiration is unchanged.

Labour

The number and strength of contractions affect the pattern and depth of respiration during labour. Breath holding should be discouraged and deep breathing between contractions should be encouraged to maintain oxygenation amidst considerable muscular activity. Breathing exercises can assist the woman both physically and psychologically. Maternal hyperventilation can lead to decreased fetal oxygenation (Blackburn 2007).

Postnatal period: maternal

Respiration returns swiftly to its pre-pregnant rate, volume and pattern once labour is completed. This is due to the decrease in intra-abdominal pressure that allows increased movement of the diaphragm. The effects of progesterone on the respiratory tract, for example, rib cage elasticity, take 1–3 weeks to resolve completely (Blackburn 2007).

Postnatal period: baby

Respiration is initiated as the baby is born and the fetal circulation adapts to the extrauterine circulation. A mature, patent respiratory tract is needed for oxygenation of the lungs. The first breath requires high negative intrathoracic pressure (30–40 cmH$_2$O) but thereafter, due to the action of surfactant, a pressure of only 5 cmH$_2$O is required. Respiration is established by a number of factors:

- stimulation (light, tactile and temperature)
- compression and decompression of the chest as it passes through the vagina
- reflex stimulus of the respiratory centre from the chemoreceptors
- changes within the cardiovascular system to perfuse the lungs.

Factors influencing normal respiration

- Exercise: an increase in oxygen demand causes an increase in respiration.
- Emotions: the respiration rate and depth can be consciously controlled, which can be useful, e.g. breathing patterns in labour. Anxiety, nervousness,

stress, excitement, fear and other emotions can also affect respiration.

- Pain: hyperventilation is a physiological response to pain.
- Insult or injury: complications such as pulmonary embolism or amniotic fluid embolism can cause infarction of the lung tissue and respiration may cease. The preterm infant might lack maturity of the respiration centre in the brain or have structural/physiological deficiencies, e.g. lack of surfactant.
- Infection: infections that impair lung function cause the lungs to work harder to oxygenate the body. Fever (wherever the infection is) also increases the body's oxygen demands.
- Reduced number of red blood cells: anaemia or haemorrhage reduces the oxygen-carrying capacity of the blood. To overcome this hypoxia, the respiration rate increases to supply the body with extra oxygen.
- Acidosis/alkalosis: respiration adjusts automatically to maintain acid–base balance in conjunction with other body systems. Changes in respiration can shift the balance, e.g. hyperventilation creates alkalosis.
- Medications: opiate analgesics depress respiration; they are unlikely to have this effect in a healthy woman experiencing small doses (e.g. pethidine) but transplacental passage and therefore respiratory depression for the fetus/ baby at birth is well documented (Siney 2004). The woman undergoing a general anaesthetic will require mechanical ventilation as paralysis of her respiratory function is induced. Mechanical ventilation controls the rate, depth and regularity according to need.

Indications

Mother: respiration assessment

Although a recognised part of the vital signs assessment, the respiration rate is usually only counted if observed to be abnormal in rate, depth or regularity upon initial observation. The woman's colour and behaviour should also be noted: cyanosis might be seen in the mucous membranes (e.g. lips or nail beds), and shortage of oxygen can result in confused behaviour and speech. Respirations should be assessed in the following circumstances:

- Admission to hospital with any respiratory complaint (e.g. asthma, chest infection, tuberculosis), chest pain, breathlessness, cyanosis, after a road traffic accident or with any serious disorder (e.g. major haemorrhage, pre-eclampsia).
- During active resuscitation.
- Before, during and after surgery (presurgery assessment provides a baseline against which later observations are compared): the National Institute of Health and Clinical Excellence (NICE 2004) is clear that, among other vital sign observations, the respiratory rate should be assessed every 5 minutes after caesarean section for 30 minutes. Thereafter, it should be assessed every ½ hour for 2 hours and then hourly providing that the observations are satisfactory.
- Following intrathecal opioids: if diamorphine has been used it should be assessed hourly for at least 12 hours, 24 hours if morphine has been used (NICE 2004).
- Patient-controlled analgesia with opioids or epidural with opioids: hourly monitoring throughout is indicated, and for at least 2 hours following discontinuation of the treatment (NICE 2004).
- Any signs of altered breathing pattern associated with psychological upset.

Baby: respiration assessment

- At birth, as part of the Apgar score.
- Any signs of cyanosis, sternal recession, nasal flaring, noisy breathing (e.g. grunting) or laboured breathing, where the baby is using obvious energy to breathe.
- After meconium-stained amniotic fluid or administration of naloxone at delivery.
- During active resuscitation (see Chapter 56).

PROCEDURE: assessment of maternal respiration

- This is probably the only procedure when the consent of the woman is not sought: making her aware of the action of counting her respirations will undoubtedly cause her to think about them and thus give a false reading.
- A respiration assessment is made at the same time as counting the pulse: if the wrist is supported

across the woman's chest, it is possible to count the pulse and then to either feel the rise and fall of the chest, or observe it, counting respiration.

- Other factors (e.g. sound, depth, regularity, symmetry of both sides of the chest) are observed at the same time, along with the woman's colour and condition.
- Signs of increased respiratory effort should be noted: nasal flaring, pursed lips, use of accessory muscles (e.g. shoulder/neck) and any audible cough/wheeze.
- All findings should be documented.
- The respiration rate should be counted for 60 seconds.
- Records are completed and the result should be acted on accordingly.

As for pulse assessment (see Chapter 4), the findings can be recorded pictorially on an observations chart or written in prose. The findings are discussed with the woman.

PROCEDURE: assessment of baby's respiration

- Informed consent must be gained from the parent(s).
- A crying or excited baby should be calmed before respiration can be counted accurately.
- When assessing the respiration rate of a baby, it is better to expose the chest and abdomen, and observe/feel, listen and count for 1 minute, due to the irregularity of respiration.
- Signs of increased respiratory effort should be noted – nasal flaring, grunting, sternal, subcostal or supracostal recession/retraction.
- Record the findings and discuss them with the baby's parent(s).

Pulse oximetry

Pulse oximetry is used in conjunction with respiration assessment, particularly when a woman is seriously ill or after surgery. Approximately 98–99% of the oxygen breathed is carried by the haemoglobin in the blood to the body tissues and organs (arterial haemoglobin saturation: SaO_2). The other 1–2% is dissolved in the plasma and is known as the partial pressure of oxygen (PaO_2). Sufficient amounts of oxygen in the plasma result in more being carried by the haemoglobin and vice versa: less in plasma means that there is less in haemoglobin. Pulse oximetry measures the arterial saturation, referred to as SpO_2. Pulse oximetry uses two lights – red and infrared – which have different wavelengths. The lights are passed through peripheral tissue and the oxyhaemoglobin and haemoglobin without oxygen attached absorb the emitted lights differently. The probe is able to calculate the difference in the amount of light wavelengths absorbed and convert this into a percentage (Chandler 2000, Kelly 2006).

Although technologically complicated, pulse oximetry is straightforward to use and has good reliability (Moyle 1999). Kelly (2006) suggests the monitors are accurate within 2–4% of oxyhaemoglobin levels measured in arterial blood gas samples and that the machines maintain this accuracy rate within the SpO_2 range 70–100%; below 70%, the reliability is poor. Normal oxygen saturation in women and babies would be in the range of 92–98% (Coull 1992), Docherty & Coote (2006) advise that a saturation level of 95% or above is acceptable for an adult; it is unlikely to be 100%. It is clear, however, that O_2 saturation assessments do not take the place of arterial blood gas assessments (Moyle 1999). The UK Department of Health (DH 1996) suggests that failure to use pulse oximetry postoperatively constitutes substandard care.

Informed consent is gained. For adults, the monitor (Fig. 6.1A) is placed over a finger, toe or earlobe; for babies a hand or foot is the most likely site for the probe (Fig. 6.1B). The light should pass from the top of the probe to the bottom of the probe (switch on and check direction before applying the monitor).

Accuracy and safety

- Accuracy and safety are maintained only if the correct type of probe is applied correctly, hence the need to understand the different manufacturers' instructions.
- Accuracy also depends on the flow of blood through the light being adequate. Poor circulation in a limb, or too much extraneous light (poorly fitted probe), can affect the reliability of the results.

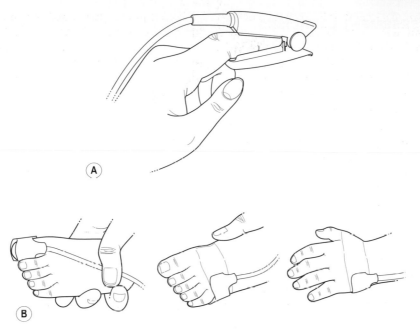

Figure 6.1 • A Adult pulse oximetry probe (Adapted with kind permission from Jamieson et al 2002). B neonatal pulse oximetry probe

- Thermal damage, possibly leading to necrosis, can occur to the skin of neonates if a probe is left in position for too long without a change of site. According to the Medicines and Healthcare Products Regulatory Agency (MHRA 2001), they should be re-sited every 4 hours. This is particularly relevant in a preterm infant.
- Accuracy is also affected by movement, shivering, dirt, dark nail polish, poor circulation, vasoconstriction, bright or fluorescent lighting and an inaccurately sized probe, e.g. never use an adult probe on a baby.
- Neonatal probes are supplied with their fixative (tape or Velcro); applying additional tape can also affect the results.
- Pulse oximetry is unaffected by skin colour or by jaundice (Moyle 1999).
- The midwife must be familiar with the equipment, noting correct storage, use and maintenance, and knowing too, when to refer. Pulse oximetry use and findings must be documented.

ROLE AND RESPONSIBILITIES OF THE MIDWIFE

These can be summarised as:

- recognising when respiration assessment is indicated and when other interventions such as pulse oximetry are required
- undertaking the techniques correctly
- referral if indicated
- contemporaneous record keeping.

Summary

- Assessing respiration is completed unobtrusively and includes the rate, depth, regularity and sound.
- The general condition of the woman or baby is assessed simultaneously.
- Pulse oximetry is an accurate, non-invasive technique that measures oxygen saturation via a correctly fitted peripheral probe.

SELF-ASSESSMENT EXERCISES

The answers to the following questions may be found in the text:

1. Discuss how pregnancy, labour and the puerperium affect respiration. What would be the accepted normal values during these times?
2. Define external respiration.
3. Describe when the midwife is likely to complete a respiration assessment:
   a. for a woman
   b. for a baby.
4. Which factors affect the accuracy of pulse oximetry?
5. Summarise the role and responsibilities of the midwife when undertaking respiration assessment.

References

Bailey M, Crossen S, Hofland J, et al: Observations. In Dougherty L, Lister S, editors: *The Royal Marsden Hospital manual of clinical nursing procedures*, ed 7, Oxford, 2008, Blackwell Science, pp 504–511.

Blackburn ST: *Maternal, fetal and neonatal physiology: a clinical perspective*, ed 3, St. Louis, 2007, Saunders.

Chandler T: Oxygen saturation monitoring, *Paediatr Nurs* 12(8): 37–42, 2000.

Coull A: Making sense of pulse oximetry, *Nurs Times* 88(32):42–43, 1992.

DH (Department of Health): *Report on Confidential Enquiries into Maternal Deaths in the United Kingdom 1991–1993*, London, 1996, The Stationery Office.

Docherty B, Coote S: Respiratory assessment as part of track & trigger, *Nurs Times* 102(44):28–29, 2006.

Gardner SL, Johnson JL: Initial nursery care. In Merenstein GB, Gardner SL, editors: *Handbook of Neonatal Intensive Care*, ed 6, St. Louis, 2006, Mosby, pp 79–121.

Hogan J: Why don't nurses monitor the respiratory rate of patients? *Br J Nurs* 15(9):489–492, 2006.

Jamieson EM, McCall J, Whyte L: *Clinical nursing practices*, ed 4, Edinburgh, 2002, Churchill Livingstone.

Kelly P: Pulse oximetry and capnography. In Schell HM, Puntillo KA, editors: *Critical Care Nursing SECRETS*, ed 2, St. Louis, 2006, Mosby, pp 284–290.

MHRA (Medicines and Healthcare Products Regulatory Agency): SN 2001(08) – Tissue Necrosis Caused by Pulse Oximeter Probes, 2001, Online. Available: http://www.mhra.gov.uk/Publications/Safetywarnings/MedicalDeviceAlerts/Safetynotices/CON0088417April2009.

Michaelides S: Physiology, assessment and care. In Henderson C, Macdonald S, editors: *Mayes' midwifery: a textbook for midwives*, ed 13, Edinburgh, 2004, Baillière Tindall, ch 31.

Mooney GP: Respiratory assessment, 2007: Online. Available: http://www.nursingtimes.net/ntclinical/respiratory_assessment.html 18 March 2009.

Moyle J: Pulse oximetry, *J Neonatal Nurs* 5(2):24–26, 1999.

Nelson CL, Schell HM: Respiratory assessment. In Schell HM, Puntillo KA, editors: *Critical Care Nursing SECRETS*, ed 2, St. Louis, 2006, Mosby, pp 241–246.

NICE (National Institute for Health and Clinical Excellence): *Caesarean section*, London, 2004, NICE.

Siney C: Drugs and the midwife. In Henderson S, Macdonald S, editors: *Mayes' midwifery: a textbook for midwives*, ed 13, Edinburgh, 2004, Baillière Tindall, ch 71.

Assessment of maternal and neonatal vital signs: neurological assessment

7

CHAPTER CONTENTS

Neurological assessment is undertaken on any woman when there are concerns about actual or possible alterations in her levels of consciousness (e.g. postseizure, magnesium toxicity, meningitis, head injury). A complete neurological assessment encompasses the level of consciousness, pupillary reaction, motor (including reflexes), sensory and cerebellar function and vital signs. This is the remit of the doctor with neurological experience and is completed initially and then as needed to determine the woman's condition. The midwife's involvement is to undertake a reduced assessment of level of consciousness, motor signs (limb movement), pupillary assessment and vital signs: respiration, heart rate, blood pressure, temperature and oxygen saturation. This chapter focuses on the principles of neurological assessment and the midwife's role in relation to undertaking this assessment.

LEARNING OUTCOMES

Having read this chapter the reader should be able to:

- describe the different components of the Glasgow Coma Scale (GCS)
- discuss how the midwife can complete the GCS
- identify the other observations that should be undertaken in conjunction with the GCS to gain a thorough neurological assessment.

Frequency of observations

The midwife must be able to complete a neurological assessment competently because it provides invaluable information regarding the woman's condition. The observations recorded should reflect the condition of the woman, and Cree (2003) recommends this should be carried out every 30 minutes until her condition has stabilized or the GCS score is 15 to enable any changes in condition to be identified early. However, the National Institute for Health and Clinical Excellence (NICE 2007) recommends that the observations should be completed every 30 minutes until the GCS is 15, when they can be recorded hourly for 4 hours, then every 2 hours, reverting to 30-minute assessments if the condition deteriorates.

Glasgow Coma Scale

The GCS was developed in 1974 and revised in 1979 to provide a quick and objective assessment of eye opening, verbal response and motor ability enabling the level of consciousness to be monitored effectively and is recognised as the 'gold standard' assessment tool (Palmer & Knight 2006). Each of these three categories has four to six different responses and each response is scored. The three scores are totalled to score between 15 (fully conscious) and 3 (no response) to provide a rapid assessment of the woman's condition and response to treatment. The score should be recorded as a fraction using 15 as the denominator (e.g. 10/15).

Eye opening

Eye opening is the first GCS measurement of consciousness as without this cognition does not occur; however, it does not indicate the neurological system is intact (Iankova 2006).

The midwife should look at the woman to see if her eyes are opening spontaneously (score 4).

If the eyes remain closed, the midwife should speak to the woman, which should provoke the eyes to open (score 3).

If the eyes continue to remain closed, the midwife will need to use painful peripheral stimuli, such as using a pen to apply pressure against the lateral outer aspect of the second or third fingers, using the alternate finger for the next evaluation (Iankova 2006, Waterhouse 2005) (score 2). Painful stimulation should be applied slowly up to a maximum of 10 seconds and should be stopped if no response has been elicited after 30 seconds. Central stimulation might elicit a response but can cause the woman to grimace whilst keeping her eyes closed, and so is not generally used unless the midwife has been appropriately trained. Jevon (2008) recommends squeezing the trapezium muscle using a thumb and two fingers, although this is difficult on large or obese women, or applying pressure to the suborbital ridge (but not if there is suspected or confirmed facial fracture or glaucoma; Palmer & Knight (2006)). The latter might cause bradycardia. Sternal rubs are used with caution because they can cause bruising. It is important to use the same stimulus on each assessment. If the eyes remain closed, a score of 1 is given. Painful stimuli should be stopped after 30 seconds if no response is achieved.

If damage has been sustained to the eyes, resulting in swelling, it is unlikely the eyes will open easily, rendering this unreliable until the swelling subsides; this should be recorded as 'C' (Jevon 2008).

Verbal response

The midwife should ascertain the level of verbal response by asking questions that require answers to show clarity and understanding – What is your name? Where are you? What day is it? – for which an accurate answer scores 5.

If the woman is able to speak using full sentences but the answers are incorrect, a score of 4 is given.

If only words and incomplete sentences are given, the score is 3, regardless of whether the words are appropriate.

A score of 2 is given if incomprehensible sounds (e.g. grunts, groans) are made.

If no sound is made in response to verbal or painful central stimuli, 1 is scored.

It is important to take into account the language spoken by the woman; if she does not speak English, an interpreter should be used.

Motor ability

The response of the upper limbs is tested to determine brain function, as the lower limbs can also be affected by spinal function. The midwife should ask the woman to bend then hold out her arms and squeeze the midwife's hands with both of her hands. The midwife can then determine that both arms can be moved, and the elbows flexed, and the power and release of grip from each hand can be noted.

A score of 6 is given if the woman is able to complete these movements and 1 if there is no response despite painful central stimuli.

Scores of 2–5 are given according to the degree of movement and flexion occurring as a result of painful stimulus: the arm moving towards the stimuli to try to remove it (5), arm bends at the elbow without rotation of the wrist (4) or with wrist rotation and forearm rotation (3), the arm extends at the elbow while the wrist flexes (2).

Pupillary assessment

The size and shape of each pupil and reaction to light are assessed by the midwife. The midwife should look at the pupils to determine if they are the same shape and whether the eyes are working together. The diameter of each pupil is then measured – the normal range is 2–6 mm (Dawson 2000) – and they are usually equal in size (unequal pupils are a late sign associated with raised intracranial pressure, but may be of little significance if the woman is alert and orientated and small differences in pupil size is often normal). Pupil reaction is assessed by shining a bright light from a pen torch into one eye, then the other. The pupils should decrease in size and the speed at which this is achieved is recorded. If there is no response, the pupil is fixed. Pupils that are slow to respond or which dilate suddenly and unequally indicate that cerebral oedema or haematoma is worsening (Waterhouse 2005). The level of sedation administered to the woman will affect pupil reaction – pupils measuring 1–2 mm can occur when barbiturates, fentanyl or opiates have been used.

The findings of the neurological assessment should be recorded on a neurological observation chart (Fig. 7.1) in conjunction with vital signs including temperature (see Chapter 3), pulse (see Chapter 4), blood pressure (see Chapter 5) and respiratory rate (see Chapter 6). Blood oxygen

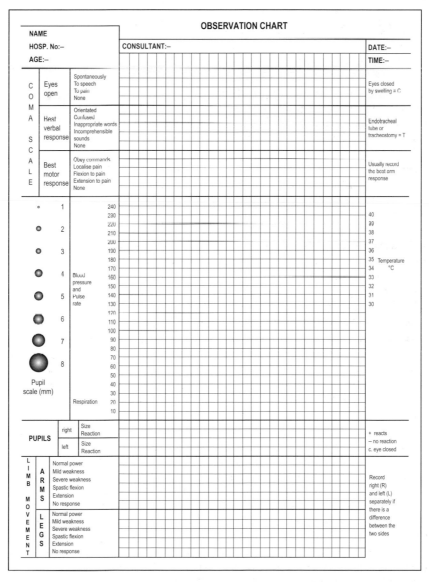

Figure 7.1 • Neurological observation chart (Adapted with kind permission from Jamieson et al 2002)

saturation should also be monitored (NICE 2007) (see Chapter 6).

As well as making a recording of the total GCS score, it is important to record – separately – the scores of the three different categories, as each one is assessing different areas of the brain. A woman with a decreasing score or one of 8 or less should always be referred to the neurologist.

The doctor should be informed if there is a severe or increasing headache, persistent vomiting, new or evolving neurological signs and symptoms (e.g. pupil inequality), a reduction to 3 or less points in eye opening or verbal responses or 2 in motor responses, agitation or abnormal behaviour as these can indicate deterioration of the woman's neurological status. If the woman's condition appears to be deteriorating, it is important for a second member of staff who is competent in performing neurological observations to confirm the deterioration before calling the doctor.

PROCEDURE: neurological assessment

- Gather equipment and take to the bedside:
  - ○ pencil torch
  - ○ observation chart
  - ○ thermometer
  - ○ sphygmomanometer
  - ○ pulse oximeter.
- Wash and dry hands.
- Inform the woman of the procedure and gain consent if conscious and responsive.
- Complete vital signs: temperature, blood pressure, pulse, respiration and blood oxygen saturation estimation.
- Assess level of consciousness by talking with the woman and asking her who she is, what day it is and where she is; use central stimuli if no response.
- Assess motor function by asking the woman to bend and lift her arms and to squeeze both your hands; use central stimuli if no response.
- Assess the size and shape of the pupils and movement of the eyes.
- Assess pupillary reaction by:
  - ○ darkening the room if necessary
  - ○ holding one eyelid open, move the pen torchlight towards and across the eye, moving the light from side to side

- ○ assess the degree and speed at which the pupil constricts
- ○ repeat with the other eye
- ○ then with both eyelids held open, shine the light into one eye: the pupil in the other eye should also be observed to constrict
- ○ repeat with the other eye.
- Ensure the woman is covered and comfortable.
- Document all findings on the observation chart.
- Act on findings accordingly.

ROLE AND RESPONSIBILITIES OF THE MIDWIFE

These can be summarised as:

- undertaking a competent examination in which all of the information is gained
- recognising deviations from the norm and instigating referral
- appropriate record keeping.

Summary

- Neurological assessment is undertaken where there are actual or potential altering levels of consciousness.
- The GCS determines the level of consciousness by assessing the woman's response to the three categories of eye opening, verbal response and motor ability.
- The midwife can undertake the GCS and estimation of vital signs as part of the woman's neurological assessment to determine any changes to her condition.
- Additionally, the doctor will evaluate motor and sensory function as required.

SELF-ASSESSMENT EXERCISES

The answers to the following questions may be found in the text:

1. What are the three categories of the Glasgow Coma Scale?
2. What observations should you undertake in conjunction with the Glasgow Coma Scale?
3. How does the midwife assess eye opening?
4. If there is no response, how are central stimuli applied?
5. How can the midwife determine the verbal response?
6. How does the midwife assess motor response?

References

Cree C: Acquired brain injury: acute management, *Nurs Stand* 18(11): 45–53, 2003.

Dawson D: Neurological care. In Sheppard M, Wright M, editors: *Principles and practices of high dependence nursing*, Edinburgh, 2000, Baillière Tindall, pp 145–182.

Iankova A: The Glasgow coma scale, *Emerg Nurse* 14(8):30–35, 2006.

Jamieson EM, McCall J, Whyte L: *Clinical nursing practices*, ed 4, Edinburgh, 2002, Churchill Livingstone.

Jevon P: Neurological assessment Part 3 – Glasgow coma scale, *Nurs Times* 104(29):28–29, 2008.

NICE (National Institute for Health and Clinical Excellence): *Head injury triage, assessment, investigation and early management of head injury in infants, children and adults*, London, 2007, NICE.

Palmer R, Knight J: Assessment of altered conscious level in clinical practice, *Br J Nurs* 15(22): 1255–1259, 2006.

Waterhouse C: The Glasgow coma scale and other neurological observations, *Nurs Stand* 19(33):56–64, 66–67, 2005.

Principles of infection control: standard precautions

8

CHAPTER CONTENTS

Healthcare professionals are widely exposed to large numbers and varieties of microorganisms. Human immunodeficiency virus (HIV) and other blood-borne contagious infections have increased the need to protect both women and midwives from infection. The term 'standard precautions' (previously having incorporated 'universal precautions') refers to the measures taken universally, i.e. by all health professionals for all women and babies, all the time, (whatever the clinical environment) to achieve mutual protection. As an important area of care, the reader is required to keep up to date with developing protocols, both for self-protection and to provide the best possible care. The 'cost' of infection to individuals (service users and staff), the NHS and the community as a whole is large and the increasing incidence of healthcare-acquired infections (HCAIs) all mean that complacency cannot be permitted. This chapter reviews the use of standard precautions and the principles of isolation nursing.

LEARNING OUTCOMES

Having read this chapter the reader should be able to:

- discuss the nature and significance of standard precautions, indicating the midwife's role and responsibilities
- describe source and protective isolation nursing
- briefly discuss the principles of protective isolation.

Standard infection control precautions

Childbearing women are considered to be in a high risk category for standard precaution use because:

- unprotected sexual intercourse is likely to have taken place
- there is exposure to large amounts of blood and body fluid during care.

It is almost impossible to appreciate who may be infected and who is not. Applying precautions to everyone maintains safety and prevents any individual feeling isolated or 'singled out'. Confidentiality might be compromised if some procedures are perceived to be used for some women and not for others. Although there might be times when wearing protective clothing is potentially disruptive to the relationship that a midwife has built up with a woman, the midwife must consider the significance of protection, both for the woman and midwife, and that of other women too.

Standard precautions should be used when there is (or expected to be) contact with blood, vaginal and seminal secretions, urine or faeces, amniotic fluid, cerebrospinal fluid, saliva, breast milk or any other bodily fluid. Sweat is the only exception. The principles need to be applied correctly and the midwife needs to be alert to the following situations:

- examination *per vaginam*, use of amnihook, fetal scalp electrodes, etc.
- childbirth, of whatever type
- theatre work, including suction/aspiration of body fluids
- disposal of administration sets, blood transfusion sets, etc.
- specimens, including neonatal capillary sampling
- injections
- newborn babies prior to bathing
- postnatal observations of lochia and perineum
- perineal repair
- cannulation and venepuncture.

Principles of standard precautions

Hand decontamination

This should be practised routinely and thoroughly before and after every episode of direct contact or care (before applying and removing gloves), when hands are visibly soiled and after several consecutive applications of alcohol hand rub (Pratt et al 2007) (see Chapter 9 for more detail). Hand decontamination should be subjected to regular audit.

Cuts or abrasions on the skin should be covered with a waterproof dressing that is an effective barrier to viruses and bacteria.

Personal protective equipment

Personal protective equipment (PPE), that is, gloves, gowns, aprons, masks, goggles, visors, caps and theatre footwear, should be selected following a risk assessment. Questions that should be asked include: What is the likelihood of transmission of microorganism to woman or midwife? What is the risk of the midwife being contaminated by any of the woman's body fluids? Determining the risk will aid the midwife in their choice of protection; Nicol et al (2008) offer a flow-chart to aid selection of PPE. The items should all be readily available at the point of use.

Properly fitting gloves should be selected and worn for appropriate procedures. Raybould (2001) found that gloves were often worn inappropriately, e.g. for washing someone's skin. This leads to staff being complacent about glove use, sometimes wearing one pair for many tasks and going from woman to woman wearing the same pair. Pratt et al (2007) are clear that gloves are single-use items put on for an aspect of care, changed for a different aspect of care and discarded as clinical waste when the procedure is completed. On removing the first glove, it is pulled off so that it becomes inside out. The gloved hand holds this while the fingertips of the ungloved hand are placed inside the cuff of the other glove in order to take it off. This is also turned inside out, with the first glove contained too. This action prevents the hands from becoming directly contaminated.

The choice of sterile or non-sterile gloves is determined by the task. Raybould (2001) gives an indication of this, but it should be interpreted in the light of newer asepsis guidelines (see Chapter 10).

Disposable plastic aprons

These should be worn when close contact with a woman or equipment is anticipated and when there is a risk that any clothing can be contaminated by body fluids (Pratt et al 2007). Like gloves, they are single-use items, worn for one task and then removed. Hart (2008) indicates that an apron should not touch the hair when being put on and it should be worn loosely. At the end of the procedure it should be removed after the gloves, by breaking the cleaner parts (e.g. neck ties and sides). It is then folded 'in' so that the potentially contaminated area does not touch the clothing. Hand decontamination should then be undertaken.

Masks and eye protection

These are necessary when body fluids can be splashed, for example during surgical procedures.

Fluid-repellent sterile gowns

These are recommended when there is a risk of extensive splashing. Pratt et al (2007) suggest that childbirth is such a situation. Hart (2008) recommend their use for invasive procedures such as siting epidurals and central catheter lines. Caps and footwear are mainly needed for theatre work, the aim is again to protect both women and staff.

Sharps

The handling of sharps must be kept to a minimum, used needles must never be resheathed but all sharps should be placed directly into an approved sharps box at the point of care. It should only be filled to the indicated level then secured and disposed of correctly.

Isolation

Isolation for known infections is necessary, this will be according to local protocol. It is discussed in greater detail below.

Infection control

The control of infection is also undertaken at service provider level. Protocols exist locally to cover issues such as cleanliness of the environment, equipment hygiene, sterile supplies, prevention of overcrowding or excessive transferring of clients between areas, disposal of clinical waste, managing accidents and spillages (discussed below) and postexposure prophylaxis, all of which the reader needs to be familiar with.

Management of spills or accidents

A specific protocol will be available in each area. The following are general guidelines:

- Skin that is accidentally exposed should be washed immediately with soap and water.

- If the conjunctiva or any mucous membrane is splashed the areas should be irrigated with copious amounts of water. Avoid swallowing if the splash is into the mouth, then rinse several times with cold water.

- In the event of a needlestick injury (or other percutaneous injury, e.g. a bite) the area should be encouraged to bleed (but do not suck the wound) under running water for at least 5 minutes (Boyle 2000). It should then be washed thoroughly (but not scrubbed) with soap and water and covered with a waterproof dressing. The agreed local protocol should be followed; this is likely to include reporting the incident to a manager and to occupational health, completing an accident form and being involved in a risk assessment.

- Spillages of body fluids should be cleared up using gloves, an apron and disposable wipes as soon after the event as possible. The local protocol will suggest which detergents are to be used, often chlorine releasing granules are used which need to be left in place for at least 2 minutes before being cleared away.

ROLE AND RESPONSIBILITIES OF THE MIDWIFE

These can be summarised as:

- recognising the significance of standard precautions and PPE, risk assessing and utilising them appropriately on every occasion
- the ability to adapt them to each area of work, maintaining safety for all
- the need to be familiar with up-to-date reports and protocols
- universal use to protect dignity and confidentiality
- the need to report and act on spillages or accidents.

Isolation nursing

Source isolation

Standard precautions aim to contain any infections, restricting their transmission between individuals. Sometimes, for specific infections such as hepatitis B, tuberculosis, *Salmonella* species or methicillin-resistant *Staphylococcus aureus* (MRSA), stricter isolation is necessary. The decision to isolate someone

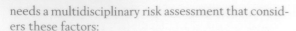

needs a multidisciplinary risk assessment that considers these factors:

- the known pathogen
- suitability of the environment, with specific regard to hygiene and domestic services support
- the anticipated length of time of the isolation
- the immune status of other ward occupants (Hart 2008).

Standard precautions and PPE are indicated as for any other clinical situation, but additional measures (depending on the causative organism and its mode of transmission) will be included. Masks may be worn; for example, if the organism is spread by droplet infection. The woman might find isolation daunting, lonely and stressful. Her understanding and cooperation are needed to achieve the desired outcome.

General principles

- In a hospital environment the use of an en suite side room is the most likely means of isolation; it is helpful if it has an anteroom where necessary items can be kept. The room should ideally have negative-pressure ventilation, i.e. air is drawn in from the ward but leaves the room externally, away from the ward (Cutter & Dempster 1999).
- The room should be equipped with all the materials required (sphygmomanometer, washing equipment, water jug and glass, sharps box, antibacterial soap and disposable towels, linen skip, infectious waste refuse sack, Pinard stethoscope, etc.). The refuse sack is sealed in the room and then removed, but otherwise none of the equipment is removed from the room until cleaned or disposed of appropriately after the woman's departure. Unnecessary furniture is removed and a visible indication is placed on the door – often a colour-coded sign – to remind all staff. Instructions should be given to friends and relatives as to how to maintain the isolation principles.
- A trolley outside the room contains items that are needed when entering the room: gloves, disposable gowns, masks, goggles, overshoes, plastic aprons and antibacterial hand rub. This should not cause an obstruction.
- The midwife should recognise the value of the multidisciplinary team: the infection control nurse, microbiologist, obstetrician and midwife

will all need to work in close communication and partnership to provide appropriate care for the woman. The woman may also remain in her side room for delivery and additional precautions should be instigated accordingly.

- Ideally, specific members of staff may be assigned to care for infected women; they should then have restricted access to other women, especially any that may be considered vulnerable to infection.

PROCEDURE: entering, attending the woman and leaving the room

- Gather any necessary additional equipment.
- Wash hands. Apply apron and any other necessary protective clothing necessary for the procedure. Use alcohol hand rub (apply gloves only if expecting to handle body fluids).
- Knock, enter the room and close the door.
- Complete the necessary care, containing all of the tasks within the room:
  ○ crockery may be brought out of the room, providing that it will be decontaminated in a dishwasher
  ○ domestic services are required to clean the room and bathroom daily; other spillages should be cleaned according to standard precaution guidelines
  ○ used linen should be placed in a red alginate bag in the room. This must be sealed before leaving the room.
- On preparing to leave the room, remove (gloves if worn), apron and use hand rub. Any other items are disposed of in the room, wash hands.
- Close the door on leaving; use antibacterial hand rub once outside the room.
- On discharge, the room is thoroughly cleaned using approved solutions; steam cleaning may be required. All furniture and equipment is washed and dried, curtains are sent to the laundry; carpeted floor may be steam cleaned.

Protective isolation

The midwife is unlikely to be involved in this type of care. It is usually applicable to severely immunosuppressed patients where it is vital that they are protected from infection. All unnecessary visitors are prohibited and extreme care is taken to ensure that no infection is taken into the room. A positive pressure environment is needed where clean air is drawn into the room from outside and forced out into the general ward area. Clearly, the ventilation systems need to be properly understood so that the opposite does not happen (Cutter & Dempster 1999). Hands are washed and protective clothing is applied before entering and removed after leaving the room.

ROLE AND RESPONSIBILITIES OF THE MIDWIFE

These can be summarised as:

- taking an active role in the multidisciplinary team to ensure that isolation is an appropriate component of care for the woman
- carrying out isolation regulations correctly, and assisting the woman and her relatives to understand their significance too
- maintaining the woman's confidentiality
- contemporaneous record keeping.

Summary

- Standard precautions aim to protect all staff, women, babies and visitors from potentially

serious infections, by recommending hand hygiene, personal protective equipment, correct management of spills, accidents, waste and sharps, and protocols that cover other issues such as environmental hygiene. It is an important aspect of the midwife's role.

- Midwives work with a high-risk client group and should include a risk assessment for standard precautions and PPE use in every situation.
- Source isolation aims to contain infection by carrying out all procedures within the woman's single room, keeping all equipment and materials within that room.
- Protective isolation prevents infection from entering the room by use of protective measures before entering and after leaving; visitors are restricted.

SELF-ASSESSMENT EXERCISES

The answers to the following questions may be found in the text:

1. Describe what constitutes standard precautions.
2. In which situations is a risk assessment necessary to appreciate which of the standard precautions or PPE are indicated?
3. Describe how to correctly apply and remove a plastic apron.
4. Discuss the principles of source and protective isolation nursing.

References

Boyle M: Blood borne infections, *Pract Midwife* 3(7):48–50, 2000.

Cutter M, Dempster L: Cover notes, *Nurs Times* 95(31):25–27, 1999.

Hart S: Barrier nursing. In Doughty L, Lister S, editors: *The Royal Marsden Hospital Manual of Clinical Nursing Procedures Student Edition*, Oxford, 2008, Wiley Blackwell, pp 117–204.

Nicol M, Bavin C, Cronin P, Rawlings-Anderson K: *Essential Nursing Skills*, ed 3, Edinburgh, 2008, Mosby.

Pratt RJ, Pellowe CM, Wilson JA, et al: epic2: National evidence-based guidelines for preventing healthcare-associated infections in NHS hospitals in England, *J Hosp Infect* 65S:S1–S64, 2007.

Raybould LM: Disposable non-sterile gloves: a policy for appropriate usage, *Br J Nurs* 10(17):1135–1141, 2001.

Principles of infection control: hand hygiene

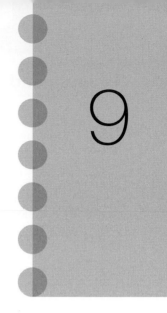

9

CHAPTER CONTENTS

This chapter focuses on the principles of hand hygiene, an important means of infection control. Hand hygiene encompasses both hand care and hand decontamination:

> Hand decontamination is the most effective and certainly the most cost effective method of preventing health-related infection.
>
> (Gould 2002)

Healthcare-acquired infections (HCAIs) are infections acquired when in hospital as a result of health-care intervention; they are caused by a wide variety of microorganisms, many of which are commensals. Approximately 30% of the population has *Staphylococcus aureus* living on their skin or in their nose with no ill effects. The methicillin-resistant *Staphylococcus aureus* (MRSA) strain of this microorganism is found in 3% of the population and is difficult to treat because of its resistance to antibiotics. MRSA is spread by direct contact with a contaminated surface/material or skin-to-skin. Hand washing and the use of alcohol hand rub help to reduce the incidence. Another bacterium that is a source of HCAIs is *Clostridium difficile*, which lives in the intestine of approximately 3% of the population. Usually, the normal gut bacteria prevent C. *difficile* from affecting the person; however, if these are destroyed by antibiotics, C. *difficile* multiplies, producing toxins that can cause diarrhoea. These spores are not killed by alcohol hand rub.

HCAIs are troublesome to those affected because they are likely to stay in hospital three times longer than those who are not affected and they will require longer-term follow-up and care; from a financial perspective, HCAIs cost up to three times more to treat (Gould et al 2007). The Department of Health (DH) estimates that it costs £4000–10 000 more to treat a patient who develops an infection and adds between 3 and 10 days on the length of stay (DH 2008).

LEARNING OUTCOMES

Having read this chapter the reader should be able to:

- discuss the principles of general hand care
- identify the occasions when the midwife should undertake hand decontamination
- describe the main differences between 'medical' and 'surgical' scrub
- discuss the role and responsibilities of the midwife in relation to hand hygiene.

General hand care

- Examine the hands for cuts, grazes and torn cuticles: these increase the risk of infection to the midwife and should be covered with a waterproof dressing.
- Keep nails short and filed: long or ragged nails can scratch women and babies or tear gloves and introduce infection. Dirt and secretions might be found under the nails, which can harbour microorganisms.
- Avoid using false nails or nail extensions: bacteria can flourish in the ridge that appears as the nail grows. Additionally, Ward (2007) suggests the percentage of Gram-negative bacteria found on false nails is higher than on natural nails.
- Apply an emollient hand cream/moisturizer to the hands on a regular basis to prevent them from drying out and cracking.

Hand decontamination

Hand washing refers to both social and clinical situations where hands are washed. Social hand washing is generally ineffective in destroying bacteria due to incorrect washing technique or inappropriate cleansing agents used. Hand decontamination is a more accurate term that refers to the removal of blood, body fluids, microorganisms and their debris by mechanical means or their destruction (Gould 2002, Pratt et al 2007).

Cleansing agents

The use of soap and water removes almost all transient microorganisms but does not reduce the number of resident microorganisms (e.g. *Staphylococcus aureus*) by any significant amount (Mallett & Dougherty 2000). Although this is acceptable in non-invasive situations with a low-risk population, there are many situations where the resident microorganisms also need to be reduced (e.g. aseptic procedures). Antiseptics (e.g. chlorhexidine) reduce the transient and resident microorganisms at the time of application, with some residual activity keeping bacterial counts low over several days as the chlorhexidine binds to the stratum corneum (Gould 2002, Gould et al 2007). Pratt et al (2007) reviewed the effectiveness of different hand washing preparations and concluded that soap was as effective as antiseptic agents.

Both soap and antiseptics usually involve the use of running water following one of two procedures: the 'medical/social' or the 'surgical' scrub. The former is used for normal hand washing and prior to aseptic techniques, whereas the latter is used when scrubbing for an operative procedure; this is a lengthier procedure involving the hands and arms.

Products containing alcohol are inexpensive, have very good bactericidal activity and are effective against most Gram-negative and Gram-positive bacteria (Gould et al 2007). Alcohol-based hand rubs can be used without water and are applied to the hands and wrists. This is much quicker as the hand rub often dries within 15 seconds; however, the action of the hand rub is short lived, has no effect on spores and some enteroviruses and has no detergent effect. Thus, alcohol-based hand rubs are recommended for use only when the hands are visibly clean [Gould et al 2007, Royal College of Nursing (RCN) 2000]. When used effectively, hand rubs remove transient microorganisms and significantly reduce the number of resident microorganisms but are not effective against some microorganisms such as C. *difficile* (Pratt et al 2007). Hand rub does not remove organic material or dirt.

Alcohol hand rubs are as effective as aqueous scrubbing in preventing surgical site infections; chlorhexidine gluconate-based aqueous scrubs are more effective than povidone–iodine-based aqueous scrubs as they result in less bacteria on the cleaned hands (Tanner et al 2008). Tanner et al (2008) found no evidence regarding the use of brushes and sponges for the surgical brush. However, Hsieh et al (2006) suggest that frequent and prolonged use of a brush/sponge might cause deterioration in skin condition, removal of the outer layer of epidermis and lead to potentially undesirable changes in colonizing skin flora such as increased colonization with Gram-negative bacteria. They further suggest the use of an alcohol-based hand rub was more effective in reducing microbial counts than the more traditional surgical scrub of 6 minutes using chlorhexidine gluconate.

Indications for hand decontamination

- Prior to putting on gloves.
- Before and after contact with the skin of the woman or baby or body fluids.

- Prior to undertaking an aseptic technique.
- Prior to handling food.
- When visibly soiled.
- After going to the toilet.
- After contact with soiled or potentially contaminated equipment.
- After removing gloves.
- After several consecutive applications of hand rub.

Principles of hand decontamination

- Consider all equipment as being contaminated: minimal handling of taps, soap dispenser, sinks, drying equipment, especially after washing; the use of foot-operated pedal bins and elbow taps is advised.
- Avoid wearing jewellery and watches: rings (particularly stoned rings) increase the number of microorganisms found on the hand; jewellery and watches also make it difficult to clean the hands thoroughly.
- Use warm running water, with the flow regulated for comfort: hot water opens the pores, predisposing to skin irritation; avoid splashing water, especially over clothes, as microorganisms can be transferred and multiply in moisture.
- Use appropriate soap and work up a lather: soap will emulsify fat and oil and lower the surface tension, making cleaning easier.
- Use a circular motion, encouraging rubbing and friction: this loosens and removes dirt and transient microorganisms.
- Use good-quality disposable paper towels to dry hands as microorganisms are removed by friction and the spread of microorganisms is minimised compared with hot air driers and towels (Blackmore 1987, Pratt et al 2007).

PROCEDURE: medical/social scrub

The hands should be rubbed vigorously together under tepid running water for a minimum of 15 seconds (NICE 2003, Pratt et al 2007). If an alcohol hand rub is used, 2×5 mL applications should be rubbed in following the steps in Figure 9.1 to ensure all surfaces of the hand come in contact with the hand rub. The hands should be rubbed until the hands and wrists are dry:

- Remove all jewellery (except for plain gold band), including wrist watch.
- Turn the taps on and adjust the water temperature and flow, taking care not to splash the water, and wet the hands (Fig. 9.1A).
- Using an appropriate cleansing agent, rub the palms together vigorously (Fig. 9.1B), then rub the palm of one hand along the top of the other hand and along the fingers, using the fingers on the top hand to rub along the edge of the lower hand; repeat for the other hand (Fig. 9.1C).
- Wash the fingers by interlacing together, rubbing them back and forth, ensuring the inner aspects of both sides of all the fingers are rubbed together (Fig. 9.1D).
- Wash the fingertips of one hand by rubbing them against the palm of the other hand; repeat for the other hand (Fig. 9.1E).
- Wash the thumb of one hand by using the fingers of the other hand wrapped around it, washing in a circular motion; repeat for the other thumb (Fig. 9.1F).
- Grasp the left wrist with the right hand, rubbing around the wrist; repeat for the right wrist (Fig. 9.1G).
- Rinse all the surfaces of the hand and wrist.
- Repeat hand washing if hands are heavily contaminated.
- Dry each hand and wrist separately.
- Turn off the taps using the elbows or the paper towel.
- Dispose of the towel using a foot-operated pedal bin.

PROCEDURE: surgical scrub

This involves washing the hands and forearms to remove as many bacteria as possible from these areas and maintain the lowest possible microbial count throughout the surgical procedure; washing should take at least 2 minutes.

- Remove all jewellery, including wrist watch.
- Turn the taps on and adjust the water temperature and flow, taking care not to splash the water.
- Keeping the hands above the level of the elbows, wet the hands and forearms to the elbows.

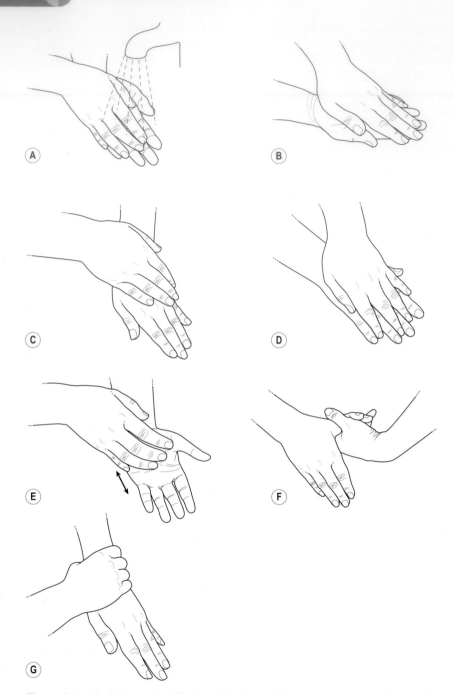

Figure 9.1 • Medical scrub. **A** Rinsing with water. **B** Washing the palms. **C** Washing the top surfaces of the fingers. **D** Interlacing the fingers. **E** Washing the fingertips. **F** Washing the thumbs. **G** Washing the wrists

- Using an antiseptic soap, e.g. 4% chlorhexidine solution, povidone–iodine, wash fingers and hands as for medical scrub and extend washing to include forearms (this may require several applications of antiseptic soap) using brush/sponge if first surgical scrub of the day.
- Rinse the soap from hands and elbows, keeping the hands above the level of the elbows, allowing the water to run from the fingertips down to the elbows.
- Turn off the taps using elbows.
- Dry each hand and arm separately with a disposable towel, drying from the fingertips towards the elbows, keeping the hands above waist level.
- Dispose of the towel using a foot-operated pedal bin.

- The use of soap and water will remove almost all transient microorganisms, blood, body fluid and dirt but does not significantly reduce the number of resident microorganisms.
- Hand rubs remove almost all transient microorganisms and significantly reduce the number of resident microorganisms but do not remove blood, body fluid and dirt.
- A 'medical scrub' involves washing for a minimum of 15 seconds.
- A 'surgical scrub' involves washing with a brush/sponge for at least 2 minutes, with the hands above the elbows.

ROLE AND RESPONSIBILITIES OF THE MIDWIFE

These can be summarised as:

- recognising when hand decontamination should be undertaken
- being able to undertake a medical or surgical scrub correctly.

Summary

- Hand decontamination is an important means of infection control.

SELF-ASSESSMENT EXERCISES

The answers to the following questions may be found in the text:

1. What are the general principles of hand care?
2. When should the midwife undertake decontamination?
3. What hand washing agent should be used for a 'medical' scrub?
4. Describe how the hands are washed for a 'medical' scrub.
5. What are the main differences between a 'medical' and a 'surgical' scrub?

References

Blackmore M: Hand drying methods, *Nurs Times* 83(37):71–74, 1987.

Department of Health (DH): *Clean, safe care. Reducing infections and saving lives*, London, 2008, DH.

Gould D: Hand decontamination, *Nurs Times* 98(46):48–49, 2002.

Gould D, Hewitt-Taylor J, Drey N, et al: The clean your hands campaign: Critiquing policy and evidence base, *J Hosp Infect* 65(2):95–101, 2007.

Hsieh HF, Chiu HH, Lee FP: Surgical hand scrubs in relation to microbial counts: systematic literature review, *J Adv Nurs* 55(1):68–74, 2006.

Mallett J, Dougherty C: *The Royal Marsden NHS Trust manual of clinical nursing procedures*, ed 5, Oxford, 2000, Blackwell Science.

NICE (National Institute for Clinical Excellence): Clinical guideline 2: infection control, *Prevention of healthcare-associated infection in primary and community care*, London, 2003, NICE.

Pratt R, Pellow C, Wilson J, et al: epic2: National evidence-based guidelines for preventing healthcare-associated infections in NHS hospitals in England, *J Hosp Infect* 65S:S1–S64, 2007.

RCN (Royal College of Nursing): *Good practice in infection control*, London, 2000, RCN.

Tanner J, Swarbrook S, Stuart J: Surgical hand antisepsis to reduce surgical site infection, *Cochrane Database Syst Rev* Issue 1, Art. No.: CD004288. DOI: 10.1002/14651858.CD004288.pub2, 2008.

Ward D: Hand adornment and infection control, *Br J Nurs* 16(11):654–656, 2007.

Principles of infection control: principles of asepsis

10

Asepsis – the absence of sepsis or infection – is a critical component of care. Women, babies and staff all need to be protected. Among other things, infections – and particularly those arising from health care (i.e. healthcare-associated infections; HCAIs) – result in mortality, morbidity and expense. This chapter reviews the current position with regard to the principles of asepsis.

LEARNING OUTCOMES

Having read this chapter the reader should be able to:

- discuss the principles of asepsis, including equipment used, non-touch technique and establishing a sterile field
- summarise the role of the midwife.

It is recognised that an aseptic technique is important, but that it is largely based on repeated practice rather than researched evidence; it is also noted that staff perform poorly in this area (Hartley 2005). There is therefore debate around which procedures need an aseptic technique (Aziz 2009), whether gloves should always be sterile (Flores 2008) and whether asepsis or a clean technique can be used (Gilmour 1999). An initiative called ANTT (aseptic non touch technique) is a best-practice guideline endorsed by the Department of Health (DH 2009) and epic2 (Pratt et al 2007). It is a means of standardizing the technique and applying it across healthcare providers. Guidelines are provided for different procedures (intravenous practice, urinary catheterisation, wound care, cannula insertion and central venous catheter insertion), training is expected and audit is perpetual (ANTT 2008). It should also be noted that, whereas asepsis is one of the key components in reducing HCAIs, Pratt et al (2007) also put significance on hospital environmental hygiene, hand hygiene, use of personal protective equipment and the safe use and disposal of sharps. The DH (2009) places these things within the context of the whole of healthcare provision (prescribing, laboratory and mortuary services etc.).

The term 'surgical asepsis' describes the depth to which pathogens are removed from an environment, for example in operating theatres; 'medical asepsis' refers to that which is often used for generally ward-based procedures, such as catheterisation or inserting cannulae, when the transmission of pathogens is reduced as much as possible. It is accepted that an ANTT is used when referring to medical asepsis. Gilmour (2000), however, also describes a clean technique in which some of the non-touch principles are upheld but non-sterile gloves are worn.

Which procedures need an aseptic technique?

There is a lack of consensus as to which procedures need an aseptic technique. Whereas ANTT (2008) provide their guidelines for specific situations (listed above), Hart (2008) suggests that an aseptic procedure should be used for any situation that touches the mucous membranes or breaks the skin. Any invasive procedure qualifies, examples include:

* venepuncture and intravenous cannulation
* urinary catheterisation
* examination *per vaginam*
* childbirth, of whichever mode
* perineal suturing
* siting of epidural analgesia
* wound dressing
* any surgical procedure in theatre or on the ward.

They are, however, very different procedures and therefore it is the principles of asepsis that should be constantly upheld. Elements of aseptic principles are included in almost every chapter of this text, such is its importance. The reader should also read Chapters 8 and 9 to fully understand the practice.

Principles of asepsis

Preparation

Hart (2007) suggests that some element of risk assessment is necessary each time a procedure is to be undertaken. This involves the:

* woman/baby: What are their main risk factors for infection? Is their level of personal hygiene good?
* procedure: How invasive is it?
* environment: Is it cluttered? Is it disturbed (e.g. after bed making)? Is it contaminated?

Questions such as these encourage the midwife to plan and undertake care appropriately to minimise the risks. Consent also needs to be gained and the procedure carried out in a dignified way in a private

place. Environmental disturbances such as open windows, curtains wafting, use of fans and doors opening all increase the levels of airborne bacteria and so should be reduced.

Use of sterile packs and equipment

Equipment that is sterilised centrally is usually autoclaved. The colour change on the packet indicates sterility but the pack should be inspected to ensure that it has not been damaged or wet in the meantime. Sterile items should be used within their expiry date. Sterile lotions, syringes, cannulae, etc. are all supplied for single-use only (unless otherwise stated) and are disposed of after use. Increasingly, a system operates that allows sterile packs to be traced through the system, from central sterilising through to which operator used them for which woman. A label (or something similar) is placed in the woman's record after the equipment has been used and the same verification returns to the sterile supplies department.

Dressings trolleys should be used purely for aseptic procedures and should be washed daily (using detergent and dried with paper towels) and at any time if visibly contaminated. They should be wiped with an alcohol-impregnated wipe prior to each use.

Using an assistant

During an aseptic procedure a sterile field is established on the trolley/surface as well as around the woman, for example, under her buttocks and over her abdomen when catheterizing. This field must remain sterile and therefore only decontaminated hands covered in sterile gloves should touch it. Frequently in practice the midwife will undertake aseptic procedures alone. However, Hart (2007) notes that the use of an assistant is helpful in maintaining the asepsis. The assistant needs to:

* have decontaminated hands
* handle/open the external wrappers and pass the sterile contents to the sterile field or directly to the midwife (Fig. 10.1)
* aid the woman to be comfortable and 'uncovered' at the correct time
* appreciate the presence of a sterile field around the woman, taking care not to decontaminate it
* be prepared to collect additional items if necessary.

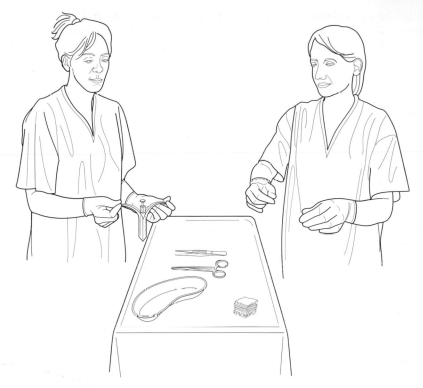

Figure 10.1 • Assistant passing items to maintain sterility of sterile field

If working alone, a midwife can adapt these principles by opening the pack, adding the other sterile items, applying hand rub, applying gloves and then continuing with the procedure. This is less efficient, leaving the sterile field and the woman exposed for longer.

Hand hygiene

Hand hygiene is the most important principle of asepsis (for greater detail, see Chapter 9). Briggs et al (1996) state that hand hygiene is one aspect of asepsis that is 'vital, well researched and uncontroversial'. Hart (2007) considers that most HCAIs are thought to be transmitted by healthcare workers' hands. The use of an alcohol-based hand rub is acceptable mid-procedure in many circumstances. It is only acceptable, however, when hand hygiene initially has been thorough and when the items handled subsequently have not been heavily contaminated. Hand hygiene is as important after a procedure as before – microorganisms can grow in gloved hands.

Use of protective clothing

Microorganisms can also be carried on clothing. The use of a clean plastic apron is indicated; this protects the clothing from bacteria, and thus the spread from one situation to another. Other personal protective equipment may be worn depending on the situation and risk assessment made.

Use of non-touch technique

Hart (2008) indicates that it is only decontaminated hands in sterile gloves with or without the use of sterilised instruments that may undertake the procedure. The susceptible site should not be touched by anything that is not sterile. No touching of ungloved hands should occur at any time, and care should be taken that the sterile gloves do not become contaminated. Kocent et al (2002) demonstrated that in 83% of cases they did. Consequently, Pratt et al (2007) reiterate that any sterile item used for any part of the procedure must not touch anything unsterile, e.g. the tip of a urinary catheter remains inside the sterile polythene on the sterile field until it enters the urethra. It does not touch the woman's leg or labia or anywhere else prior to insertion. The Luer end of a sterile syringe would be inserted directly into the end of a sterile needle; it would not touch anything else prior to the woman.

PROCEDURE: aseptic technique

- Ensure that the woman has given consent and is in an appropriate place for the procedure.
- Clean hands with alcohol hand rub, locate a clean trolley, wipe it with an alcohol impregnated wipe.
- Place the items needed on the lower shelf (checking sterility, expiry, etc.).
- Take the trolley to the woman, position her accordingly, keeping her covered until ready.
- Decontaminate hands by washing them and put on an apron.
- Taking hold of the outer wrapper of the sterile pack (whatever sort it is), open it carefully (not touching any part of the inner wrapper) onto the trolley.
- Open out the sterile inner wrapper by using only the corners or edges of the paper/cloth to create the sterile field (Fig. 10.2).

- Slide or 'drop' on all other items needed without any touching of hands on sterile items.
- Decontaminate hands with hand rub, than apply sterile gloves.
- Arrange the sterile field so that items that may be needed quickly are towards the edge, easily accessible, e.g. cord clamps.
- Ensure that the woman is comfortable and ask her to remove any covers, etc. Establish a sterile field around her, placing the drapes appropriately.
- Undertake the procedure. A gentle touch creates less contamination on the gloves (Kocent et al 2002) and is more comfortable for the woman.
- Nothing contaminated is returned to the sterile field unless absolutely necessary. It should then be placed at the far end of the field away from sterile items.
- The principle of a 'dirty' and a 'clean' hand can be upheld: this is unresearched and currently infrequently mentioned, but often seen in practice. The midwife uses one hand (the dirty hand) for initial direct contact with the woman, while the other (the clean hand) is retained over the sterile field, ready to be used for the cleaner part of the procedure. Items are passed from the clean hand to the dirty hand and then disposed of when used, preventing the dirty hand from

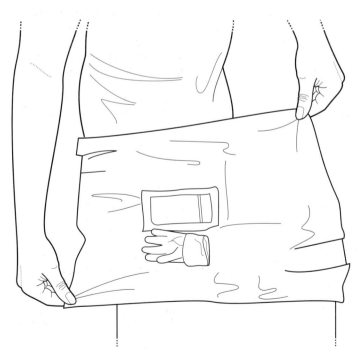

Figure 10.2 • Opening a sterile field (Adapted with kind permission from Nicol et al 2000)

contaminating anything on the sterile field. The clean hand is often the dominant or examining hand. This is illustrated in the video demonstration on the Nottingham University website (Nottingham University 2007).

- Once completed, the woman is made comfortable, the sterile field is disposed of by wrapping the remaining contents (if disposable) in the paper and placing them into the infectious waste refuse sack.
- Gloves and apron are removed and hands are washed.
- The trolley may be taken to a sluice area (non-sterile gloves are worn) where the non-disposable items are prepared for return to the sterile supplies department in the agreed format and the trolley is washed ready for the next procedure.
- Decontaminate hands and complete the woman's records.

Variations

If an assistant is available the midwife should decontaminate their hands and put on sterile gloves while the assistant adds the other items to the sterile field (see Fig. 10.1). This reduces the time that the field is exposed.

A new pack should be used if a procedure takes longer than 30 minutes (Hart 2007), the previous one having been exposed to possible contamination in that time.

Some procedures include an obviously unsterile activity, for example removing a wound dressing or swabbing the labia prior to catheterisation. Hand decontamination must take place after that part of the procedure and new sterile gloves should be worn before continuing. If it is possible to undertake such activities before the sterile field is established, e.g. using the ungloved hand inside the polythene bag to remove the wound dressing (Hart 2007), this should be done.

ROLE AND RESPONSIBILITIES OF THE MIDWIFE

These can be summarised as:

- appreciating the significance of asepsis and undertaking the procedure thoroughly and consistently
- educating the woman when caring for herself and her baby, in the light of available evidence.

Summary

- The principles of asepsis should be included (adapted if necessary) for every invasive procedure.
- Hand hygiene is essential; a non touch technique is advocated.
- Further research is indicated.

SELF-ASSESSMENT EXERCISES

The answers to the following questions may be found in the text:

1. Give four examples of the circumstances in which asepsis is indicated.
2. List the principles of asepsis.
3. Describe how to establish a sterile field, both on a trolley and around the woman, using a non-touch technique.
4. Summarise the role and responsibilities of the midwife when undertaking an aseptic procedure.

References

ANTT (Aseptic non-touch technique): 2008, Online. Available: http://antt.co.uk/ 3 February 2009.

Aziz AM: Variations in aseptic technique and implications for infection control, *Br J Nurs* 18(1):26–31, 2009.

Briggs M, Wilson S, Fuller A: The principles of aseptic technique in wound care, *Prof Nurse* 11(12): 805–810, 1996.

DH (Department of Health): *The Health and Social Care Act 2008*, London, 2009, DH.

Flores A: Sterile versus non-sterile glove use and aseptic technique, *Nurs Stand* 23(6):35–39, 2008.

Gilmour D: Redefining aseptic technique, *J Community Nurs* 13(7):22–26, 1999.

Gilmour D: Is the aseptic technique always necessary? *J Community Nurs* 14(4):32–35, 2000.

Hart S: Using an aseptic technique to reduce the risk of infection, *Nurs Stand* 21(47):43–48, 2007.

Hart S: Aseptic technique. In Doughty S, Lister S, editors: *The Royal Marsden Hospital Manual of Clinical Nursing Procedures Student*

Edition, Oxford, 2008, Wiley Blackwell, pp 83–116.

Hartley J: Handwashing needed every 3 minutes in ICU, *Nurs Times* 101(2):7, 2005.

Kocent H, Corke C, Alajeel A, et al: Washing of gloved hands in antiseptic solution prior to central venous line insertion reduces contamination, *Anaesth Intensive Care* 30(3):338–340, 2002.

Nicol M, Bavin C, Bedford-Turner S, et al: *Essential nursing skills*, ed 2, Edinburgh, 2000, Mosby.

Nottingham University: *ANTT Video demonstration*, 2007, Online. Available http://www.Nottingham. ac.uk/nursing/sonnet/rlos/places/antt/index.html [3 April 2009].

Pratt RJ, Pellowe CM, Wilson JA, et al: epic2: National evidence-based guidelines for preventing healthcare-associated infections in NHS hospitals in England, *J Hosp Infect* 65S:S1–S64, 2007.

Principles of infection control: obtaining swabs

11

The midwife might be required to obtain a swab from the woman or the baby when infection is suspected. By culturing the microorganisms obtained by the swab, specific antibiotics can be prescribed to prevent them multiplying and so stop the infection. Swabs might be required even if there is no evidence of infection (e.g. a pregnant woman with a history of vaginal group B streptococcus infection) to help inform care. This chapter focuses on obtaining swabs from the more common sites of the eye, ear, nose, throat, umbilicus, vagina, wound and placenta.

LEARNING OUTCOMES

Having read this chapter the reader should be able to:

- describe how a swab is obtained from the eye, ear, nose, throat, umbilicus, vagina, wound and placenta
- discuss the role and responsibilities of the midwife in relation to obtaining swabs.

Obtaining the swab

To increase the likelihood of isolating a microorganism, it is important that the swab is coated all over and an aseptic technique used to prevent the risk of cross-contamination. This can be achieved by rotating the swab around the area to be swabbed. Different organisms thrive and die in different cultures, thus it is important to use the correct swab stick and transport medium. For the majority of swabs, a dry swab and transport medium is sufficient. It is important to check that the swab is still sterile and has not expired, as this may affect the results. It is also important to ensure that alternative swabs and mediums are used where indicated; for example, *Trichomonas vaginalis*, *Chlamydia* spp. and *Bordetella pertussis* need charcoal-based swabs and medium. Thus, the midwife should be aware of which microorganisms are being considered as the causative organism for the presenting symptoms in the woman or baby and, if unsure, the midwife should verify with the doctor in order to use the correct swabs, media and bottles. The woman should also be aware of why several swabs are undertaken.

In some situations, the midwife might need to collect pus, exudates, moisture, etc. from the woman or baby (e.g. from the umbilical stump). These may need collecting via a swab stick, although where pus is being collected, a sterile spatula or syringe can be used to collect the pus and place it in a specimen container.

Once obtained, the swab should be placed in the transport medium, the lid secured and it should be correctly labelled, including the woman's name, hospital number, date of birth, specimen taken, time and date, all of which should correspond with the pathology form (this should also indicate if the woman is taking antibiotics). The swab should be placed in a transport bag that is sealed to prevent spillage and contamination with the pathology form.

The swab should be sent for laboratory analysis as soon as possible. The microscopy, culture and sensitivity (MC&S) analysis comprises a microscopic examination for a quick initial report of the microorganism(s) present, culture of the microorganism(s) to identify exactly which are present, a microbial count to determine if they are the result of colonisation or infection and an analysis of sensitivity to antibiotics that can prevent further growth and replication. If delay is anticipated, refrigeration may be necessary (although some swabs can be kept at room temperature); it is therefore important the midwife is aware of how to store swabs and specimens that cannot be transported quickly.

In high-risk situations, the swab should be double wrapped and labelled accordingly and the midwife should ensure she is wearing gloves and apron and, if appropriate, goggles. Standard precautions should be followed for obtaining all swabs (Chapter 8).

If swabs are required from more than one site (e.g. both eyes, ears, nostrils), a separate swab should be used for each site to minimise the risk of cross-infection from an infected to a non-infected area. Usually only one swab is required; the area that appears most affected is swabbed.

The midwife should record in the notes which swabs have been taken and the time and date. This will ensure that all staff are aware the swabs have been obtained and will serve as a reminder to check the results as soon as they are ready.

Eye

To obtain a swab from a woman, she should be sat up, with her head supported. If the swab is from a baby, the baby should be supported, with the head held steady. The lower eyelid should be pulled down gently. The swab should be held parallel to the cornea and rubbed very gently against the conjunctiva in the lower eyelid. Usually just one swab is sufficient.

Ear

To obtain a swab from the ear of a woman, she should be sat up with her head tilting to the unaffected side. If the swab is from a baby, one of the parents or another midwife should hold the baby with the head up and tilted to one side. A baby who is too ill to be moved can be laid on the good side. The external canal of the exposed ear is straightened by gently pulling the pinna upwards and backwards and the swab is inserted gently into and rotated around the external canal. It is also important to withhold medication administered via the ears for 3 hours prior to obtaining the swab as the medication can interfere with the growth of the microorganism.

Nasal swab

To obtain a nasal swab from a woman, she should be sat up with her head tilting back or lying in a supine position. If the swab is from a baby, the baby can be cradled in someone's arms or laid on his or her back. The procedure may be easier if there is someone to hold the baby's arms; alternatively wrap the baby in a blanket. The end of the swab should be moistened with sterile water. The swab should be inserted gently into the nose, moving it upwards towards the tip of the nose and rotating it.

Throat

The woman should be sitting or lying facing a strong light source and asked to open her mouth widely. The tongue should be depressed using a disposable spatula and the swab inserted to the back of the throat. The swab is then rotated quickly around the back of the throat, using the faucial tonsils as the boundary, to ensure it is coated (this is likely to make the woman gag). When removing the swab, ensure it does not come into contact with any part of the mouth, tongue or saliva.

Umbilicus

The baby should be positioned to allow easy access to the umbilicus (e.g. cradled in someone's arms or lying in a cot) and undressed to expose the umbilicus. The swab is moved gently around the umbilicus, rotating it. The baby should be redressed following the procedure.

High vaginal swab

This is an aseptic procedure, and it is undertaken following the insertion and opening of a speculum (see Chapter 28). The swab should be inserted through the speculum to the top of the vagina and rotated around. When the procedure is completed the speculum should be removed and the woman assisted into a comfortable position.

Low vaginal swab

The swab is inserted into the lower vagina for 2–4 cm (a speculum should not be used) and the swab rubbed around the front, side and back walls of the vagina.

Wound

Donovan (1998) recommends using normal saline (at room temperature) to irrigate the wound prior to swabbing (to remove surface contamination), and to moisten the swab. The swab should be rotated across a 1 cm^2 area of the wound (Levine's technique) using sufficient pressure to release exudate or fluid from the wound; the tissue should be clean, not necrotic (Gardner et al 2006).

Placental swab

The swab should be moved around the placenta (fetal side) in a zigzag direction and the placenta disposed of appropriately.

PROCEDURE: obtaining a swab

- Gain informed consent and gather equipment:
  - ○ disposable gloves and apron (if required)
  - ○ sterile swab and appropriate transport medium
  - ○ speculum and lubricating jelly, e.g. KY Jelly® (high vaginal swab only)
  - ○ sterile water (nasal swab only)
  - ○ sterile normal saline (wound swab only).
- Wash hands and apply apron and gloves.
- Position the woman or baby appropriately and obtain the swab specimen.
- Remove the swab and insert into the transport medium, sealing securely.
- Label the container with the name, hospital number (if applicable) and date of birth of the woman or baby, date and time the swab was obtained, nature of specimen, whether right or left (if applicable) and signature. Place into transport bag.
- Assist the woman or baby into a comfortable position.
- Remove and dispose of gloves and apron.
- Wash hands.
- Arrange transportation of the specimen to the pathology laboratory.
- Document findings and act accordingly.

ROLE AND RESPONSIBILITIES OF THE MIDWIFE

These can be summarised as:

- recognising the need for a swab to be taken
- ensuring the procedure is undertaken correctly, with minimal discomfort to the mother or baby and with the use of appropriate standard precautions/personal protective equipment
- correct documentation.

Summary

- Obtaining a swab is a significant, simple, but invasive procedure that may be undertaken on either the woman or the baby.

SELF-ASSESSMENT EXERCISES

The answers to the following questions may be found in the text:

1. How would the midwife obtain a swab from:
   a. the ear?
   b. the eye?
   c. the nose?
   d. the throat of a woman or baby?
2. How is an umbilical swab obtained?
3. Describe how a wound swab is obtained from a small wound.
4. What are the differences in procedures for obtaining high and low vaginal swabs?

References

Donovan S: Wound infection and wound swabbing, *Prof Nurse* 13 (11):757–759, 1998.

Gardner SE, Frantz RA, Saltzman CL, et al: Diagnostic validity of three swab techniques for identifying chronic wound infection, *Wound Repair Regen* 14(5):548–557, 2006.

Principles of hygiene needs: for the woman

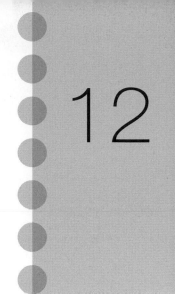

12

This chapter considers the skills required to meet the complete range of hygiene needs of the woman. Cleanliness and attention to physical appearance can be significant in promoting psychological wellbeing, as well as physical health. The principles of bed making are considered as well as personal, vulval and oral hygiene.

LEARNING OUTCOMES

Having read this chapter the reader should be able to:

- discuss the ways in which the midwife facilitates personal hygiene

- describe the ways in which vulval and oral toilets are undertaken
- identify the principles applied for the making of an occupied or unoccupied bed
- discuss the midwife's role and responsibilities in relation to each of these aspects of care.

Personal hygiene

Cleanliness is a basic human right. It is something for which individuals will set their own standards; Downey & Lloyd (2008) suggest that it is inappropriate for health professionals to apply their own standards to the women that they care for. However, the Healthcare Commission (2007) found that approximately one-third of the complaints received related to failures in meeting personal hygiene and standards of privacy for inpatients in NHS Trust hospitals.

Meeting hygiene needs

Midwives work with women for whom their level of independence is generally sufficient for them to care for their own hygiene needs. The occasions when assistance may be required include:

- immobility: epidural or spinal analgesia, surgery or existing mobility problem
- intensive or high dependency care
- prescribed bed rest, e.g. antepartum haemorrhage.

Maintaining personal hygiene affects several aspects of care. Psychologically, most people feel 'better' when clean, in particular knowing that there are no offensive odours around them. This is especially the case with postnatal women and their perineal care. In addition, the skin itself is the largest body organ and needs to be kept free from breaks and infection in order to protect the inner organs. Where a wound does exist, good standards of hygiene are often the means of preventing colonisation and so aiding healing. Perineal trauma is one such example (Steen 2007). Vulval toilet is discussed below. Pressure-area care (see Chapter 53) – particularly when incontinence is also an issue – is an important aspect of care that maintains the skin's integrity and is hindered by poor hygiene.

In ensuring that the woman's hygiene needs are met the midwife should consider facilitating as much independence as is possible. Many people will feel embarrassed to have someone else undertaking very personal aspects of care. Mobility is also encouraged (when appropriate) to reduce the thromboembolic risks that accompany child bearing (see Chapter 54). Consequently, the following measures are often preferable to being bathed in bed:

- assisting a woman to sit with a bowl, or at the sink, midwife assisting as necessary
- assisting a woman into a bath or shower, remaining with her or returning after a few minutes to assist as required.

When assisting a woman to facilitate her own needs, care should be taken to ensure that all that she needs is with her (clean clothes, toiletries, pads, etc.) and that she has access to a call bell.

Assisting with hygiene needs (in whatever way) does necessitate a risk assessment. The use of infection control strategies (standard precautions and personal protective equipment) and moving and handling guidelines should be employed accordingly (Pegram et al 2007). Consideration should also be given to upholding individual preferences and dignity with privacy. Analgesia may be given and allowed to take effect before the procedure begins.

Bed bathing

Bed bathing aims to meet the complete hygiene needs of a woman if she is confined to bed, although Baker et al (1999) indicate that bed bathing is the least effective method of patient hygiene. If required, it is a task that can bring psychological wellbeing from the period of uninterrupted individualised care, it is also a time in which holistic care is completed. The following aspects of care should accompany a bed bath:

- observation of consciousness and levels of pain (on both resting and moving)
- observation of the skin, particularly areas of pressure (see Chapter 53), inflammation, infection or allergy
- general health and nourishment, oral intake of diet and fluids
- ante- or postnatal examination
- assessment of vital signs
- wound care
- catheter or bladder care, vulval toilet
- bowel care
- attention to circulation, passive or active exercises, observations for varicosities or oedema, prevention of complications associated with immobility (see Chapter 54)
- care of intravenous infusion and fluid balance
- oral hygiene
- hair washing, pedicure or manicure
- therapeutic touch, communication, education
- attention to a safe and aesthetic environment including changes of sheets and bedding.

Principles

- Ideally, the midwife is assisted by another practitioner, this enables the woman to be exposed for a shorter time and reduces the moving and handling risks.
- The procedure should be carried out in a warm environment. Informed consent is obtained. All equipment that is needed should be gathered before commencing in order to reduce the risks of interruption.
- Own or single-use toiletries should be used and areas such as the perineum should be cleansed using disposable cloths. Attention is paid to changes in water so that dirty water (after cleansing the perineum) is not then used for cleaner areas, e.g. the feet.
- A coordinated approach is used so that there is minimal exposure of the body. Washing and drying the areas nearest to each practitioner prevents leaning over the woman and dampening areas that have already been dried (Pegram et al 2007).

- A nearby linen skip allows for the correct disposal of the used sheets once the bed has been changed.
- All care and observations are documented contemporaneously.

Modified bed baths

If the woman is able, a modified bed bath allows her to wash as much as she can, with the midwife completing any outstanding areas afterwards. If the woman is seriously ill or too uncomfortable, a partial bed bath may be performed, using the same principles but washing only the hands, face, axillae and genital area.

Vulval toilet

This is particularly appropriate for women in the early postnatal period, especially after caesarean section or instrumental delivery. While it attends to the hygiene of the perineum, it also acts as a soothing analgesic. Plain warm water is used, Sleep & Grant (1988) indicated that water was comparable to salt or Savlon® in its soothing and healing effects. Soaps and other substances can be irritant to the delicate tissues of the perineum. The midwife records this aspect of care as for any other and adheres to standard precaution and infection control protocols. The midwife may carry out the procedure or advise the woman how to undertake it herself. There are three methods of vulval toilet:

1. Assist the woman onto a bedpan, pour warm water over the vulva and perineum, pat dry with disposable wipes.
2. Sit the woman on the toilet and pour warm water over the vulva and perineum from a jug.
3. Sit the woman on the bidet (facing either direction, depending on her mobility and the comfort of her perineum). It is important that:
   a. the water is warm, not hot
   b. the sprinkle rather than jet is used, gently, so that water does not enter the vagina
   c. the perineum is dried carefully afterwards using disposable wipes.

Oral hygiene

Silk et al (2008) discuss the significance of oral care in pregnancy. Oral hygiene cleans and freshens the mouth, teeth and gums. It may aid the flow of saliva and prevent dental caries. Poor oral health can cause poor systemic health (e.g. bacterial endocarditis) and psychological wellbeing is also increased if the mouth, teeth and breath are all clean and fresh (Jones 1998). The majority of women that the midwife works with will attend to their own oral hygiene. If the woman is not able to do this, for whatever reason, the midwife must carry out this aspect of care. Likely occasions when the midwife will need to assist include:

- when nil by mouth:
  - pre- or postsurgery
  - nasogastric tube *in situ*
  - unconscious, receiving intensive or high-dependency care
- nausea and vomiting
- oxygen therapy
- mouth breathing, e.g. labour, use of inhalational analgesia.

Undertaking oral hygiene

A toothbrush and paste are considered to be the most effective tools for oral hygiene (Jones 1998). A toothbrush should be of a soft texture and used with a pea-sized amount of fluoride toothpaste (Bowsher et al 1999). The toothbrush should be correctly positioned (bristles pointing towards the roots of the teeth; Fig. 12.1) and moved gently,

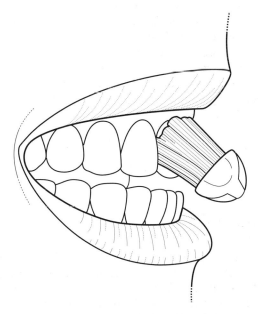

Figure 12.1 • Correct position of toothbrush for cleaning teeth (Adapted with kind permission from Jones 1998)

slightly from side to side, systematically around the top and then the lower jaw, on all surfaces of the teeth (Jones 1998). The mouth should be rinsed thoroughly to prevent any burning sensations from the toothpaste residue (Turner 1996). Foam sticks are considered to be less effective than a toothbrush, but can be useful in situations where the mouth is sore. Sodium chloride 0.9% or chlorhexidine gluconate 0.2% may be prescribed if mouthwash is indicated (Quinn 2008). Vaseline® or lip balm may be applied to dried lips (Jones 1998).

Bed making

Changing sheets or remaking a bed is indicated if the sheets are soiled, sweaty or dishevelled. The aim is to ensure that the bed is crease free, protecting skin integrity and increasing comfort. It is a difficult and time-consuming procedure to complete alone. Standard precautions use and correct disposal of used linen both reduce the risks of infection transmission. The timing of bed making should fit in with the individualised plan of care. This is particularly important if a wound is to be redressed (see Chapter 52) as the disturbance of used sheets

in the environment increases atmospheric microorganisms. The babies of postnatal women also often have contact with the woman's bed clothes (e.g. use of pillows when breastfeeding), this also necessitates that bed linen is changed frequently and that babies are exposed to minimal sources of infection.

Principles

- All equipment needed should be gathered before commencing. The bed should be at a suitable working height for both practitioners and should be easily accessible.
- If in any way contaminated the mattress is cleaned according to the agreed protocol before the bed is made.
- Care is taken to ensure that none of the bedding touches the floor; the pillows or other items that will be reapplied to the bed should be carefully stacked on an empty chair or the shelf (it pulls out) at the end of the bed.
- Working in a coordinated way, e.g. lifting the mattress at the same time allows the sheets to be anchored correctly. Mitring the corners (Fig 12.2)

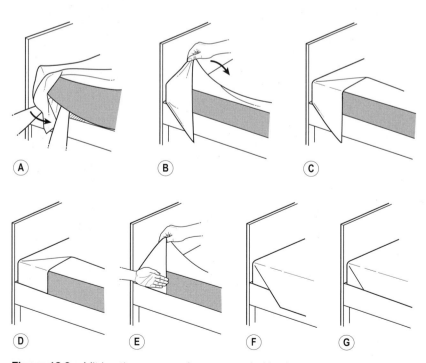

Figure 12.2 • Mitring the corners of an unoccupied bed (Adapted with kind permission from Lammon et al 1995)

also helps the sheets to stay in place and crease free (Bloomfield et al 2008).

- The woman's preference is considered when deciding how many layers of bedding are added.

Making an occupied bed

This is undertaken in one of two ways, from side to side or top to bottom. An assistant is required and, if able, the woman helps too. Care is taken to maintain her temperature and dignity. She needs to be aware of what will happen and of the fact that at some point there will be a linen 'lump' to ease over. Any appliances, catheters, drains, infusions, etc. should be handled with care.

Side to side

The woman is rolled onto her side facing the assistant. The old sheet is untucked from the bed and rolled up next to the woman's back (Fig. 12.3). The new sheet is tucked in at the top, bottom and side of the bed. It is then also rolled up next to the woman's back. The woman is assisted to roll over the 'lump' to now face the midwife on her other side. The assistant removes the old linen, unrolls the new and tucks it in. The woman is repositioned.

Top to bottom

The woman is assisted to sit up as far forwards as she is able. The old sheet is untucked at the head of the bed and rolled up so that it sits beside the woman's buttocks. The new sheet is tucked in and rolled up next to the old one. Using an overhead hoist the woman is asked to lift her buttocks whilst the two sheets are pulled through. The old one is removed, the new one is tucked in.

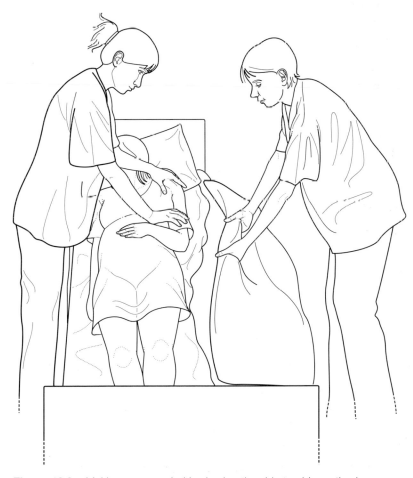

Figure 12.3 • Making an occupied bed using the side-to-side method

ROLE AND RESPONSIBILITIES OF THE MIDWIFE

These can be summarised as:

- completing the procedures safely with the maintenance of dignity and privacy, applying infection control and safe environment protocols
- offering an individualised approach, encouraging independence and mobility where possible
- contemporaneous record keeping.

Summary

- Attention to all types of hygiene benefit the physical and psychological wellbeing of the woman.
- The midwife should adapt care according to the individual woman's needs and level of dependence.

- Vulval hygiene can be both cleansing and soothing, particularly after a vaginal birth.
- Toothbrush and paste are the recommended cleaning agents for oral toilet.

SELF-ASSESSMENT EXERCISES

The answers to the following questions may be found in the text:

1. Discuss the significance of personal hygiene.
2. Identify the ways in which a woman may be assisted to wash when mobility is restricted.
3. Describe the different ways that a vulval toilet may be completed.
4. Demonstrate bed making: occupied and unoccupied.
5. Summarise the midwife's responsibilities in relation to the complete hygiene needs of the woman.
6. What equipment is used for an effective oral toilet?

References

Baker F, Smith L, Stead L: Giving a blanket bath – 1, *Nurs Times* 95 (3):40ff, 1999.

Bloomfield J, Pegram A, Jones A: Recommended procedure for bedmaking in hospital, *Nurs Stand* 22(23):41–44, 2008.

Bowsher J, Boyle S, Griffiths J: Oral care, *Nurs Stand* 13(37):31, 1999.

Downey L, Lloyd H: Bed bathing patients in hospital, *Nurs Stand* 22(34):35–40, 2008.

Healthcare Commission 2007 State of Healthcare: *Improvements and Challenges in England and Wales*, London, 2007, Commission

for Healthcare Audit and Inspection.

Jones CV: The importance of oral hygiene in nutritional support, *Br J Nurs* 7(2):74–83, 1998.

Lammon CB, Foote AW, Leli PG, et al: *Clinical nursing skills*, St Louis, 1995, Mosby.

Pegram A, Bloomfield J, Jones A: Clinical skills: bed bathing and personal hygiene needs of patients, *Br J Nurs* 16(6):356–358, 2007.

Quinn B: Personal hygiene: mouth care. In Doughty L, Lister S, editors: *The Royal Marsden Hospital Manual of Clinical Nursing Procedures Student*

Edition, Oxford, 2008, Wiley Blackwell, pp 853–870.

Silk H, Douglass AB, Douglass JM, Silk L: Oral health during pregnancy, *Am Fam Physician* 77 (8):1139–1144, 2008.

Sleep J, Grant A: Routine addition of salt or Savlon bath concentrate during bathing in the immediate postpartum period: a randomised controlled trial, *Nurs Times* 84(21):55–57, 1988.

Steen M: Perineal tears and episiotomy: how do wounds heal? *Br J Midwifery* 15(5):273–280, 2007.

Turner G: Oral care, *Nurs Stand* 10(28):51–54, 1996.

Principles of hygiene needs: for the baby

13

CHAPTER CONTENTS

The midwife has a pivotal role in educating and advising new parents on aspects of caring for their baby and helping them adjust to their new role. Women are often keen to develop the skills of caring for the baby and quickly have to learn how to change the nappy and bath the baby. However, Wray (2006) found that two thirds of women (50% were primiparous women) were not shown how to change their baby's nappy or undertake a 'top and tail' and that 34% were not shown how to bath their baby. Although this may not be a requirement for all women, primiparous women may not have pre-existing knowledge and experience of these subjects to help them, which might add to their anxieties and insecurities of becoming a new mother. This chapter focuses on the hygiene needs of the baby, specifically bathing and washing, and cleaning of the genital area, the cord and the eyes. While oral hygiene is important for the baby who is unwell, it is rarely needed for the healthy baby and will not be discussed further.

LEARNING OUTCOMES

Having read this chapter the reader should be able to:

- discuss the role and responsibilities of the midwife in meeting the hygiene needs of the baby
- discuss the rationale for not using soap or bath additives
- discuss the principles of bathing and washing the baby
- describe the methods used for applying a non-disposable nappy.

Newborn skin

The skin of the term newborn baby differs from that of an adult in a number of ways and is more delicate, increasing the risk of allergic and irritant reactions occurring. In particular, the epidermis is thinner, the protective lipid film changes after a few weeks and the secretion of sebum lessens as it is replaced by lipids of cellular origin. The lipid structure of the epidermis allow the skin to be semi-permeable thus water can pass through the skin from the baby and substances can be absorbed from the outer surface of the skin (Atherton 2005, Hale 2007, Hopkins 2004). During the neonatal period both the epidermis and dermis develop further, and there is a change in the skin's desquamation and pH surface (Steen & Macdonald 2008). Trotter (2006) agrees that the newborn skin can be easily damaged and compromised, suggesting two main causes are the destruction of the skin's barrier from delipidization (removal of lipid or fat molecules) within the top layer of the epidermis and the stimulation of an inflammatory immune response. A damaged epidermis allows more fluid to pass through the skin, which can result in dry skin further increasing the risk of sensitisation and infection (Trotter 2006).

Some babies, particularly postmature ones, have dry skin, which can crack. Although there is a temptation to rub in substances such as olive oil or emollients in an attempt to 'moisturize' the skin, Trotter (2004) cautions against this practice as the dry layer will peel off within a few days revealing a healthy layer of skin underneath, which will then require 2–4 weeks to gain its protective barrier. Steen & Macdonald (2008) agree, advising against the use of emollients or creams on the skin during the first 2–4 weeks. A further concern is that the effects of absorbing creams and emollients at such a young age are unknown. Walker et al (2005) warn that olive oil has been found to reduce the skin barrier function in mice, although it is not known if this is true for humans.

Skin cleansers/bath additives

Although water will wash away the majority of matter accumulating on the baby's skin, some substances may be fat soluble, and are more easily removed by water once they have been emulsified by a mild cleanser. Thus there is a place for using cleansing agents when washing or bathing adults and children. However, the cleansers work by suppressing the surface tension keeping the fatty substances on the skin; if this is excessive there is a risk of trauma occurring to the skin surface which is increased for the newborn baby's more delicate skin and can result in allergic and/or irritant dermatitis (Steen & Macdonald 2008, Trotter 2006).

Frequent bathing, particularly if alkaline soaps or lotions are used, may also predispose the baby to infection. An acidic skin surface – the 'acid mantle' – affords some protection against infection; a pH <5.0 has bacteriostatic properties (Blackburn 2007). At birth the baby's skin is alkaline, with a pH of 6.34, reducing to 4.95 within 4 days (Lund et al 1999). Following a bath in which an alkaline soap or bath additive is used, the skin pH increases, becoming less acidic and it may take up to an hour to regain the acid mantle (Blackburn 2007) during which time the skin is more vulnerable to microorganisms. It is advisable to undertake a bath using just warm water, as this is usually sufficient to clean the baby.

There is a lack of good researched evidence evaluating the effects of soaps and cleansers on the newborn skin (Walker et al 2005) and consequently NICE (2006) advise that cleansing agents should not be added to bath water or medicated wipes or lotions used when cleaning the baby during the first 2–4 weeks. Hale (2008) suggests it can take 2–4 weeks for the term baby's skin to develop the protective barrier with premature babies needing longer. Substances added to the bath may also be absorbed through the skin, which may increase the risk of future allergic sensitisation to topical agents (Blackburn 2007, Lund et al 1999). Simon & Simon (2004) suggest that the use of soaps and cleansers may increase the risk of omphalitis. Thus, if cleansers, wipes or soaps are to be used, they should have a neutral pH, with little or no perfume or dye added and be specifically designed for babies (never use an adult product). Hopkins (2004) suggests a compromise when parents want to use bath additives or cleansers of alternating between bathing with water only and the use of cleansers. However, bathing babies in hard water may also increase the risk of eczema occurring (Hopkins 2004, Steen & Macdonald 2008).

Baby bathing

There is no consensus about the timing of the first bath; it is in part dependent on the condition of the baby and the staffing levels of the maternity unit. A healthy term baby may be bathed shortly after birth, although in many maternity hospitals this is delayed until the baby and woman are transferred from the delivery suite to the postnatal ward or home. The rationale for the timing of the first bath centres mainly on concerns over the risks of the baby becoming cold and the risk of transferring infection.

Johnston et al (2003) recommend delaying the first full bath until feeding is established to minimise the risks of the baby becoming cold, which they suggest may be towards the end of the first week. Steen and Macdonald (2008), however, suggest that bathing can take place once the baby's temperature has stabilized above 36.8°C. Newell et al (1997) advise delaying the bath until the baby has acquired his own skin flora, considering that this may reduce the risk of infection (although this will be affected by the use of cleansers). Equally, early bathing may be advocated to reduce the risk of transmission of blood-borne infection (e.g. human immunodeficiency virus; Penny MacGillivray 1996). Trotter (2006) advises delaying the bath until the cord has separated as she considers this can interfere with the physiological process of cord separation.

The parents should be involved as much as possible, and be given the opportunity to bath their baby if they choose to, or be shown how to bath their baby if they have not had prior experience. Parents with little or no experience of handling babies may not feel confident to bath them until they are more confident holding them, thus it is important that the midwife considers the needs of the parents and supports them accordingly. Often, a big concern of the parents is that they may drop the baby in the water. If they express this concern, the midwife should ask them what they would do if this happened. Invariably the response is 'I'd pick the baby up'. This can then lead to a discussion of how to bath the baby safely and help the parents recognise what they would do if something unexpected occurred.

Whereas it is important to minimise the risk of infection, it is not necessary to bath babies every day, nor is it necessary to wash the baby's hair with each bath. For some parents, daily bathing may be an easier and more pleasurable option than washing the baby. However, Steen & Macdonald (2008) advise that when the baby is immersed in water the superficial layers of the skin hydrate and thicken with an associated reduction in cellular cohesion. Thus, skin that is overhydrated from frequent or prolonged bathing becomes more fragile increasing the risk of trauma occurring to it (Hale 2007, Hopkins 2004). Consequently Steen & Macdonald (2008) recommend that immersion in the bath should last no longer than 5 minutes.

There is no right or wrong way to bath a baby, although it is important to adhere to certain principles:

- keep the baby warm
- keep the baby secure and safe

- use warm water: the temperature should be neither too hot (which risks scalding the baby) nor too cold.

Keeping the baby warm

As babies lose heat quickly when undressed or wet, both the room and water temperature should be warm and the baby bathed quickly, without unnecessary exposure. Additionally, convective heat loss can be minimised by closing windows and switching off fans to stop draughts. Warming clothes, towel and surfaces (e.g. changing mat) minimises conductive heat loss. Drying the baby quickly, particularly the head, reduces evaporative heat loss, and ensuring the baby is not bathed close to cold surfaces such as windows minimises heat loss via radiation.

Security and safety

The bath should be filled initially with cold water to prevent the bottom of the bath from becoming too hot. Also, it reduces the risk of other children scalding themselves should they play with the bath water as it is filling. The bath should not be more than half full. The baby should never be left unattended and should always be held to prevent the head from submerging. A woman with epilepsy should place the bath on the floor rather than on a stand and should not be alone. Following a caesarean section, the woman will have difficulty lifting the baby and equipment and will require help. It may be advisable to use a jug to fill and empty the bath as lifting even a small bath half full with water may result in muscular damage.

When washing the face and hair, the baby is wrapped securely in a towel and held under the non-dominant arm, secured between the arm and body, with the head and neck supported by the non-dominant hand. To place the baby in the bath, support the baby's head and neck across the forearm and wrist of the non-dominant hand, encircling the forefinger and thumb around the top of the baby's arm. The dominant hand grasps the ankles to lift the baby in and out of the water (Fig. 13.1). The baby can be sat up to wash his back by supporting his head across the wrist or forearm of the dominant hand (Fig. 13.2), then returning the baby to the original position.

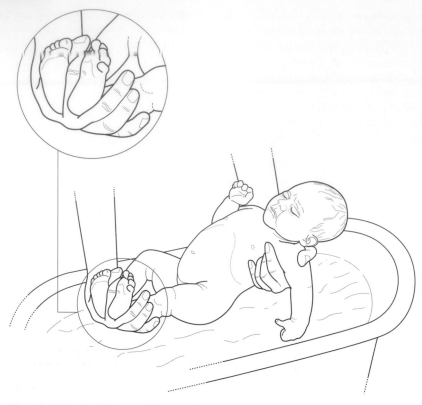

Figure 13.1 • Positioning of the hands when placing a baby in the bath

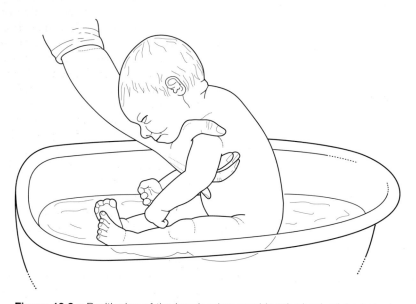

Figure 13.2 • Positioning of the hands when washing the back of the baby in the bath

Water temperature

The water should feel warm, not hot, no more than 37.0°C (Steed & MacDonald 2008) and is often between 34 and 36°C. This can be tested using the inner aspect of the wrist or the elbow. It is inadvisable to use fingers to test the heat of the water, as fingers are able to tolerate quite hot water and so are less sensitive to heat. Alternatively a bath thermometer can be used.

Equipment

- Baby bath: a large bowl will suffice provided it is only used for bathing the baby; the bath or sink can be used, although the latter may be more tiring for the woman's back.
- Towel: some towels have an integral hood, useful for drying the baby's head (if using an ordinary towel, fold over about 25 cm of towel lengthways; this can then be pulled up to dry the head).
- Sponge or flannel.
- Nappy-changing equipment and nappy.
- Baby clothes.
- Plastic apron (non-slip).
- Non-sterile gloves, if necessary.

PROCEDURE: bathing a baby

Although this procedure is written as if the midwife is bathing the baby, it can also be used as the basis for instructing the parents on how to bath their baby:

- Gain informed consent from the parents.
- Gather equipment and prepare room.
- Wash and dry hands and apply apron (put on gloves if contact with bodily fluids is likely).
- Fill the bath (no more than half full) and check the water temperature.
- Undress the baby, leaving the nappy on and wrap the baby in the towel.
- Wash the baby's face with plain water, using the sponge or flannel to wipe over the face but avoiding the eyes.
- Dry the face with the towel, using gentle patting motions.
- Wash the hair if required with water, rubbing gently over the baby's hair and dry.

- Remove the nappy, cleaning the genitalia if necessary (see pp 102–104).
- Place the baby in the water as discussed earlier, using the dominant hand to gently wash the body and limbs with water.
- Wash the baby's back.
- Lift the baby out of the water using both hands, taking care as the baby may be slippery.
- Wrap the baby in the towel.
- Dry the baby quickly using gentle patting motions, with particular attention to skin folds (use either the changing mat or midwife's lap).
- Put on a clean nappy and dress the baby.
- Give the baby to one of the parents, or place in the cot.
- Empty the bath water and dispose of equipment.
- Wash and dry hands.
- Document the findings and act accordingly.

Nappy changing

Nappies should be changed as soon as possible following soiling with urine or faeces. The skin should be cleaned at this time with either warm water or a baby wipe/mild cleanser to minimise the risk of the skin becoming excoriated and nappy rash occurring (Atherton 2005, Trotter 2006). Nappy rash is generally a result of irritant contact dermatitis rather than infection (Blincoe 2006). Ammonia-producing bacteria help to increase the skin's alkalinity; additionally, the presence of the excretory by-products of microbial proliferation in the skin folds act as irritants and sensitisers (Hale 2008). Hale (2007) suggests that faecal enzymes attack and erode the skin surface; this is more likely to occur as the skin pH becomes less acidic. Atherton (2005) suggests this is most likely to occur when urine and faeces are present together as the urease in the faeces break down the urea in the urine which results in an increase in pH. It is important that the midwife can demonstrate to the parents how to change the baby's nappy, using whichever method the parents will use at home.

Nappies

Nappies are either reusable or disposable. Reusable nappies are usually made of towelling or cloth, in a variety of styles. The traditional terry towelling nappy is square shaped, requiring folding prior to use. A nappy liner can be placed in the nappy to reduce the amount of urine and faeces coming into contact with the skin and minimise the risk of nappy rash. Manufacturers' instructions should be followed when disposing of the nappy liners; they should be used once only and not disposed of down the toilet. Waterproof overpants may be used to prevent urine and faeces seeping onto the baby's clothes. Alternatives are the all-in-one reusables (self-fastening fitted cloth nappies, covered with a waterproof shell), two-piece reusables (cloth nappies that fit into special waterproof pants with self-adhesive fastenings) and wrap-around nappies (cloth nappies with ties, used in conjunction with waterproof overpants). All reusables require laundering. A thin layer of a barrier cream can be used to protect the genitalia and buttocks and reduce the risk of nappy rash, but may be contraindicated with some nappy liners.

There are three ways to fold a towelling nappy: the triangle, the kite and the triple-fold method. The triple-fold is useful for boys as it provides extra thickness and absorbency at the front of the nappy where urination is likely to occur.

1. The triangle method (Fig. 13.3)

- Place the nappy in a diamond shape, fold in half to make a triangle shape with the longest side at the top and the point at the bottom.
- Place the baby on the nappy, bringing up the top layer between the baby's legs.
- Wrap one side of the nappy across the baby, then the other side.
- Bring up the lower layer of the nappy between the baby's legs and secure with a safety pin.

2. The kite method (Fig. 13.4)

- Place the nappy in a diamond shape; fold the outer two points to the centre to make a kite shape.
- Fold the top corner down and the bottom corner up towards the centre; the latter fold can be adjusted to suit the length of the baby.
- Place the baby on the nappy, bringing up the nappy between the baby's legs.
- Wrap one side of the nappy across the baby, then the other side, securing with two safety pins.

3. The triple-fold method (Fig. 13.5)

- Place the nappy in a square shape and fold into half lengthways from bottom to top.
- Fold in half again, from left to right, to make into a four-thickness square shape.
- Take hold of the bottom right hand corner of the first layer of the nappy and open it to the left.
- Turn the nappy over carefully, keeping the layers in position so that the point lies to the left.
- Take hold of the next two layers forming the square shape and fold the outer third over towards the centre and then in half, creating a triangle shape with an extra thick pleat in the centre.
- Place the baby on the nappy, bringing up the nappy between the baby's legs.
- Wrap one side of the nappy across the baby, then the other side, securing with a safety pin.

Disposable nappies

Disposables are paper nappies (made from fluffed wood pulp) containing absorbent crystals that form a gel when they become wet from urine. Many now use super-absorbent polymers, which increase their absorbency resulting in the nappies staying drier against the baby's skin for longer and consequently less incidence of nappy rash (Hale 2007). Breathable nappies are also available, which allow more airflow around the baby's skin regardless of whether the skin is wet or dry. Hale (2007) advises that this reduces the risk of nappy rash by inhibiting the growth of *Candida albicans*. Certain brands of nappies may also contain nappy liners impregnated with a barrier cream (e.g. petroleum) and are considered to be an additional way of reducing the incidence of nappy rash (Hale 2007). The barrier cream is hydrophobic and, in response to the warmth of the skin and movement by the baby, the cream should transfer from the nappy to the baby's skin to serve as a protective barrier.

Disposable nappies have an outer plastic layer, fitted elasticated leg bands and sticky tapes at the sides to fasten the nappy. Some disposables also have elasticated waists; some have a hole for the umbilical cord, to allow it to remain dry. They come in a variety of sizes, from newborn to toddler size. Disposables are used once only and should not be disposed of down the toilet.

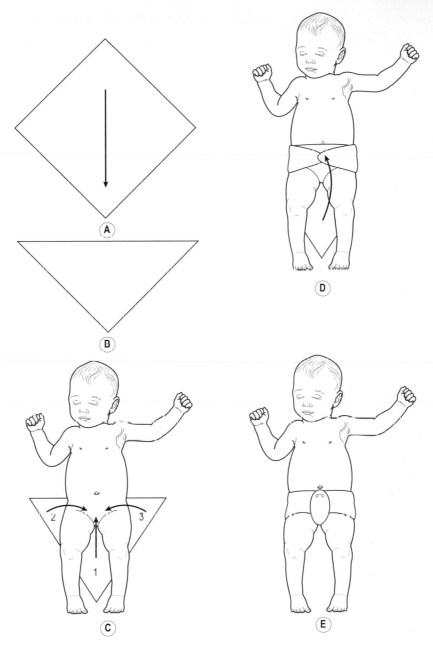

Figure 13.3 • Triangle method of nappy folding

Use of barrier creams

Barrier creams applied in a thin layer at each nappy change can reduce the effect of friction between the nappy and the skin and minimise contact between the skin and urine or faeces (Atherton & Mills 2004). This, in conjunction with prompt changing and thorough cleansing of the area, can help to reduce the incidence of nappy rash. The cream should allow water vapour to pass through the barrier from the baby but prevent fluid passing the opposite way to the baby's skin. Atherton & Mills (2004) suggest that creams containing zinc or titanium oxides should be avoided as they are difficult to remove and white soft paraffin is less effective at allowing transfer from the skin to the nappy. Hale

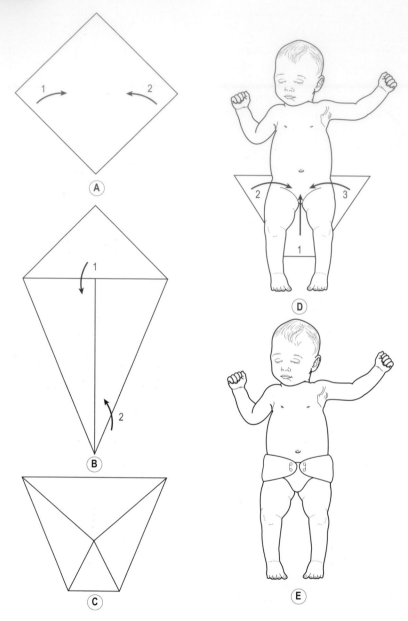

Figure 13.4 • Kite method of nappy folding

(2007), however, recommends the use of petroleum based lubricant or a cream containing zinc oxide; further research is required into this area. Bacterial preparations are unnecessary as nappy rash is not caused by infection and the cream may interfere with the resident skin flora. Atherton & Mills (2004) recommend the use of Bepanthen ointment, a mixture containing dexpanthenol and lanolin.

Barrier cream used as a protective layer should:

- allow the transfer of fluid from the skin to the nappy
- prevent the transfer of fluid from the nappy to the skin
- contain no antibiotics, steroids, perfumes, zinc or titanium oxides
- use lanolin rather than white soft paraffin as the emollient.

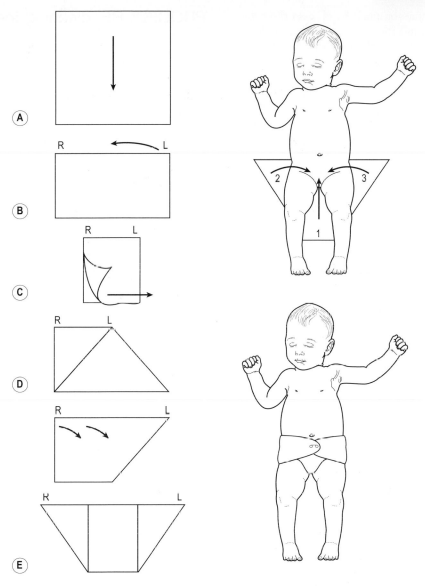

Figure 13.5 • Triple-fold method of nappy folding

PROCEDURE: changing a nappy

- Gain informed consent from the parents.
- Gather equipment:
  - non-sterile gloves and apron
  - changing mat or towel
  - small bowl and cotton wool balls or dry wipes
  - nappy bag or nappy bucket and disposable bag for used nappy and wipes
  - clean nappy
  - nappy liner (optional)
  - barrier cream (optional).
- Wash hands, put on apron and gloves.
- Put warm water into the bowl.
- Lay the baby on a safe, flat surface (e.g. cot mattress, changing mat), with the towel under the baby if required.
- Undress the baby sufficiently to gain access to the nappy.
- Remove the dirty nappy and put to one side.

- Using the non-dominant hand, hold the baby securely around the ankles, enabling the legs to be straightened and the buttocks raised slightly to facilitate cleansing of the genital area.
- With the dominant hand, using either a cotton wool ball or wipe moistened with water, clean the genitalia from front to back before the perianal area to reduce the risk of infection:
  ○ females: wipe one side of the labia then the other, moving from front to back
  ○ males: wipe around the penis, towards the scrotum.
- Place the cotton wool ball/wipe in nappy bag and repeat on the other side until the genitalia are clean.
- Clean between the folds of the groin and thigh, then the buttocks.
- Pat the area dry with the towel or dry cotton wool balls/wipes.
- If a barrier cream is used, apply a thin layer to the genitalia and buttocks.
- Place the nappy under the baby and secure, ensuring a boy's penis points down and the cord is outside the nappy.
- Redress the baby.
- Dispose of equipment correctly.
- Wash hands.
- Document the findings and act accordingly.

Cleaning the eyes

The baby's eyes should not be cleaned unless they are discharging, in order to minimise the risk of trauma and infection. Sticky eyes are commonly due to blocked tear ducts and usually are not infected. The discharge is a yellowish colour and may be seen as crusting on the eyelid. A profuse or offensive discharge, or a discharge of a different colour, is most likely due to infection and may be accompanied by erythema and localised oedema of the eye. If infection is suspected, a swab may be taken (see Chapter 11), referral made and antibiotics commenced. To reduce the risk of cross-infection, each eye is cleaned separately; the cotton wool ball is used to wipe the eye once from the inner part outwards, and then disposed of. While sterile water can be used if available, cooled boiled water usually suffices. The midwife should demonstrate this procedure to the parents to enable them to clean the baby's eyes themselves.

PROCEDURE: cleaning the baby's eyes

- Gain informed consent from the parents.
- Gather equipment:
  ○ cotton wool balls
  ○ clean container and cooled boiled water
  ○ non-sterile gloves if infection suspected
  ○ paper towel/bag or disposable tray.
- Wash hands, apply gloves.
- Using a cotton wool ball moistened with water, wipe from the inner edge of the eye outwards, using the wipe once only placing the used wipe in the paper bag or on the disposable tray/paper towel.
- Dispose of the wipe and repeat with another cotton wool ball.
- Repeat until the eye is clean then undertake for the other eye.
- Dispose of the equipment correctly.
- Wash hands.
- Discuss ongoing care with the parents e.g. when to repeat the procedure, signs to be aware of.
- Document the findings and act accordingly.

Cord care

At birth, the umbilical cord is clamped to leave 2–5 cm of umbilical cord that has no further function. Following birth, the cord vessels fibrose, the Wharton's jelly dries and the cord separates over the next 5–15 days by a process of dry gangrene (it will dry, harden, shrivel and blacken); finally, it detaches (this can occur more quickly with a lotus birth, see Chapter 32). During this process, leucocytes infiltrate the base of the cord to digest the cord, which can result in cloudy mucoid material appearing at the base of the cord (Trotter 2004). This might be mistaken for pus but it is part of the normal physiological process of cord separation and not due to infection (although omphalitis can also occur). Trotter (2004) advises that a moist or sticky cord is also part of the physiological process and thus should not cause alarm. However, the cord is a potential site of infection, providing ideal conditions for colonization and replication of organisms. *Staphylococcus aureus* commonly colonizes the cord

(Newell et al 1997). There is insufficient evidence to suggest the use of antiseptics or antibiotics have any additional advantage over keeping the cord clean and dry; cord separation time was shorter when no topical care was used (Zupan et al 2004). Evens et al (2004) suggest that the cord should be left dry for preterm babies as they found the cord detached more quickly, there was less exposure of alcohol and skin breakdown with no increase in infection rate. The current management for the baby not at high risk of infection, including those who have had a lotus birth, continues to revolve around scrupulous hand hygiene, keeping the cord clean and using water when bathing or nappy changing. In areas where the risk of infection to the baby is high, Zupan et al (2004) suggest the use of topical antibiotics may be prudent but caution that further research is required to determine what is the best regimen and treatment for such cords.

ROLE AND RESPONSIBILITIES OF THE MIDWIFE

These can be summarised as:

- completing the procedures safely and correctly
- educating the parents
- referral, if required
- correct documentation.

Summary

- Meeting the hygiene needs of the baby is an important skill for the midwife, who not only undertakes this but also educates the parents on how to do this.

- The baby does not need to be bathed every day.
- Bathing the baby can be an enjoyable process for all involved but attention must be paid to keeping the baby warm, safe and secure.
- The use of alkaline soaps and bath additives disrupts the acid mantle of the skin, predisposing to infection; the use of plain water is recommended.
- Nappies may be disposable or reusable, with three ways of folding the latter.
- The baby's eyes should not be cleaned unless discharging.
- The cord should not be cleaned routinely as this can delay separation and increase the risk of infection.

SELF-ASSESSMENT EXERCISES

The answers to the following questions may be found in the text:

1. What advice can a midwife provide to parents who are enquiring which cleansing agent to use?
2. How can the midwife ensure the safety of the baby during bathing?
3. Describe how a baby bath is undertaken.
4. Demonstrate the different ways to apply a reusable nappy.
5. When would the midwife clean the baby's eyes and how is this done?
6. What advice can be given regarding cord care?

References

Atherton D: Maintaining healthy skin in infancy using prevention of irritant napkin dermatitis as a model, *Community Pract* 78(7):255–257, 2005.

Atherton D, Mills K: What can be done to keep babies' skin healthy? *Midwives* 7(7):288–290, 2004.

Blackburn ST: *Maternal, fetal and neonatal physiology: a clinical perspective*, ed 3, St. Louis, 2007, Saunders.

Blincoe AJ: Protecting neonatal skin: cream or water? *Br J Midwifery* 14(12):731–734, 2006.

Evens K, George J, Angst D, et al: Does umbilical cord care in preterm infants influence cord bacterial colonization or detachment? *J Perinatol* 24(2):100–104, 2004.

Hale R: Newborn skin care and the modern nappy, *Br J Midwifery* 15(12):784–787, 2007.

Hale R: Maintaining healthy infant skin, *Br J Midwifery* 16(6):403–406, 2008.

Hopkins J: Essentials of newborn skin care, *British Journal of Midwifery* 12(5):314–317, 2004.

Johnston PGB, Flood K, Spinks K: *The newborn child*, ed 9, Edinburgh, 2003, Churchill Livingstone.

Lund C, Kuller J, Lane A, et al: Neonatal skin care: the scientific basis for practice, *J Obstet Gynaecol Neonatal Nurs* 28(3):241–254, 1999.

Newell SJ, Miller P, Morgan I, et al: Management of the newborn baby: midwifery and paediatric perspectives. In Henderson C, Jones K, editors: *Essential midwifery*, London, 1997, Mosby, pp 229–264.

NICE (National Institute for Health and Clinical Excellence): *Clinical guideline 37 postnatal care*, London, 2006, NICE.

Penny-MacGillivray T: A newborn's first bath: when? *J Obstet, Gynaecol Neonatal Nurs* 25(6):481–487, 1996.

Simon NP, Simon MW: Changes in newborn bathing practices may increase the risk of omphalitis, *Clin Pediatr (Phila)* 43(8):763–767, 2004.

Steen M, Macdonald S: *A review of baby skin care*. Midwives online. Available: http://www.rcm.org.uk/ magazines/web-only-papers/a-review-of-baby-skin-care/ 6 April 2009, 2008.

Trotter S: Care of the newborn: proposed new guidelines, *Br J Midwifery* 12(3):152–157, 2004.

Trotter S: Neonatal skincare: why change is vital, *RCM Midwives* 9(4):134–138, 2006.

Walker L, Downe S, Gomez L: Skin care in the well term newborn: Two systematic reviews, *Birth: Issues in Perinatal Care* 2(3):224–228, 2005.

Wray J: Seeking to explore what matters to women about postnatal care, *Br J Midwifery* 14(5): 246–254, 2006.

Zupan J, Garner P, Omari AAA: Topical umbilical cord care at birth, *Cochrane Database Syst Rev* (3) Art. No.: CD001057. doi: 10.1002/ 14651858.CD001057.pub2, 2004.

Principles of elimination management: micturition and catheterisation

14

CHAPTER CONTENTS

Care of the urinary tract, supporting normal micturition or using a catheter, is an important aspect of care for the childbearing woman. This chapter reviews the factors that influence micturition, the direct effects of child bearing on the urinary tract, the safe use of bedpans and correct (short term) indwelling catheter care.

LEARNING OUTCOMES

Having read this chapter the reader should be able to:

- define micturition, describing the adult normal urine volumes
- discuss the changes to the urinary tract that child bearing brings
- describe how to facilitate normal micturition, including the correct use of a bedpan
- describe, with rationale, the equipment chosen for urinary catheterisation
- describe how to insert and remove a urinary catheter.

Micturition

Micturition is the voiding of urine from the bladder via the urethra. It requires a correctly functioning renal system as well as coordination between the brain and nervous system. Inability (for whatever reason) to pass urine is an acute emergency; acute urinary retention is very painful and can cause complications such as renal failure. The urinary system consists of the bladder (a pelvic organ but displaces out of the pelvis when full), two ureters that connect the bladder to the kidneys, two kidneys that (amongst other things) are responsible for urine formation and filtration and one urethra that carries urine out of the body from the bladder. The bladder fills at approximately 0.5 mL/kg/hour; the sensation of needing to empty the bladder occurs in adults at a 200–400 mL volume. An adult normally voids 1500–6000 mL per day (minimum 30 mL per hour). An understanding of fluid balance (see Chapter 48) is also fundamental to appreciating elimination care. Various factors influence micturition, including:

- anxiety/stress
- personal habits: distraction (e.g. reading), privacy, time, etc.
- poor muscle tone due to damage or increasing age
- pain
- position
- disease
- urinary infection
- obstruction, e.g. compression from the enlarging uterus, presenting part, faecal impaction
- damage to the nervous pathway due to trauma, disease or age
- surgery
- childbirth (discussed below) (Dolman 2007)
- poor bladder care antenatally, intrapartum and postnatally (Blackburn 2007)
- stress incontinence
- drugs: anticholinergics (e.g. atropine), antihypertensives (e.g. methyldopa), antihistamines (e.g. pseudoephedrine), beta-adrenergic blockers (e.g. propranolol).

Changes related to childbirth

Pregnancy

During pregnancy, a number of structural and functional changes occur within the renal system, some of which continue into the postnatal period. Blackburn (2007) summarises the changes, some of which are discussed below.

During the first trimester, the renal calyces, renal pelvis and ureters begin to enlarge, resulting in physiological hydroureter and hydronephrosis becoming more pronounced during the second half of the pregnancy. During the last trimester, the enlarging uterus displaces the ureters laterally; they elongate, becoming more tortuous. The volume of the ureters increases, possibly up to 25 times, resulting in up to 300 mL of urine being stored in the ureters (Blackburn 2007). This has implications for the accuracy of 24-hour urine collections and increases the risk of urinary tract infection (UTI).

Progesterone relaxes the smooth muscle of the bladder, resulting in decreased tone; oestrogen predisposes vesicourethral valve incompetence (and therefore reflux of urine) and the glomerular filtration rate increases by 40–60% (Blackburn 2007). Bladder capacity doubles by term, holding up to 1000 mL. The bladder mucosa becomes more oedematous, predisposing it to trauma or infection. McCormick et al (2008) cite that the incidence of UTI in pregnancy is 8%. The National Institute of Health and Clinical Excellence (NICE 2008) suggests that all women should be routinely offered mid-stream urine (MSU) screening in early pregnancy (booking visit) to screen for asymptomatic bacteriuria. UTI in pregnancy affects morbidity and can lead to preterm labour.

During the first trimester, the enlarging uterus compresses the bladder, increasing the desire to micturate, resulting in urinary frequency. During the second trimester, the bladder is displaced upwards, allowing bladder capacity to return to normal. However, during the third trimester, pressure from the presenting part, particularly following engagement, can once again result in urinary frequency or stress incontinence. As the bladder is displaced into the abdomen the urethra is elongated and bladder emptying is affected. Nocturia may also occur during pregnancy due to increased excretion of sodium and water occurring when the woman lies down (Blackburn 2007).

Labour

Pressure may be exerted on the sacral plexus by the presenting part during its descent through the pelvis, resulting in increased frequency or retention of urine; this is also associated with an occipitoposterior position.

Retention of urine occurs when the pressure on the sacral plexus results in inhibition of impulses. The bladder fills but there is no associated desire to void urine, compounded by the distension-inhibiting nerve receptors within the bladder wall. Pressure from the descending presenting part is exerted on the bladder and urethra, particularly at their junction. The resulting compression prevents the passage of urine, even with the desire to void. Lack of privacy and poor posture also contribute to retention of urine. Women should be encouraged to void urine every 1–2 hours during labour to minimise these risks, and particularly at the onset of second stage.

Decreased awareness of the need to void urine occurs if regional anaesthesia is used (e.g. epidural or pudendal block) as the drugs temporarily paralyse the nerves supplying the bladder.

A full bladder may be traumatised in labour and may also affect the course of labour in several ways:

- delayed descent of the presenting part, particularly when above the ischial spines (Gee & Glynn 1997, Walsh 2004)
- reduced efficiency of uterine contractions (Walsh 2004) and therefore delayed cervical dilatation: may predispose to postpartum haemorrhage (Verralls 1993)
- unnecessary pain (Verralls 1993)
- dribbling of urine during expulsive second stage contractions (Verralls 1993)
- delayed delivery of the placenta (Gee & Glynn 1997).

Postnatal period

During the early postnatal period, a marked diuresis occurs. Between the second and fifth postnatal day, up to 3000 mL of urine may be produced daily, with 500–1000 mL being voided at a time (Blackburn 2007). Proteinuria may be evident as a result of autolysis (Abbott et al 1997). The structural changes that occurred during pregnancy slowly return to normal during the puerperium, although in some women this may take longer (up to 16 weeks).

Women should pass urine within 6–8 hours of delivery (Blackburn 2007). However, some women may experience a delayed sensation to void urine. The risk of partial or complete inability to void urine is increased in the presence of:

- trauma to the bladder or urethra
- decreased bladder sensation arising from the use of regional anaesthesia, catheter use or an overdistended bladder
- haematoma formation within the genital tract.

Incomplete emptying of the bladder and urinary stasis increase the risk of UTI.

Stress incontinence may also occur following delivery as a result of damage to the perineal branches of the pudendal nerves (Abbott et al

1997). If this persists beyond the puerperium medical attention should be sought.

An important part of the midwife's role and responsibilities is record keeping, especially if the woman is experiencing difficulty with micturition (dysuria). Records should show the amount of urine passed and the frequency, with any symptoms associated with dysuria, e.g. stinging (NMC 2005).

The baby

A baby's bladder is an abdominal organ, it being too large for the small pelvis to accommodate it. Consequently, a full bladder can compress the diaphragm and affect respiration. Micturition is an involuntary process with no control over when and where to void urine. Babies usually pass urine within the first 48 hours of life, with approximately 66% of babies passing urine in the first 12 hours, 93% by 24 hours and 99% by 48 hours (Blackburn 2007). It is important that the midwife records that the baby has passed urine following birth (NMC 2005). Urinary output is variable, depending on gestational age, fluid and solute intake, the ability of the kidneys to concentrate urine and perinatal events. Urinary output increases during the neonatal period; for example, breastfed babies pass around 20 mL of urine during the first 24 hours, increasing to 200 mL by the tenth day (Johnston et al 2003). Usually, small amounts are passed on a frequent basis, and by the second week of life the baby may produce up to 20 wet nappies a day.

Facilitating normal micturition

Given that the changes to the urinary tract and the effects of childbirth are significant, the midwife has a responsibility to ensure good bladder care for all women. Wherever possible, the woman should be encouraged to void normally, namely on the toilet. However, at times the use of a bedpan is indicated and urinary catheters, in particular circumstances, are also used. Catheterisation of the bladder is not without risks and so should be used only when there is a clinical indication. The midwife should facilitate normal micturition wherever possible; three factors influence this:

1. stimulating the micturition reflex
2. maintaining elimination habits
3. maintaining adequate fluid intake (Potter & Perry 2003).

Stimulating the micturition reflex

Position

- An upright position, leaning forwards, facilitates contraction of the pelvic and intra-abdominal muscles, forced glottis expiration, bladder contraction and sphincter control.
- This is difficult to achieve in bed: use of a bedpan or commode by the bedside or use of the toilet should be encouraged.

Reduce anxiety

Anxiety can cause a sense of urgency and frequency, resulting in voiding small amounts of urine and the bladder may not empty completely as the abdominal and perineal muscles and external urethral sphincter do not relax. Anxiety can result from lack of privacy, embarrassment, fear of passing urine and the use of cold bedpans. It can be reduced by the following:

- Staying with a woman while she attempts to pass urine may inhibit micturition; however, if she feels unsteady she may prefer someone with her. Her needs should be ascertained.
- Warming the bedpan prior to use encourages relaxation. Use of the toilet can increase the sense of privacy.
- Allowing sufficient time to relax and pass urine is also important.
- Warm water poured over the perineum may help the woman to relax (measure amount of fluid first if recording fluid balance).

Use of sensory stimuli

- Ludwick (1999) recommends the sound of running water using the power of suggestion. If the woman is embarrassed by the noise made during micturition, particularly if others are close by, the sound of running water may mask the sound of her passing urine.
- Stroking the inner aspect of the woman's thigh, placing her hand in warm water or offering a drink may stimulate the sensory nerves to stimulate the micturition reflex (Potter & Perry 2003).

Reduce fear of pain

- Pain, or fear of pain, often has an inhibitory effect on micturition. This is not unusual

following delivery with perineal trauma. Concentrated urine may increase pain; additional fluid intake should be encouraged.

- Use of the bidet during micturition may reduce discomfort.
- Strategies to minimise actual pain should be used, e.g. analgesia.

Encourage regular emptying of the bladder

- This is important, especially in the absence of the desire to void (caused by prolonged use of an indwelling catheter, damage to the nervous pathways, following surgery, use of drugs, etc.).

Encourage muscle tone

- Weakness of the pelvic floor muscles (e.g. following vaginal birth), indwelling catheter or severe constipation can affect micturition.
- Dolman (2007) recommends undertaking regular pelvic floor exercises to increase muscle volume. This increases the maximum urethral closure pressure, promoting stronger reflex contractions that follow a rise in intra-abdominal pressure.
- Prevent severe constipation that can obstruct the flow of urine.

Maintaining elimination habits

- Supporting the woman to adopt the position and routine (including habits such as reading) that she is used to, assist with micturition.

Maintaining an adequate fluid intake

- Normal renal function requires 2000–2500 mL per day and the midwife should encourage a regular fluid intake.

Bedpans

The majority of women would prefer not to use a bedpan, the embarrassment factor and difficult issues concerned with its use (discussed above) mean that sensitive care is required for those that will need to use one. There are two main types of bedpan (Fig. 14.1), standard (deeper) and slipper (smaller and shallower). Whilst cardboard liners

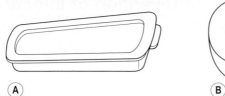 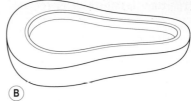

Figure 14.1 • Different types of bedpan. A Non-disposable slipper. B Bedpan with disposable lining

are available, local infection control protocols are upheld whichever type of pan is used.

PROCEDURE: use of a bedpan

- Gain informed consent, prepare the environment to facilitate micturition (discussed above) and gather equipment:
  - ○ bedpan
  - ○ non-sterile gloves and apron
  - ○ liner (if used)
  - ○ bedpan cover
  - ○ toilet paper
  - ○ sanitary towel disposable bag and clean sanitary towel (if required)
  - ○ handwashing facilities.
- Wash hands, apply apron and gloves.
- If possible, warm the bedpan prior to administration.
- Consider moving and handling issues (bed at correct height, need for second midwife, etc.).
- Take the bedpan to the woman and ensure privacy.
- Help the woman to remove her knickers and sanitary towel.
- Place the bedpan under the woman, assisting her into a comfortable, preferably upright position. Lying on her side and then rolling back onto the bedpan may be easier for some women. Her legs should be slightly apart.
- Stay with the woman if necessary, otherwise supply a call bell.
- When the woman has finished, allow time for her to wipe between her legs.
- Remove and cover the bedpan.
- Assist the woman with replacing her sanitary towel and knickers, ensuring she is comfortable.
- Provide facilities for hand washing.

- Undertake urinalysis and measure urine if required.
- Wash bedpan, if non-disposable, and replace.
- Dispose of remaining equipment correctly.
- Remove gloves and apron and wash hands.
- Document findings and act accordingly.

Urinary catheterisation

Definition

A sterile catheter is inserted aseptically into the bladder to drain it of urine. The most common catheterisation is urethral (via the urethra), for which the catheter may be secured in the bladder (indwelling) or inserted and immediately removed (intermittent).

An indwelling catheter can drain urine continually via a urine bag, or a catheter valve can be inserted that allows the bladder to be emptied intermittently. A drainage system can be added if necessary. The bladder can also be catheterised through the abdominal wall (suprapubic), but this is seen infrequently within the maternity setting.

Indications

Whilst a straightforward procedure, catheterisation is not without significant risks (see below) and so should only be undertaken when clinically indicated and with full consent from the woman. Clinical indicators include:

- Prior to caesarean section or other abdominal surgery.
- During labour if unable to pass urine, especially prior to instrumental delivery.
- During the third stage of labour when a full bladder may be impeding normal uterine activity,

e.g. during postpartum haemorrhage or retained placenta.

- Inability to pass urine, e.g. postsurgery (urinary retention).
- For diagnostic purposes, e.g. postnatal incontinence.
- Accurate monitoring of fluid balance when acutely ill or in shock, e.g. pre-eclampsia, major haemorrhage.
- Specific urine testing, e.g. to obtain an uncontaminated specimen for protein measurement when pre-eclamptic. Chan et al (2008) would question this. They found a clean catch in women with no history of urinary infection, vaginal bleeding or ruptured membranes to be an equally accurate method of specimen collection.
- On each occasion the clinical decision is made as to whether an indwelling or intermittent catheter is the most appropriate.

Contraindications

Urinary tract infections account for approximately 35% of all healthcare-associated infections (Hart 2008). The effects on both the woman and the health service are significant. Catheterisation is a risk factor and 2–6% of catheterised patients will develop a UTI (Pratt et al 2007). Catheters can also be bypassed or blocked and bladder spasms can be very uncomfortable. The urinary tract can be traumatized or inflamed, urinary stones can form and body image and sexual function can be affected.

Prevention of infection

The infection risk increases according to the susceptibility of the woman, type and length of time the catheter is *in situ*, and the quality of catheter care. The risk is higher for women than for men, due to the close proximity of the urethra to the anus, and the shorter length of the female urethra.

Infection-reducing measures

Strict hand hygiene and aseptic insertion technique

There is no doubt that asepsis is vital for catheterisation (Pratt et al 2007), including, as suggested by Hart (2008), decontamination of the hands at several times during the procedure. The use of alcohol hand rub is acceptable for clean hands, and Nicol et al (2008) suggest the wearing of two pairs of sterile gloves so that once anaesthetic gel has been inserted one pair can be removed prior to inserting the catheter.

Catheter care

Comprehensive catheter care, including maintaining a closed drainage system that does not allow entry to bacteria (Fig. 14.2), is crucial. All portals (e.g. catheter valve, bag emptying valve, sampling valve) should be wiped with an alcohol-impregnated wipe before and after use and sterile gloves should be worn when taking specimens, changing bags, and so on.

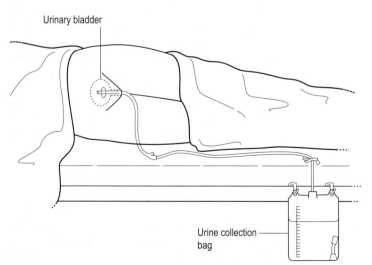

Figure 14.2 • Closed drainage system (Adapted with kind permission from Jamieson et al 2002)

Urinary bladder

Urine collection bag

Ongoing catheter care includes observing the amount, colour, clarity and smell of the urine, in conjunction with the woman's vital signs and clinical signs of illness or UTI. The woman must be given advice on all aspects of catheter care.

The catheter should be removed as soon as the woman's condition allows.

The drainage bag

This should be supported at a level lower than the bladder (maximum 30 cm; Evans et al 2001) to allow free drainage and prevent backflow of the urine. A catheter stand is used to both keep the bag away from the floor and to reduce trauma to the urethra.

The bag should be emptied when two-thirds full (Yates 2008). Occluding or kinking the catheter (e.g. in the knicker leg) can cause stasis of urine in the bladder and subsequent UTI.

Perineal hygiene

Perineal hygiene is necessary both on insertion of the catheter and on a daily basis. Pratt et al (2007) state that sterile sodium chloride should be used for urethral meatal cleansing prior to catheter insertion. If catheterisation is undertaken at the same time as examination *per vaginam* or some other perineum-related procedure then it is likely that the locally approved solution will be used for meatal/perineal cleansing; many units use warm tap water. The reader is encouraged to be aware of evolving evidence with regard to this. Leaver (2007) indicates that soap and water are adequate cleansers of the catheter and meatus on a daily basis; showering is preferable.

General health of the woman

Although largely unresearched, a daily oral fluid intake of 2 L is considered to flush the urinary tract and limit the chances of UTI (Getliffe & Fader 2007, Steggall 2007).

Choice of equipment

The choice of catheter should be made while taking into account reducing:

- tissue inflammation and trauma to the urethra (also improves comfort)
- mineral deposits that may cause the catheter to block
- bacterial growth.

Sterile PTFE latex catheters have a lifespan of 7–21 days and so are often the catheter of choice for maternity use. Caution must be taken to ensure that there is no latex allergy on the part of the recipient. A standard-length catheter (40–45 cm) is used for larger women, otherwise a female catheter (23–26 cm) is acceptable. The lumen should be large enough to drain adequately without overdistending the urethra, a size 12 Ch is suitable for most women (white valve).

Indwelling (Foley) catheters are retained in the bladder by a balloon inflated with a maximum (in adults) of 10 mL of water (Pratt et al 2007). Catheters vary, some have a self-inflating balloon and others a prefilled sterile syringe. The sterile water is squeezed from the external balloon or syringe to the internal balloon (and clamped) when the catheter is in the bladder. Catheters for intermittent use are generally made from PVC plastic with holes at the tip (no balloon). All catheters are singly wrapped, sterile and with an expiry date. Correct storage – out of sunlight, heat and humidity in original cardboard and without elastic bands (Winder 1999) – protects the quality of the catheter. Valves, drainage bags and catheter packs (containing swabs, gallipot and receivers) are also sterile and for single use only.

Analgesia

It is difficult to anaesthetize the length of the female urethra but nevertheless efforts should be made to reduce the pain and discomfort of catheter insertion. The analgesic gel (there are various sorts; preprepared 6 mL lidocaine 2% is most commonly used) acts as a lubricant as well as bringing anaesthesia. It is sterile for single use and needs to be administered 2–5 minutes before the procedure. It can be used for intermittent catheterisation (e.g. during labour) but it is important that the lidocaine does not enter the bloodstream via any lacerations; this could cause cardiac arrhythmias. Lubricant without lidocaine is available for those with lidocaine allergy (Robinson 2007).

Documentation

As well as the clinical indication for the catheterisation these details also need to be recorded in the woman's record:

- the catheter: type, length, size, manufacturer, batch number, expiry date and number of millilitres in the balloon (sometimes a label is supplied with the catheter for sticking into the woman's records)
- cleansing solution and lubricant used
- any problems encountered with the insertion
- plan of care including expected removal time
- any information relating to local or national infection control audits
- specimen taken and sent (if needed)
- name and signature of midwife.

PROCEDURE: female catheterisation using an indwelling catheter

It is helpful to have an assistant when setting up for catheterisation. If one is not available the procedure is adapted using additional hand hygiene episodes:

- Gain informed consent and ensure privacy.
- Gather equipment:
  - disposable receiver
  - sterile Foley catheter (likely size: 10–12 Ch; a second one may be helpful)
  - sterile drainage bag and stand
  - two pairs of sterile gloves and a plastic apron
  - sterile catheter pack
  - sterile analgesic gel (most likely 6 mL lidocaine 2%)
  - sterile sachet sodium chloride 0.9% or approved cleanser
  - disposable sheet
  - work at the correct height and with good light source.
- Position the woman (removing sanitary towels and underwear) on a disposable sheet, in a semi-recumbent position, ankles together, knees apart. Keep the woman covered while the remainder of the preparations are made.
- Apply apron and wash hands while the assistant opens the pack.
- Open the inner wrapper, ask the assistant to slide the gloves, catheter, drainage bag and anaesthetic gel onto the sterile field.
- Put on both pairs of gloves and arrange the contents of the pack while the assistant pours

the sodium chloride into the bowl. Expose the tip of the catheter only, place nozzle on gel.
- The assistant exposes the woman's genital area.
- Establish a sterile field by placing a sterile drape beneath the woman's buttocks and one over her abdomen.
- Using the non-dominant hand, separate the labia with gauze swabs (this minimises pressure on the labia, increases visibility and makes catheter insertion easier), cleanse the vulva using each swab once only, cleaning front to back.
- Locate the urethra, insert the anaesthetic gel and wait for this to take effect (2–5 minutes). Remove the top pair of gloves.
- Place the receiver on the sterile field between the woman's thighs.
- Using the non-dominant hand part and hold the labia with a gauze swab whilst, with the dominant hand, pass the catheter gently and smoothly in an upwards and backwards direction into the urethra until urine begins to flow. Maintain sterility by pulling back the plastic wrapper as the catheter is advanced. If the urethra is difficult to visualise, ask the woman to take a deep breath in; on expiration the urethra is easier to see (the pelvic floor relaxes).
- Once urine is seen, the catheter should be inserted a further 5 cm to ensure the balloon is in the bladder.
- If the woman is very uncomfortable or there is resistance at any stage, stop and seek experienced assistance.
- Inflate the balloon by squeezing the fluid from the external balloon or syringe, apply the clamp/remove the syringe. If there is great discomfort, the balloon may be in the urethra, and the catheter would need to be advanced further into the bladder before the balloon is inflated.
- Fully remove the plastic wrapper, placing it and the end of the catheter into the sterile receiver.
- Attach the drainage bag.
- Clear the area, assisting the woman to replace her sanitary towel and underwear as required, and to adopt a comfortable position.
- Attach the catheter bag to the stand, securing it to the side of the bed.
- Discuss ongoing care, e.g. principles of infection control, sufficient mobility, avoiding constipation.

- Undertake urinalysis if necessary (using the sample gained when the catheter was inserted).
- Dispose of equipment correctly.
- Wash hands.
- Document findings and act accordingly.

Precautions

- In the event of mistakenly placing the catheter into the vagina, it should be retained while a new one is placed into the urethra. The vaginal one is then removed. A contaminated catheter should *never* be placed into the urethra.
- If a urine specimen is needed for culture and sensitivity it should be taken from the catheter before the drainage bag is attached.
- Excessive loss of fluid from the body quickly in one episode, i.e. up to 1 L, can result in shock. The immediate drainage of urine should be observed and the flow halted with a clamp, if the volume is approaching 1 L.

Intermittent catheterisation (female)

The procedure is exactly the same as inserting an indwelling catheter, except that the catheter is a single-use residual one, which is removed once the urine has been drained. It is an aseptic procedure and the receiver should be large enough to hold the volume expected.

Emptying and changing the drainage bag

A drainage bag has a life of approximately 5 days (Winder 1999). Yates (2008) suggests the drainage bag is emptied before it is two-thirds full to minimise pressure exerted on the urethra and to promote continued drainage. It should be emptied into a disposable container. The midwife should have clean hands, wear disposable gloves and should wipe the tap with an alcohol-impregnated swab before and after the emptying (Yates 2008). Contact between the container and valve should be avoided. The urine should be measured and recorded if fluid balance is being monitored.

Removing a urethral indwelling catheter

Catheter removal should occur as soon as the woman's condition allows. Depending on local protocol a catheter specimen of urine (CSU) may be obtained before removal to screen for infection. Traditionally catheters are removed early in the morning. However, Kelleher (2002) suggests that removal at midnight allows the woman to rest and begin a normal voiding pattern in the morning. The reader is encouraged to be aware of the evolving research on this issue.

PROCEDURE: removing an indwelling catheter

- Gain informed consent and ensure privacy.
- Gather equipment:
  - disposable receiver
  - 10 mL syringe (depending on catheter design)
  - non-sterile gloves and plastic apron
  - disposable sheet
  - equipment for perineal cleansing (p 91), depending on chosen method.
- Position the woman on the disposable sheet, as for insertion, placing the receiver between her legs; keep covered.
- Apply apron, wash hands and apply gloves.
- Ask the woman to lift up the sheet that is covering her.
- Deflate the balloon by removing the clamp and allowing the fluid to drain into the external balloon or by withdrawing the water using the syringe.
- Ask the woman to take a deep breath, remove the catheter smoothly but quickly as she exhales, placing it into the receiver.
- Cleanse the perineum using one of the methods described on page 91.
- Assist the woman to replace her sanitary towel and underwear as required and to adopt a comfortable position.
- Give the woman clear explanations regarding:
  - possible frequency and urgency of micturition due to urethral irritability, or mild haematuria due to urethral trauma
  - the need to pass a good volume of urine over the next 6–8 hours

○ possible urinary retention

○ having a fluid intake of 2–3 L to flush out any bladder debris.

• Measure and record the drained urine if fluid balance is being monitored.

• Dispose of equipment correctly.

• Document findings and act accordingly, ensuring the next urine output is measured and recorded.

ROLE AND RESPONSIBILITIES OF THE MIDWIFE

These can be summarised as:

• understanding and applying the measures necessary to facilitate normal micturition, including advising and educating the woman

• undertaking all the clinical procedures described correctly, particularly in relation to prevention of infection

• recognising deviations from the norm, managing them and if necessary referring

• correct documentation of all care.

Summary

• All aspects of child bearing can affect and be affected by the urinary tract.

• Micturition can be influenced in three main ways: stimulating the micturition reflex, maintaining normal habits and ensuring adequate fluid intake.

• Catheterisation of the bladder is indicated in certain clinical circumstances. Infection is one of the greatest risks, the midwife must be aware of all the care that contributes towards reducing the risk.

SELF-ASSESSMENT EXERCISES

The answers to the following questions may be found in the text:

1. What factors influence micturition?
2. Describe how child bearing affects micturition and therefore the measures that the midwife can undertake to promote good urinary care.
3. Describe the advantages and disadvantages of bedpan use.
4. List the situations in which a midwife is likely to undertake catheterisation for a childbearing woman.
5. Discuss the similarities and differences between indwelling and intermittent catheterisation.
6. Which is the most likely complication to occur from catheterisation and how may this be prevented in all stages of care?

References

Abbott H, Bick D, MacArthur C: Health after birth. In Henderson C, Jones K, editors: *Essential midwifery*, London, 1997, Mosby, pp 285–318.

Blackburn ST: *Maternal, fetal and neonatal physiology: a clinical perspective*, ed 3, Missouri, 2007, W B Saunders, ch 11.

Chan B, Parviainen K, Jeyabalan A: Correlation of catheterized and clean catch urine protein/creatinine ratios in preeclampsia evaluation, *Obstet Gynecol* 112(3):611–620, 2008.

Dolman M: Mainly women. In Getliffe M, Dolman M, editors: *Promoting continence: a clinical and research resource*, ed 3, Edinburgh, 2007, Elsevier, ch 3.

Evans A, Painter D, Feneley R: Blocked urinary catheters: nurses' preventative role, *Nurs Times* 97 (1):37–38, 2001.

Gee H, Glynn M: The physiology and clinical management of labour. In Henderson K, Jones K, editors: *Essential midwifery*, London, 1997, Mosby, pp 171–202.

Getliffe K, Fader M: Catheters and containment products. In Getliffe K, Dolman M, editors: *Promoting continence: a clinical and research resource*, ed 3, Edinburgh, 2007, Elsevier, ch 10.

Hart S: Urinary catheterisation, *Nurs Stand* 22(27):44–48, 2008.

Jamieson EM, McCall J, Whyte L: *Clinical nursing practices*, ed 4, Edinburgh, 2002, Churchill Livingstone.

Johnston PGB, Flood K, Spinks K: *The newborn child*, ed 9, Edinburgh, 2003, Churchill Livingstone.

Kelleher M: Removal of urinary catheters: midnight vs.

0600 hours, *Br J Nurs* 11(2):84–90, 2002.

Leaver RB: The evidence for urethral meatal cleansing, *Nurs Stand* 21 (41):39–42, 2007.

Ludwick R: Urinary elimination. In Potter A, Perry A, editors: *Fundamentals of nursing*, ed 4, St Louis, 1999, Mosby, pp 972–1008.

McCormick T, Ashe R, Kearney P: Urinary tract infection in pregnancy, *Obstet Gynaecol* 10(3):156–162, 2008.

NICE (National Institute for Clinical Excellence): *Antenatal care Routine care for the healthy pregnant woman*, London, 2008, NICE.

Nicol M, Bavin C, Cronin P, Rawlings-Anderson K: *Essential Nursing Skills*, Edinburgh, 2008, Mosby.

NMC (Nursing and Midwifery Council): *Guidelines for records and record keeping*, London, 2005, NMC.

Potter PA, Perry A: *Basic nursing*, ed 5, St Louis, 2003, Mosby.

Pratt RJ, Pellowe CM, Wilson JA, et al: Epic 2: National evidence based guidelines for preventing healthcare-associated infection in NHS Hospitals in England, *J Hosp Infect* 65S(Suppl):S1–S64, 2007.

Robinson J: Female urinary catheterisation, *Nurs Stand* 22(8):48–56, 2007.

Steggall MJ: 2007, Acute urinary retention:causes, clinical features and patient care. *Nurs Stand* 21 (29):42–46.

Verralls S: *Anatomy and physiology applied to obstetrics*, ed 3, Edinburgh, 1993, Churchill Livingstone.

Walsh D: Care in the first stage of labour. In Henderson C, Macdonald S, editors: *Mayes midwifery: a textbook for midwives*, ed 13, London, 2004, Baillière Tindall, pp 428–457.

Winder A: Female urinary catheterisation, *Community Nurse* 5(10):33–34, 36, 1999.

Yates A: Urinary Catheters Part 5 Catheter drainage and support systems, 104(43):22–23, 2008.

Principles of elimination management: urinalysis

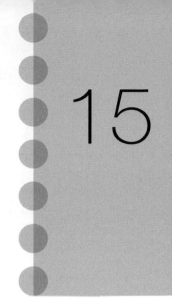

15

CHAPTER CONTENTS

This chapter considers 'normal' urine, changes that may occur during childbirth, the significance of abnormal findings and the procedure for undertaking urinalysis. Although pregnancy tests can also be undertaken using a specimen of urine, this is not discussed within this chapter. Whilst urinalysis is an effective screening tool, it should not be used in isolation when considering whether or not treatment is required (Steggall 2007).

LEARNING OUTCOMES

Having read this chapter the reader should be able to:

- discuss the midwife's role and responsibilities in relation to urinalysis, identifying when and how it is undertaken
- recognise 'normal' urine and gain some understanding of the significance of the findings of urinalysis.

Definition

Urinalysis is the testing of both the physical characteristics and the composition of freshly voided urine. It is undertaken for the purposes of:

- screening: for systemic and renal disease
- diagnosis: of a suspected condition
- management: to monitor the progress of a particular condition (Getliffe & Dolman 1997), e.g. pregnancy-induced hypertension.

Urinalysis can be undertaken by laboratory testing or, for immediate results, by using a chemical reagent strip, in addition to assessing the physical characteristics of colour, clarity and odour of urine.

The physical characteristics of urine

- Colour: urine ranges from pale straw to amber colour, depending on its concentration. The colour results from urochrome, a by-product of haemoglobin breakdown. Urine voided in the morning is usually more concentrated and darker than urine voided throughout the day when fluids are taken in.
- Clarity: urine is usually transparent when freshly voided.
- Odour: urine has a characteristic inoffensive odour.

Composition of urine

Urine has a pH of 4.5–8, specific gravity of 1.003–1.030 and is mainly water (96%) with 4% dissolved substances:

- urea (2%)
- uric acid, creatinine, sodium, potassium, phosphates, sulphates, oxalates and chlorides
- cellular components, e.g. epithelial cells, leucocytes
- protein and glucose are present in negligible amounts, normally undetectable by routine testing.

Normal changes during childbirth

- Pregnancy: glycosuria is more common due to changes in renal function (Blackburn 2007).
- Labour: proteinuria may occur following rupture of the membranes or as a result of contamination by the vaginal discharge or the operculum.
- Ketonuria: may occur and, provided it is mild, is insignificant.

Indications for urinalysis

- As part of the antenatal examination.
- Throughout labour.
- On admission to hospital for any reason as a baseline observation.
- Specific maternal disorders or treatment, e.g. hypertensive disease, diabetes mellitus, anticoagulant therapy.

- Clinical symptoms, e.g. stinging on micturition.
- Altered micturition.

Significance of findings

Colour

Dark yellow urine is associated with concentrated urine, pale urine with dilute urine. Bilirubinuria colours the urine very dark amber or brown–green; this should also be suspected if the urine develops yellow foam when shaken. Haematuria also affects the colour: dark red if bleeding is within the kidneys or ureters, bright red if bleeding is from the bladder or urethra. Diet may also influence the colour, with beetroot and rhubarb causing a deep red colour, as can drugs (e.g. sulfasalazine causes orange-coloured urine).

Clarity

Urine becomes cloudy (turbid) if left to stand for several minutes due to precipitation of some of the dissolved substances (e.g. uric acid). Proteinuria may cause the urine to appear cloudy or foamy and bacteriuria may cause it to appear cloudy and thick. Infection can also cause urine to appear cloudy (Smyth et al 2006).

Odour

The odour becomes stronger as the concentration of the urine increases. Stagnant urine smells of ammonia due to the breakdown of urea into ammonium carbonate. A sweet odour could indicate the presence of ketones, a by-product of fat metabolism. Infection may cause the urine to smell offensive. The smell of urine can also be affected by the ingestion of fish, curry and other strongly flavoured food.

Specific gravity

This reflects the kidneys' ability to concentrate or dilute urine, normal levels in a healthy adult are 1.001–1.035. Low levels are associated with water diuresis, hypercalcaemia, hypokalaemia, high levels with dehydration. High levels of proteinuria and glycosuria also increase specific gravity.

pH

Urine usually has a pH between 5 and 8. A low pH indicates the urine is more acidic than normal and may predispose to the formation of calculi (stones) within the bladder or kidney. The type of diet ingested can also influence pH with a protein-rich diet causing the urine to be more acidic and one with a high intake of vegetables or dairy products can result in the urine becoming more alkaline (Steggall 2007). Stale urine will cause a high pH (Wilson 2005).

Bilirubin

This is due to hepatic or biliary disease, particularly if the flow of bile into the duodenum is obstructed and may be found in conjunction with urobilinogen. A false-positive result may occur when certain drugs are taken (e.g. chlorpromazine) and a false-negative result if the urine is stale, particularly if the sample is exposed to sunlight.

Blood

Blood should not appear in the urine. Its presence might be indicative of infection, trauma, tumour or calculi, or may be due to contamination by blood from another part of the body (e.g. vaginal discharge, haemorrhoids). A positive result warrants further investigation.

Glucose

Glucose appears in the urine when blood glucose levels rise (hyperglycaemia) or if renal absorption lowers. It may be indicative of diabetes mellitus, stress or, less commonly, acute pancreatitis or Cushing's syndrome.

Ketones

These may occur due to fasting, vomiting and uncontrolled diabetes mellitus. Some drugs, e.g. captopril, may give a false-positive result.

Leucocytes

Leucocytes in the urine are suggestive of pyuria, indicating a urinary tract infection (UTI); however, the urinalysis test is less sensitive than microscopy and the specimen may be contaminated by leucocytes from an alternative source (e.g. vaginal discharge). A positive test does not diagnose UTI, although, when found with nitrites, it makes the diagnosis more probable. Equally, a negative result does not exclude UTI as pyuria is not always present with a UTI.

Nitrites

Nitrates from the diet are converted to nitrites in the presence of bacteria, particularly Gram-negative bacteria (e.g. *Escherichia coli*). Nitrites in the urine are indicative of a UTI and a mid-stream urine (MSU; see Chapter 17) specimen should be sent for laboratory analysis. A false-negative result can occur if the bacteria have had insufficient time to convert the nitrates; for example, if the woman is experiencing frequent micturition (common with cystitis). The urine should be in the bladder for at least 4 hours prior to obtaining a sample. Additionally, if the urinary reagent strip has been exposed to air, the nitrite test can become inactive and lead to a false-negative result. A false-positive result can be obtained in the presence of hyperbilirubinaemia (Watts et al 2007).

Protein

This may indicate a contaminated specimen, infection or underlying renal disease. Transient positive tests are usually insignificant, due to the presence of small amounts of albumin and globulin in the urine; to detect larger amounts of protein an early morning specimen is required. To exclude infection, an MSU specimen (see Chapter 17) should be obtained, tested and sent for laboratory analysis (if necessary).

Urobilinogen

Normally present in small quantities, larger amounts may be indicative of liver abnormalities or excessive haemolysis.

Equipment for urinalysis

Urinary reagent strips or 'dipsticks' are the current method used for testing the composition of urine. They are quick and easy to use with good reliability, particularly for detecting proteinuria (Craver & Abermanis 1997), although Walerstein (2005) considers them to be unreliable and recommends

24-hour urine collection for hypertensive pregnancies. Accuracy for detecting glycosuria increases as the plasma glucose level increases (Li & Huang 1997); glycosuria may not be detected when hyperglycaemia is mild. Use of an automated strip reader will reduce observer error and increase the sensitivity of the reagent strips, resulting in a more accurate analysis of the components of the urine sample (Cronin 2008, Patel et al 2005).

The strips can degenerate with time, compounded by storage at temperature extremes or exposure to excessive humidity. Storage should be according to the manufacturer's instructions, in a cool, dry, dark area. The lid should be tight and the desiccant should not be removed from the bottle.

PROCEDURE: urinalysis

- Obtain a fresh specimen of urine for testing (if refrigerated, allow it to warm to room temperature prior to testing; invert the sample to ensure even distribution of constituents).
- Gather equipment:
  ○ reagent strips (ensure they are still in date)
  ○ non-sterile gloves
  ○ apron (if contact with urine is likely)
  ○ watch with second hand if reading manually.
- Examine the reagent strip to ensure it is not contaminated.
- Wash hands, put on gloves and apron.
- Observe the colour, clarity and odour of the urine.
- Insert the reagent strip into the urine to cover the reagent areas, remove immediately.
- Tap the edge of the strip against the side of the urine container to remove excess urine, keeping the strip horizontal to avoid it running down the strip and mixing the colours.
- If reading the reagent strip manually, follow the manufacturer's instructions for timing, hold the strip close to the colour charts and read the results in good lighting (alternatively a urine

chemistry analyser may be used in accordance with the manufacturer's instructions and the results printed off)
- Dispose of urine and equipment correctly.
- Wash hands.
- Discuss the findings with the woman.
- Document the findings and act accordingly.

ROLE AND RESPONSIBILITIES OF THE MIDWIFE

These can be summarised as:

- undertaking the procedure correctly, using an appropriate urine specimen and equipment
- recognising deviations from the norm, referring if necessary
- correct documentation
- education of the woman.

Summary

- Urinalysis may be undertaken for the purpose of screening, diagnosis or assessment of management.
- It is quick and easy to do, with instantaneous results, detecting abnormal constituents in the urine.
- False-negative and false-positive results may occur; these can be minimised if the correct procedure is followed.

SELF-ASSESSMENT EXERCISES

The answers to the following questions may be found in the text:

1. What are the normal constituents of urine?
2. For what reasons might urinalysis be undertaken?
3. What observations are undertaken on urine prior to urinalysis and why?
4. List the substances that may be found on urinalysis and discuss the significance of each.

References

Blackburn S: *Maternal, fetal and neonatal physiology: a clinical perspective*, ed 3, St. Louis, 2007, Saunders.

Craver RD, Abermanis JG: Dipstick only urinalysis screen for the pediatric emergency room, *Paediatr Nephrol* 11(3):331–333, 1997.

Cronin M: Automated urinalysis technology improves efficiency and patient care, *Med Lab Obs* 40 (10):30–31, 2008.

Getliffe K, Dolman M: Normal and abnormal bladder function. In Getliffe M, Dolman M, editors: *Promoting continence: a clinical and research resource*, London, 1997, Baillière Tindall, ch 2.

Li K, Huang H: Comparing urinary reagent strips for detecting glycosuria in patients with diabetes mellitus, *Lab Med* 28(6):397–401, 1997.

Patel H, Livsey S, Swann R, et al: Can urine dipstick testing for urinary tract infection at point of care reduce laboratory workload? *J Clin Pathol* 58(9):951–954, 2005.

Smyth M, Moore J: Goldsmith C: Urinary tract infections: role of the clinical microbiology laboratory, *Urol Nurs* 26 (3):198–203, 2006.

Steggall MJ: Urine samples and urinalysis... clinical skills: 29, *Nurs Stand* 22(14–16):42–45, 2007.

Walerstein S: Review: point of care dipstick urinalysis has low accuracy for detecting proteinuria in pregnancy, *Evid Based Med* 10(1):25, 2005.

Watts S, Bryan D, Marill K: Is there a link between hyperbilirubinemia and elevated urine nitrite, *Am J Emerg Med* 25(1):10–14, 2007.

Wilson LA: Urinalysis, *Nurs Stand* 19(35):51–54, 2005.

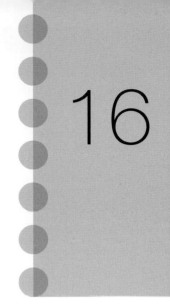

Principles of elimination management: defecation

16

Women experience a number of changes with their bowel habits during pregnancy and the postnatal period that might lead them to feel constipated or have loose stools, both of which can be uncomfortable and embarrassing. The midwife plays an important role in promoting normal bowel habits and preventing complications. This chapter focuses on defecation: the passage of faeces through the anal sphincter. Relevant physiology, factors influencing defecation and a discussion on how the midwife promotes defecation are all included.

LEARNING OUTCOMES

Having read this chapter the reader should be able to:

- describe the physiology of defecation
- discuss the factors that influence defecation
- discuss the ways in which the midwife can promote defecation.

Physiology

Faeces are normally semi solid in consistency, containing 70% water. The remaining constituents are the end products of digestion, the residue of unabsorbed food, bile pigments, epithelial cells, mucus, bacteria, cellulose and some inorganic material. Faeces are propelled through the large intestine to the sigmoid colon by peristalsis, and water is absorbed from the faeces. The longer the faeces remain in the large intestine, the greater the amount of water absorbed, the harder the faeces become, and vice versa. Faeces usually stay in the sigmoid colon until the stimulus for defecation occurs.

The stimulus to defecate arises in response to the presence of faeces in the sigmoid colon, causing the faeces to pass from there to the rectum. This stimulus can vary from person to person and is often related to habit (Crisford 2008). The rectum is very sensitive to changes in pressure and, as the faeces enter the rectum, the pressure rises by 2–3 mmHg. As the rectal walls distend, the internal anal sphincter relaxes, reducing anal pressure – the inhibitory reflex – creating an awareness of the need to defecate. The puborectalis muscle contracts, decreasing the anorectal angle – the inflation reflex (Edwards 1997). If it is appropriate to defecate, the diaphragm, abdominal and levator ani muscles contract and the glottis closes. This results in a rise in pressure within the rectum and a decrease in pressure exerted by the internal and external sphincters. The pelvic floor lowers as the puborectalis muscle relaxes, increasing the anorectal angle, facilitating the passage of faeces into the anal canal by peristalsis. The posture adopted can assist this process by increasing the action of the abdominal muscles and pushing the walls of the sigmoid colon and rectum inwards. A sharp increase followed by a decrease in blood pressure can occur during defecation.

This reflex stimulus can be ignored and inhibited; defecation is, to a limited extent, under conscious control. When ignored, the external anal sphincter contracts, increasing the anal pressure. As a result, the rectal pressure decreases and the puborectalis muscle contracts. The anorectal angle is reduced as the rectum is pulled backwards and the faeces move back to the rectum from the anal canal (retroperistalsis). The stimulus will disappear and return several hours later. If the stimulus continues to be inhibited, suppression of the reflex occurs and constipation ensues.

If it is inconvenient to defecate, impulses pass to the cerebral cortex to inhibit defecation. In babies and young children this ability is absent, and defecation becomes a reflex response to faeces in the rectum.

Factors inhibiting defecation (possibly resulting in constipation)

- Diet, e.g. inadequate bulk.
- Dehydration.
- Drugs, e.g. opiates, iron supplements.
- Disease, e.g. Hirschsprung's disease, paralysis.
- Lack of exercise or immobility.
- Changes to normal lifestyle and routines, e.g. hospitalization.
- Psychological: unfavourable conditions (e.g. lack of privacy, shared toilet facilities, bedpans), fear of damaging a sutured perineum.
- Pain: may be associated with haemorrhoids.
- Psychiatric disorders, e.g. depression.
- Pregnancy: progesterone relaxes the smooth muscle of the bowel, slowing down the movement of faeces through the large intestine, allowing more water to be absorbed.

Factors increasing defecation (possibly causing diarrhoea)

- During the onset and early part of labour (this could result in defecation being delayed in the first 48 hours after delivery).

- Diet: excessive intake of certain food, e.g. very spicy food.
- Drugs, e.g. antibiotics, iron supplements, laxatives.
- Disease, e.g. carcinoma, diverticulitis.
- Infection.
- Damage: lax pelvic floor muscles provide little support for the anal sphincter; as the abdominal pressure rises, faeces will be forced down the anal canal and pass out through the sphincter.

Principles: promoting defecation

- Posture: sitting forwards in a crouched position with the forearms supported on parted knees allows the diaphragm to move down and facilitates the action of the contracted abdominal muscles; the glottis should be closed, the jaw should be relaxed, lips open and teeth apart. The use of a footstool to raise the legs may facilitate this position.
- Diet: a high-fibre diet with an adequate fluid intake will prevent the stools becoming too firm to pass.
- Education: advice on care of the perineum and likelihood of causing damage to a sutured perineum; reassurance of expected changes and return to normal bowel function following birth.
- Soft toilet paper: this may help psychologically.
- Conditioning: sitting on the toilet following a meal may help bowel habits be relearned.
- Mobility: constipation is associated with decreased mobility, so mild exercise will help.
- Easy access to clean toilet facilities: avoid using the bedpan which increases straining and oxygen consumption and causes embarrassment.
- Suitable barrier cream to prevent anal excoriation.
- Use of laxatives: but these should not be the first course of action.
- Suppositories and microenemas may provide immediate but short-term relief of constipation; the cause of constipation should also be treated.

ROLE AND RESPONSIBILITIES OF THE MIDWIFE

These can be summarised as:

- asking the woman about her bowel habits is part of the antenatal and postnatal examination; this should be undertaken in such a way so as not to embarrass the woman
- any difficulties with defecation should be discussed and advice given to promote defecation
- a record of any problems, advice given and evaluation of the advice should be recorded in the woman's case notes
- any drugs given to assist defecation should be in accordance with the responsibilities of drug administration
- if difficulties with defecation do not resolve, the midwife should refer the woman for further investigation.

Summary

- Defecation is primarily under conscious control (in the adult).
- Inhibition of defecation can lead to constipation.
- Defecation can be promoted by a number of different factors.

SELF-ASSESSMENT EXERCISES

The answers to the following questions may be found in the text:

1. Describe the physiology of defecation.
2. What factors influence the ability to defecate?
3. How can the midwife promote defecation?

References

Crisford M: Elimination; bowel care. In Dougherty S, Lister S, editors: *The Royal Marsden Hospital Manual of Clinical Nursing Procedures*, ed 7, Oxford, 2008, Wiley Blackwell, pp 324–347.

Edwards C: Down and away: an overview of adult constipation and faecal incontinence. In Getliffe K, Dolman M, editors: *Promoting continence: a clinical and research resource*, London, 1997, Baillière Tindall, ch 6.

Principles of elimination management: obtaining urinary and stool specimens

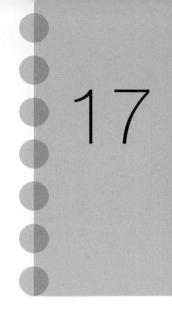

17

CHAPTER CONTENTS

Specimens should be obtained correctly to increase the reliability of the results. The midwife may be best placed to appreciate that a specimen is indicated, but care should be taken to avoid unnecessary specimen collection as it is resource heavy and can be stressful for the woman. This chapter considers how the range of urine and stool specimens is obtained.

LEARNING OUTCOMES

Having read this chapter the reader should be able to:

- describe the procedure for obtaining a catheter specimen, a mid-stream specimen and a neonatal specimen of urine

- describe how a 24-hour urine collection is taken
- describe how a stool specimen is obtained
- summarise the midwife's role and responsibility in relation to specimen collection.

Catheter specimens of urine

Urine may be taken from a catheterised woman for the purposes of urinalysis (e.g. infection screening) but occasionally a catheter may be inserted (often residual) to obtain an uncontaminated specimen (e.g. protein urinalysis when pre-eclamptic). This section focuses on obtaining a catheter specimen of urine (CSU) from an indwelling catheter. It is important that the following principles are applied:

- sterility, for both accuracy of the result and prevention of infection
- maintaining a closed drainage system, also for prevention of infection (specimens should only be taken when absolutely necessary)
- fresh urine is screened
- correct technique, sample bottle and dispatch to laboratory within the required time for the nature of the test
- recording of the test to avoid duplication
- collected in a manner that protects staff, including laboratory staff (Higgins 2008a).

Depending on the manufacturer, the type of urinary drainage bag will determine the way in which the specimen is taken:

- a resealing rubber 'window' port in the tubing
- a needle-less port in some part of the tubing or drainage bag (Fig. 17.1).

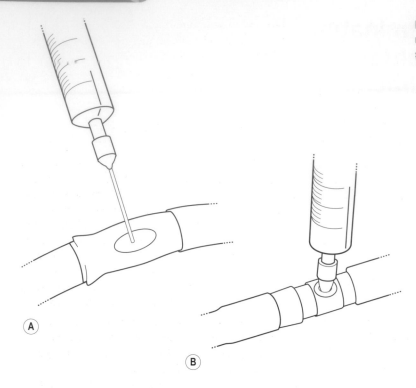

Figure 17.1 • A Rubber resealing needle sampling port. B needle-less sampling port

Wilson & Coates (1996) found that using an alcohol-impregnated wipe did not destroy bacteria. Its use is questionable, but recommended at this time. Pratt et al (2007) state that an aseptic technique must be used when obtaining a CSU.

PROCEDURE: catheter specimen of urine

- Gain informed consent and gather equipment:
  - ○ sterile specimen pot (correct one for the nature of the test required)
  - ○ sterile gloves
  - ○ 20 mL sterile syringe (and 25 g orange needle if it is a resealing port, with portable sharps box)
  - ○ alcohol-impregnated swab
  - ○ gate clamp.
- Ensure privacy.
- Examine the tubing for fresh urine; if none present apply the gate clamp below the level of the port and wait a few minutes for urine to collect.

- Wash hands and apply gloves.
- Wipe the port (both sorts) with the swab for 30 seconds (Wilson 1998) and allow to dry for 30 seconds (Steggall 2007).
- Resealing port: insert the needle into the rubber port taking care not to pierce out through the other side.
- Needle-less port: insert the syringe firmly into the port.
- Both: withdraw the required amount of urine (10–20 mL usually).
- Resealing: discard the needle (non-touch technique) using the sharps box.
- Place urine carefully into the specimen pot. Wipe the port for 30 seconds with the swab. Dispose of syringe correctly.
- Remove the clamp.
- Remove gloves and wash hands.
- Label the specimen correctly and dispatch to the laboratory, often within 1 hour; this will depend on the nature of the test (if delayed, refrigeration is sometimes acceptable).
- Document the findings and act accordingly.

Mid-stream specimens of urine

If a urine specimen is to be specifically screened for infection it is important that as much bacterial contamination as possible (from the vulva or urethra) is excluded. Consequently, the middle part of a urine specimen – a mid-stream urine (MSU) – is collected, with the initial voiding clearing the urethra of debris. The woman is required to contract her pubococcygeal muscle to 'stop and start' the urine flow, something that may be harder to achieve in late pregnancy. NICE (2008) recommend that all women are offered screening for asymptomatic bacteriuria in early pregnancy, culturing the urine following an MSU.

Meatal cleansing has traditionally been carried out prior to an MSU being taken. Lifshitz & Kramer (2000) suggested that in females cleansing makes no difference to contamination rates. However, if personal hygiene is poor or faecal contamination is suspected then meatal cleansing is recommended (Gilbert 2006). Soap and water is sufficient, using a front to back technique. However, a strong urine flow would appear to flush out the urethra when first voiding and so Leaver (2007) recommends ensuring that the bladder is at least half full prior to taking an MSU.

PROCEDURE: mid-stream specimen of urine

- Explain the procedure to the woman and gain her consent, ensure that her bladder is at least half full. If dexterity is a problem, the midwife may need to wear sterile gloves and assist.
- Gather equipment:
  - sterile specimen pot (correct for the investigation)
  - sterile receiver: usually a single-use tinfoil bowl or MSU pack that may contain a funnel.
- Ask the woman to wash her hands and part the labia (Steggall 2007).
- Ask her to void the first part of the urine into the toilet, halt the flow, void again to collect the specimen using either the funnel with the pot, or the foil bowl, then complete the voiding into the toilet, washing her hands when finished.
- Transfer the urine from the bowl to the pot if necessary (wear non-sterile gloves while doing this).

- Dispose of equipment and wash hands.
- Label the specimen and dispatch to the laboratory immediately.
- Document the findings (including the time of specimen) and act accordingly.

24-hour urine collection

The entire amount of urine passed in 24 hours is sent for analysis, usually for protein. It is important that every drop is sent, if a sample is missed the test is invalid and should be recommenced. It is important to have the correct specimen container. Some tests require the presence of nitric acid, the amount may be subtracted from the total volume on completion; local protocols will guide on this. The woman needs to have a good level of understanding and compliance to complete this test correctly.

- The collection is started in the morning and is completed and sent the following morning.
- Urine is passed and discarded, the exact time noted and the collection begins.
- The woman is supplied with a sterile jug and asked to void into the jug then transfer the urine into the correct specimen container. If testing of the urine is required this is done using the specimen in the jug prior to its transfer to the container.
- 24 hours later the woman is asked to pass urine as near to finishing time as possible. Once the last collection is added, the container(s) are sent directly to the laboratory with the request card.
- Any other specimens required are taken before or after the 24-hour collection.

Urine specimens from the baby

These are usually obtained from ill babies as part of an infection screen. The urine may be caught in a sterile bowl or directly into the specimen bottle (clean catch). This is unpredictable, but for the healthy baby it is the 'gold standard' method of urine collection (Rogers & Saunders 2008). Sterile specimen bags may be placed over the baby's genitalia and the specimen poured into the pot when collected. Repeated specimen collection can cause the skin to be damaged. Urine collection pads (placed in the nappy) are often preferred by the parents but contamination from the rectum and perineum is likely with both of these methods (Rogers & Saunders 2008).

A suprapubic bladder aspiration may be completed by the paediatrician by inserting a sterile needle through the abdominal wall into the bladder and drawing urine off. This is uncomfortable and may puncture the bladder or bowel.

Obtaining a stool specimen

Stool specimens screen for gastrointestinal (GI) infection or the presence of occult blood. *Clostridium difficile* is known to cause considerable mortality and morbidity, parasites such as hookworm can cause anaemia in infected pregnant women and other GI infections may be debilitating and infectious. Stool specimens should be assessed for their colour, consistency, odour and frequency, and the information recorded. Gill (1999) cites the Bristol stool chart (Fig. 17.2), which describes the seven main types of stool classification. If a series of specimens is required, it is important to indicate which in the series the specimen is. It is also important

to be aware of the need to send some specimens at specific times, local protocols provide guidance on this (Higgins 2008b).

PROCEDURE: stool specimen (adult)

- Explain the procedure to the woman and gain informed consent.
- Gather equipment:
  - clean bedpan or disposable liner
  - stool specimen pot with integral scoop or spatula
  - non-sterile gloves and apron.
- Ask the woman to defecate into the bedpan, but not to urinate. If incontinent, take specimen from soiled pads, without urine contamination, if possible.
- Apply apron, wash hands and apply gloves.
- Using the scoop, place the stool sample in the specimen pot, filling approximately one-third of the container, and seal the lid.
- If any parasite is visible, aim to place all of it in the pot.

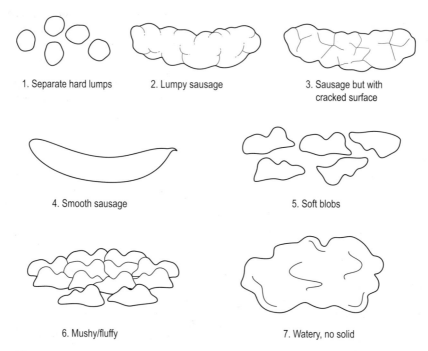

1. Separate hard lumps   2. Lumpy sausage   3. Sausage but with cracked surface

4. Smooth sausage   5. Soft blobs

6. Mushy/fluffy   7. Watery, no solid

Figure 17.2 • Bristol stool classifications. Type 1, separate hard lumps; type 2, lumpy sausage; type 3, sausage but with cracked surface; type 4, smooth sausage; type 5, soft blobs; type 6, mushy/fluffy; type 7, watery, no solid

- Dispose of equipment, wash hands, label and dispatch specimen, document findings (including stool classification) and act accordingly.

PROCEDURE: stool specimen (baby)

- Gain parental consent.
- Observe the baby for signs of straining (to obtain a fresh specimen).
- Using non-sterile gloves, fill one-third (if possible) of the stool specimen pot with the stool taken from the baby's nappy, seal the lid.
- If the stool is too wet and has been absorbed, efforts should be made to catch the sample in a sterile foil bowl on the next evacuation.
- Dispose of equipment correctly.
- Wash hands.
- Label and dispatch specimen (immediately for some screenings), indicating whether contamination with urine is a possibility.
- Document findings and act accordingly.

ROLE AND RESPONSIBILITIES OF THE MIDWIFE

These can be summarised as:

- explaining the procedure and gaining consent
- ensuring correct specimen collection and dispatch
- knowledge and application of infection control protocols
- correct documentation.

Summary

- Specimens should be obtained, labelled and dispatched correctly.
- A catheter specimen is taken from the recognised port, causing minimal disruption to the closed drainage system.
- An MSU is the middle part of the voided urine, the bladder should be at least half full before collecting the specimen.
- Urinary specimens from babies may be obtained using a specimen bag, a 'clean catch' or sterile suprapubic aspiration.
- Stool specimens from the woman are obtained from a clean bedpan; from the baby they are obtained from the baby's nappy.

SELF-ASSESSMENT EXERCISES

The answers to the following questions may be found in the text:

1. Describe how a catheter specimen of urine is obtained.
2. Why is a mid-stream specimen of urine so named?
3. List the ways a urine specimen may be obtained from a baby.
4. Describe how a stool specimen is obtained from a woman.
5. Summarise the role and responsibilities of the midwife in relation to specimen collection.

References

Gilbert R: Taking a mid-stream specimen of urine, *Nurs Times* 102(18):22–23, 2006.

Gill D: Stool specimen 1. Assessment, *Nurs Times* 95(25):40, 1999.

Higgins D: Specimen collection obtaining a mid-stream specimen of urine, *Nurs Times* 104(17):26–27, 2008a.

Higgins D: Specimen collection Part 3 – collecting a stool specimen, *Nurs Times* 104(19):22–23, 2008b.

Leaver RB: The evidence for urethral meatal cleansing, *Nurs Stand* 21(41):39–42, 2007.

Lifshitz E, Kramer L: Outpatient urine culture, *Arch Intern Med* 160 (16):2537–2540, 2000.

NICE (National Institute for Clinical Excellence): *Antenatal care Routine care for the healthy pregnant woman*, London, 2008, NICE.

Pratt RJ, Pellowe CM, Wilson JA, et al: epic2: National evidence-based guidelines for preventing healthcare-associated infections in NHS hospitals in England, *J Hosp Infect* 65S:S1–S64, 2007.

Rogers J, Saunders C: Urine collection in infants and children, *Nurs Times* 104(5):40–42, 2008.

Steggall M: Urine samples and urinalysis, *Nurs Stand* 22(14–16): 42–45, 2007.

Wilson M: Infection control, *Prof Nurse Study Suppl* 13(5):S10–S13, 1998.

Wilson M, Coates D: Infection control and urinary drainage bags, *Prof Nurse* 11(4):245–252, 1996.

Principles of drug administration: legal aspects, pharmacokinetics and anaphylaxis

18

CHAPTER CONTENTS

This chapter considers the legal regulations covering drug administration by the midwife and also discusses pharmacokinetics for both the woman and baby and the management of anaphylaxis. Errors in drug administration can have serious consequences not only for the person to whom the drug was administered, but also for the midwife who could face charges of professional misconduct and ultimately be removed from the Nursing and Midwifery Council (NMC) register. Up to 10 000 preventable deaths occur each year due to medication errors (Matthew 2007). Some drugs in the maternal circulation do not pass through to the fetus during pregnancy and labour, as the placenta acts as a barrier. However, some drugs are able to pass through the placental barrier and can have an effect on the fetus (e.g. pethidine). Drugs may also pass from the maternal circulation to the baby via breast milk. This chapter does not consider fetal pharmacokinetics or drugs and breastfeeding, and the reader is directed towards the growing number of books that look specifically at this topic if further information is required.

LEARNING OUTCOMES

Having read this chapter the reader should be able to:

- discuss the supply, storage, administration, surrender and destruction of controlled drugs
- discuss the responsibilities of the midwife in relation to drug administration
- understand how drugs are absorbed, distributed, metabolised and excreted
- identify factors that influence absorption of drugs via the oral route
- list the factors that can interfere with the metabolism of drugs
- discuss how pharmacokinetics differs for the baby
- recognise the signs and symptoms of anaphylaxis and discuss the management of this condition.

Legislation

A number of Statutory Acts and Regulations govern the use of drugs by the midwife in the UK, including the Medicines Act (1968), the Misuse of Drugs Act (1971), Misuse of Drugs Regulations (2001, which are of particular relevance when using controlled drugs) and the Health Act (2006). Rule 7 of the Midwives Rules and Standards (NMC 2004) sets out the responsibilities of the midwife in relation to the administration of medicines, and this should be followed in conjunction with the Standards for Medicine Management (NMC 2008).

Drugs are classified according to whether they are non-prescription or prescription drugs (non-controlled and controlled). Midwives can supply and administer non-prescription medicines without a prescription; however, for prescription drugs, a medicine administration chart signed by a medical practitioner is a requirement unless the medicine is covered by a patient group direction.

Drugs should be administered in line with relevant legislation and local standard operating procedures. It is important that the medicine administration chart for any drug is written in ink and is legible. It should contain details of:

* the name of the drug
* dose
* method of administration
* frequency of administration
* date of prescription
* doctor's signature.

The doctor's signature should be recognisable as that of the doctor overseeing the woman or baby. Any known allergies or medical conditions that may influence which drugs are administered (e.g. asthma) should be clearly visible. It is also important that the midwife is familiar with the drug to be administered, knowing why it is to be given, normal dosage, precautions, contraindications and side effects.

Patient group direction

A patient group direction (PGD) is a specific written instruction covering the supply and administration of a named (prescription only) medicine or vaccine drawn up locally by doctors to cover particular clinical situations (e.g. labour). This allows the midwife working both in hospital and in the community to administer named drugs without a signed medicine administration chart. Community midwives can carry and use a number of drugs which can include:

* ergometrine maleate tablets and injection
* diamorphine, morphine, pethidine and pentazocine (controlled drugs)
* promazine hydrochloride (Sparine®)
* lidocaine hydrochloride
* phytomenadione (vitamin K)
* naloxone hydrochloride (Narcan®)
* oxytocin.

Locally agreed policies may be developed to provide guidance surrounding the circumstances when a PGD may be used and administration and dosage for medicines the midwife is able to supply and administer. The consultant obstetricians or paediatricians must sign the PGDs and these should be dated; some will require reviewing each year to ensure they are up to date. They should also be replaced whenever there is a change of consultant. They are usually displayed in a prominent place close to the drugs cupboard. Students cannot supply or administer drugs under a PGD but are required to understand the principles and be involved in the process.

Controlled drugs

A controlled drug refers to narcotic drugs and those that cause drug dependence. There are five controlled drug schedules:

* Schedule 1: drugs usually used illegally (e.g. cannabis), which are available only with a controlled drugs licence.
* Schedule 2: drugs that are extremely addictive (e.g. pethidine, morphine).
* Schedule 3: some barbiturates (e.g. temazepam, pentazocine).
* Schedule 4: includes benzodiazepine tranquillizers (e.g. diazepam, nitrazepam).
* Schedule 5: medicines containing a small amount of a controlled drug (e.g. cough mixtures, analgesia).

Legislation covers the supply, storage, administration, surrender and destruction of controlled drugs.

Supply of controlled drugs

The midwife is able to supply and administer controlled drugs in accordance with the Prescription Only Medicines (Human Use) Order (1987), and requires a Midwives Supply Order to obtain these drugs. The drugs are supplied to the midwife for use within her professional practice only (NMC 2005) and relate to pethidine, morphine and diamorphine, listed on Schedule 2. Following notification of their intention to practise, midwives can be supplied with pethidine for use with home confinements using a supply order procedure. The Midwives Supply Order must be in writing, and provide details of the midwife's name and occupation, the drug, purpose for which it is required and total quantity to be supplied.

PROCEDURE: obtaining a supply of controlled drugs

- The supply order is taken to the supervisor of midwives or an Appropriate Medical Officer (a doctor authorized in writing by the local supervising authority) for signing (inspection of the midwife's drug register, record of cases and remaining stock may be undertaken prior to signing).
- The signed supply order is taken to a pharmacist who has a prior agreement to supply the drug and who has a record of the midwife's signature.
- On supply of the drug, the name, amount and form of the drug supplied and name and address of supplier are recorded in the midwife's drugs book (this also contains details of the dates the drug is administered, the woman's name and amount).

The alternative, and usually preferable, option is for the general practitioner to prescribe pethidine directly to the pregnant woman; the woman then becomes responsible for the destruction or return of any unused ampoules. Midwives working in hospital should follow their local policy for obtaining controlled drugs.

Storage of controlled drugs

Drugs on Schedules 1 and 2 are kept in a locked cupboard within a non-moveable locked cupboard that should only be opened by the midwife. The cupboard should conform to BS2881 or be approved by the pharmacy department. Drugs on Schedules 3, 4 and 5 are not kept in a controlled drug cupboard, but are locked away, with the exception of temazepam (a Schedule 3 drug).

Administration of controlled drugs

Drugs should be administered in line with relevant legislation and local standard operating procedures. In addition, it is recommended that the controlled drug is checked by two people, one of whom should be a registered midwife, nurse, doctor or operating department practitioner (ODP) although this may vary according to local standard operating practices. It is recommended that the second signatory is a registered healthcare professional – doctor, midwife, nurse or student midwife (NMC 2008). Both people should witness the drug be prepared and administered and the destruction of any surplus drug (e.g. part of the ampoule not administered). Where it is necessary to administer only part of a vial, both the amount given and the amount wasted should be recorded; for example, 'morphine 15 mg given and 5 mg wasted'. If a small amount of a controlled drug is emptied into the sharps bin, the bin must be labelled 'contains mixed pharmaceutical waste and sharps – for incineration' (DH 2007).

The controlled drugs register and medicine administration chart should be completed and signed by both the person administering the drug and the witness, indicating:

- name of person receiving the drug (controlled drug register only)
- date and time of administration
- dose administered
- route
- both signatures.

PROCEDURE: administration of a controlled drug

- Obtain the signed medicine administration chart (if not covered by a PGD) and ensure it is correctly filled out.
- Check the stock of the drug in the cupboard with the drug register total.
- Record the woman's name, amount of drug to be given, date of administration and amount remaining in the drug register.
- Check the name, amount and expiry date of the ampoule.

- Draw up the drug, take to the woman.
- Confirm her identity (ask her to verbally state her name and date of birth and confirm details on her identity band against the medicine administration chart).
- Administer the drug and dispose of equipment (see Chapters 19, 20 and 23).
- Sign the drug register, recording details of the time of administration.
- Record the amount and name of the drug, route, time and date of administration in the appropriate documentation, e.g. medicine administration chart, obstetric notes, partogram.
- Note and document the effect of the drug, e.g. good/poor response to analgesia.

Surrender of controlled drugs

Stocks of controlled drugs no longer required are surrendered to an authorized person (e.g. the pharmacist who supplied the drugs). A record of when and to whom the drugs were surrendered is made in the midwife's drugs book.

Destruction of controlled drugs

Unwanted or expired controlled drugs can be destroyed by the midwife in the presence of an authorized person, and both should sign the midwife's drugs book confirming this. An authorized person includes:

- a supervisor of midwives in England, Wales, Scotland or Northern Ireland
- a regional pharmaceutical officer in England
- a pharmaceutical officer of the Welsh Office
- chief administrative pharmaceutical officers of health boards in Scotland
- in Northern Ireland, an inspector appointed by the Department of Health and Social Services under the Misuse of Drugs Act 1971
- medical officers in England, Scotland or Wales
- an inspector of the Royal Pharmaceutical Society of Great Britain
- a police officer
- an inspector of the Home Office drugs branch.

Unused drugs supplied to a woman on prescription should be destroyed by the woman in the presence of the midwife, alternatively the woman can return the drugs to the pharmacist who supplied them (NMC 2004).

Prescription-only medicines

Midwives who have notified their intention to practise may be supplied with certain drugs (usually only available on prescription) for use in their practice (NMC 2004) (see p 136). Non-controlled drugs should have a correctly completed medicine administration chart (or PGD), which should be completed by the midwife following administration of the drug. It is advisable, wherever possible, for two midwives to check the drug prior to administration to minimise the risk of errors occurring.

PROCEDURE: administration of a non-controlled drug

- Obtain the signed medicine administration chart (if not covered by a PGD) and ensure it is legible and completed correctly.
- Ensure the label on the medicine dispensed is clearly written and unambiguous.
- Check the name, dose and expiry date of the drug (including weight-related doses where relevant) and ensure the method of administration, route and timing are appropriate to the choice of drug being administered.
- Ensure the woman is not allergic to the drug and that it is compatible with breastfeeding (where appropriate).
- Take the drug to the woman and confirm her identity (ask her to verbally state her name and date of birth and confirm details on her identity band against the medicine administration chart).
- Observe the woman taking the drug if self-administered (e.g. with oral drugs).
- Administer the drug and dispose of equipment (see Chapters 19 to 23).
- Complete and sign the medicine administration chart and record the dose given, route, date and time of administration in other relevant documentation (e.g. obstetric notes, partogram). Only one signature is required.
- If any contraindications found or a reaction develops following administration, or if the drug/route of administration is no longer suitable, contact the doctor/prescriber immediately and take appropriate action.
- Note and document the effect of the drug, e.g. good/poor response to analgesia.

ROLE AND RESPONSIBILITIES OF THE MIDWIFE

In addition to the statutory requirements laid down by Parliament, midwives are also bound by the Midwives Rules and Standards (NMC 2004). Rule 7 governs the administration of medicines and other forms of pain relief by the midwife. A midwife can only administer medicines following appropriate training in the use, dosage and methods of administration of drugs and equipment. This also encompasses the proper maintenance of equipment and only using equipment approved for use by the NMC (e.g. Entonox® apparatus).

The midwife should have a good working knowledge of both the Midwives Rules and Standards (NMC 2004) and the Standards for Medicine Management (NMC 2008). Local policy relating to drug administration should also be adhered to. Record keeping is an integral part of drug administration. The midwife should also have knowledge of pharmacokinetics.

Summary

- Legislation, the NMC and local policy govern the administration of drugs by the midwife; the midwife requires a good working knowledge of how these affect the supply, storage, administration, surrender and destruction of drugs.
- All drugs should be written on a medicine administration chart by a medical practitioner unless covered by a patient group direction.
- The midwife should receive appropriate training in the administration of drugs and use of equipment before taking on this responsibility.
- Ensuring the drug is administered correctly and knowledge of pharmacokinetics are essential.

Pharmacokinetics

Pharmacokinetics is the absorption, distribution, metabolism and excretion of drugs. As part of drug administration, an understanding of pharmacokinetics is important and may help the midwife to:

- recognise adverse reactions early
- minimise the risk of unwanted drug interactions occurring
- prevent drugs being used inadvertently during pregnancy and lactation
- educate the woman to help her make an informed choice regarding drug administration.

Adult pharmacokinetics

Absorption

Drugs administered orally are usually absorbed from the gastrointestinal (GI) tract, entering the bloodstream (some drugs bind to plasma albumin – protein binding) via the portal vein to pass through to the liver where metabolism begins. Capsules and tablets must disintegrate prior to absorption; liquid or soluble drugs are absorbed quicker than capsules and tablets. Where a rapid response is required an oral drug should be administered in a soluble form. Modified release drugs take longer to be absorbed and are inappropriate if a rapid response is required. It is important not to crush drugs that are intended to be swallowed whole as this may render them ineffective and they are not covered by the product licence (if the woman is unable to swallow drugs, the pharmacist should be consulted).

Drug absorption via the oral route is influenced by:

- gut motility and transit time: less drug is absorbed if it passes rapidly; the reverse is also true
- presence of food in the stomach: always follow the recommendations of taking the drug before, with or after food
- acid and enzymes of the GI tract
- lipid solubility (lipid-soluble drugs are easily absorbed and distributed throughout the body water compartments)
- drug formulation.

Certain drugs cannot be administered orally because the acid or enzymes of the GI tract would destroy them and so are administered parenterally (e.g. benzylpenicillin, insulin).

Drugs administered via the sublingual route enter the bloodstream directly and avoid the liver. Drugs administered intravenously enter the bloodstream immediately and can be distributed to the tissues quickly.

Drug plasma concentrations can be measured. The rate of concentration usually declines rapidly, but then slows over several hours. Administering a drug on a regular basis maintains the plasma concentration of the drug at a constant level, although a peak will still occur following administration.

Distribution

The drug is distributed around the body via the circulation until it penetrates the organs or tissues and has an effect. Drugs that distribute into body fluid can be affected by fluid balance (e.g. dehydration, oedema) and those that distribute into fatty tissues are influenced by the amount of fat (e.g. malnutrition, obesity). Different drug dosages may be required depending on the clinical condition of the person.

Metabolism

This usually occurs within the liver and may be impaired by:

- age
- severe liver disease
- respiratory or cardiac disease affecting hepatic blood flow and oxygenation
- drug interaction
- genetic factors.

Elimination

The kidneys are responsible for the majority of drug excretion. The half-life of a drug is the time taken for the plasma concentration of the drug to reduce by 50%. A drug that has a short half-life is quickly removed, necessitating frequent doses whereas a drug with a long half-life requires smaller doses as it remains in the body having an effect for longer periods. Loading doses – an initial total dose given to attain high plasma concentrations – may be needed with long half-life drugs to achieve a therapeutic plasma concentration.

Changes in pregnancy

Physiological changes occurring during pregnancy can affect pharmacokinetics. Decreased absorption in the stomach and increased absorption in the small intestine may occur due to decreased transit time. The latter may increase the time taken to attain optimal plasma concentration. The increase in plasma volume increases the volume of distribution of water-soluble drugs. The increased renal blood flow and liver activity increase drug clearance and elimination, which may necessitate higher dosages. Different doses may be required during pregnancy and their effect may be slower, thus it is important for pregnant women with pre-existing medical conditions requiring medication to have their medication requirements reviewed by their specialists/GPs on a regular basis.

Neonatal pharmacokinetics

Absorption

A variety of factors may affect drug absorption via the oral route. At birth, the pH of the term baby's stomach is 7. It becomes more acidic (pH 1.5–3.0) over the first hours of life, followed by a decrease in acid production during the first 10 days of life. Preterm babies have less ability to secrete gastric acid (Jackson 1999).

Drugs remain longer in the baby's stomach as gastric emptying time is slower. The stomach surface is less absorptive than the small intestine (Jackson 1999) thus it can take longer to achieve the desired plasma concentration of the drug. Less absorption of fat-soluble drugs occurs as bile output is reduced.

Intramuscular absorption is dependent on blood flow to the muscle, muscle activity, muscle mass and amount of subcutaneous fat. Decreased blood flow to the muscle is common during the first few days of life and absorption is unreliable.

Distribution

Drugs are more able to affect the brain due to greater membrane permeability of the blood–brain barrier. The baby, particularly preterm, has a higher percentage total body water content, necessitating higher doses (mg/kg) of water-soluble drugs to achieve an effective plasma concentration. However, lower doses of lipid-soluble drugs are required as the proportion of adipose tissue is reduced for both the term and the preterm baby.

Protein binding is decreased in the baby, possibly due to competing substances (e.g. bilirubin) attaching to the plasma albumin. Toxicity may occur as a result of high levels of the unbound drug (e.g. theophylline, diazepam) in the body; lower plasma concentrations are desirable. Drugs such as sulphonamides may displace bilirubin from its protein-bound site, increasing the risk of jaundice.

Metabolism and elimination are both reduced in the baby.

Summary

- Pharmacokinetics is the absorption, distribution, metabolism and excretion of drugs.
- Pregnancy affects pharmacokinetics and optimal plasma concentrations may take longer to attain.

- The differences with neonatal pharmacokinetics result in the oral and intramuscular routes being unreliable.

Anaphylaxis

The administration of a drug is not without risk; many drugs have known side effects and the midwife should be familiar with these. Anaphylaxis is a rare but potentially fatal hypersensitivity reaction that can occur following the administration of any drug, as well as food, fluid or topical applications (e.g. plasters, latex gloves), taking anything from several minutes to several hours to appear. Most reactions occur in people with no known risk factors, although it occurs more commonly with drugs such as antibiotics (e.g. penicillin) and whole blood. Early recognition of the signs and symptoms is essential to ensure prompt management of the condition. Mild anaphylaxis occurs more slowly, and symptoms tend to be less serious; it is managed by the administration of oral antihistamines with close observation for signs of improvement or deterioration and reassurance.

Severe anaphylaxis presents with cardiovascular collapse and is more urgent. The Resuscitation Council (2008) suggests anaphylaxis is likely when the following three criteria are all present:

- sudden onset and rapid advancement of symptoms
- life-threatening airway and/or breathing and/or circulation problems
- mucosal and/or skin changes (e.g. angioedema, flushing, urticaria), although these may be absent in up to 20% of cases.

Signs and symptoms

- Airway: pharyngeal/laryngeal oedema as the throat and tongue swell causing the woman to experience difficulty with swallowing and breathing and the feeling her throat is closing up; hoarseness; stridor.
- Breathing: tachypnoea (followed later by bradycardia), shortness of breath, wheezing, hypoxia resulting in confusion and cyanosis (late sign), fatigue; respiratory arrest.
- Circulation: shock, tachycardia, hypotension, dizziness, collapse, loss of consciousness, myocardial ischaemia and electrocardiograph (ECG) changes, cardiac arrest.
- Disability problems: the problems encountered with airway, breathing and circulation changes decrease brain perfusion and can alter the woman's neurological status causing agitation, confusion and loss of consciousness. There may also be accompanying gastrointestinal symptoms of abdominal pain, vomiting, incontinence, diarrhoea.
- Mucosal and/or skin changes: erythema, urticaria, angioedema.

Management of severe anaphylaxis (Resuscitation Council 2008)

- Call for medical assistance urgently; do not leave the woman.
- If anaphylaxis is the result of a substance being administered, stop administration immediately.
- Position the woman in the left lateral position. When this is not possible and the woman is on her back, place a wedge under her right side to prevent aortocaval occlusion (if pregnant) and raise her legs.
- Follow the principles of resuscitation (see Chapter 55) to establish an airway and resuscitate as needed whilst treating the anaphylaxis.
- Administer 100% oxygen therapy using a high flow mask (>10 L/min) with an oxygen reservoir to prevent collapse of the reservoir during inspiration.
- Administer intramuscular adrenaline (epinephrine) 1:1000 solution (1 mg/mL); repeated at 5-minute intervals if needed (adult dose 500 mg, 0.5 mL; baby 150 µg, 0.15 mL). If repeated doses are required, intravenous adrenaline may be administered only by a doctor who uses this in their everyday practice (e.g. anaesthetist). Continuous electrocardiograms (ECG) and pulse oximetry will be required with frequent monitoring of blood pressure.
- To correct hypotension, shock and vasodilatation, administer 500–1000 mL intravenous crystalloid solution (e.g. saline 0.9%) rapidly. If hypotension persists administer further doses.
- As a second line of treatment, an antihistamine (chlorphenamine) 10 mg can be administered

intramuscularly or by slow intravenous injection (baby dose 250 μg).

- Following initial resuscitation, hydrocortisone 200 mg may be administered intramuscularly or by slow intravenous injection (baby dose 25 mg).

- If bronchospasm persists, administration of a bronchodilator may be required, e.g. nebulized/intravenous salbutamol, inhaled ipratropium, intravenous aminophylline or magnesium (the latter may cause further flushes and hypotension).

- Document the cause and management clearly, informing the woman of this (to avoid recurrence).

- Closely observe the maternal or baby's condition over the next 6 hours in a clinical area able to monitor and treat life threatening conditions as a secondary reaction may occur. Observation is required for 24 hours following an anaphylactic reaction.

- Following an anaphylactic reaction, referral to an allergy clinic should be made for follow-up consultation and management.

Where an actual or suspected adverse drug reaction has occurred, the midwife should report this to the Medicines and Healthcare Products Regulatory Agency (MHRA) using the yellow card scheme. This can be undertaken online: www.yellowcard. mhra.gov.uk or by completing the yellow card at the back of the *British National Formulary*.

ROLE AND RESPONSIBILITIES OF THE MIDWIFE

These can be summarised as:

- being familiar with pharmacokinetics and the implications for drug administration
- understanding how pregnancy affects pharmacokinetics

- understanding why pharmacokinetics is different for the baby
- asking about known allergies at the booking interview and on each admission to hospital where medication may be required
- recognising and managing anaphylaxis correctly
- correct documentation
- informing the MHRA of a suspected or actual adverse drug reaction.

Summary

- Anaphylaxis is a rare but potentially fatal reaction that can result from drug administration, occurring from several minutes to several hours following administration.
- Where an actual or suspected drug reaction has occurred, the midwife should notify the MHRA who are responsible for monitoring such events.

SELF-ASSESSMENT EXERCISES

The answers to the following questions may be found in the text:

1. How does the midwife obtain a supply of pethidine?
2. What is the procedure for the administration of a controlled drug?
3. Identify three people who are authorized to destroy pethidine.
4. Discuss the responsibilities of the midwife in relation to drug administration of a non-controlled drug.
5. What are the four aspects of pharmacokinetics?
6. How does pregnancy affect pharmacokinetics?
7. How does pharmacokinetics differ for the baby?
8. How would the midwife recognise and manage anaphylaxis?
9. What is the name of the agency that monitors adverse drug reactions?

References

DH (Department of Health): *Safer management of controlled drugs: a guide to good practice in secondary care, (England)*, London, 2007, HMSO.

Jackson MP: Impact of age, pregnancy, disease and food on drug action. In Luker K, Wolfson D, editors: *Medicines management for clinical nurses*, Oxford, 1999, Blackwell Science, ch 4.

Matthew L: Injectable medication therapy: a patient safety challenge, *Nurs Stand* 21(31):45–48, 2007.

NMC (Nursing and Midwifery Council): *Midwives rules and standards*, London, 2004, NMC.

NMC (Nursing and Midwifery Council): *Midwives supply orders. NMC Circular 25/2005*, London, 2005, NMC.

NMC (Nursing and Midwifery Council): *Standards for medicine management*, London, 2008, NMC.

Resuscitation Council UK: Emergency treatment of anaphylactic reactions. Guidelines for healthcare providers, Online. Available: www.resus.org.uk 01 April 2009.

Principles of drug administration: oral administration

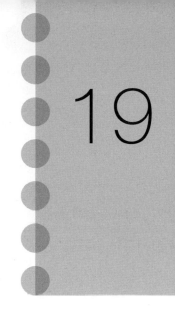

19

CHAPTER CONTENTS

This chapter considers the different preparations suitable for oral use, the procedure for administering them to an adult and a baby, and the midwife's role and responsibilities. It should be read in conjunction with Chapter 18.

LEARNING OUTCOMES

Having read this chapter the reader should be able to:

- discuss the different preparations available for oral use, giving an example of each
- describe the procedure for administering a drug orally to a woman and a baby
- summarise the role and responsibilities of the midwife.

The majority of medication taken via the mouth (orally) is absorbed by the gastrointestinal tract. The woman or baby needs to be compliant, alert and able to swallow. If this is not possible or if faster absorption is required then an alternative route should be prescribed. Many preparations can be found in alternative forms. Oral preparations may be affected by other constituents in the stomach, and so the manufacturer's directions should be followed (e.g. before, during or after a meal) for maximum effectiveness. The medication is prescribed as for any other prescription (see Chapter 18); P.O. (through the mouth) is the agreed abbreviation.

Medicine cups with gradations on the side are used; these may be disposable or washed and reused. Elixirs may be poured into a medicine cup, or 'drawn up' using an oral medicine syringe. Oral medicine syringes were originally designed for children, they are often a different colour and have a non-Luer tip so that a needle cannot be connected. This prevents accidental administration of oral medicines via intramuscular or intravenous routes. They are supplied sterile, but for older children the syringe may be washed and reused. It is supplied with a bung that fits into the bottle neck, this allows the bottle to be inverted and the correct dose drawn into the syringe at eye level.

Some inhalational drugs (e.g. Entonox®, oxygen) may be taken via the mouth, but in this chapter only the following oral medications are considered:

- Tablets: these should generally be swallowed whole. If scored they may be divided in half using a tablet cutter, according to the required dosage. Some tablets are coated to protect the stomach lining; the coating may also affect the rate of absorption, it being designed to ensure optimum therapeutic levels at the correct time. Chewing such tablets would destroy this effect.

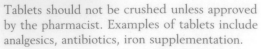

Tablets should not be crushed unless approved by the pharmacist. Examples of tablets include analgesics, antibiotics, iron supplementation.

- Granules, powders and soluble tablets: these need to be thoroughly dissolved before administration. This is generally in water, but the manufacturer's guidelines should be followed. Examples include analgesics, e.g. paracetamol.
- Capsules: these should always be swallowed whole, never chewed or opened. Examples include antibiotics and analgesics.
- Elixir: this may be supplied prepared, or require careful dilution according to the instructions. Some solutions require refrigeration. The bottle needs inverting several times to ensure thorough mixing before administration. Examples include antacids and antibiotics.
- Lozenges: these may be used specifically to treat the mouth or coat the tongue and so are sucked rather than swallowed. Examples include antifungal preparations.
- Sublingual (SL) preparations: these are absorbed in the sublingual pocket beneath the tongue. Examples include analgesics and antihypertensives. Preparations for buccal use are required to be placed between the gum and mouth, usually the cheek.

Helping the woman to understand her medication – how to take it correctly, what to expect and what to report – is a significant part of the drug administration process. If a drug is taken incorrectly it can have serious consequences including under- or overdose.

PROCEDURE: oral administration to a woman

- Ensure the woman/baby is accessible and ready for the medication prior to dispensing it.
- Undertake the thorough checking procedure as described on pages 137 and 138.
- With clean hands, select the preparation, check the expiry date and dispense the correct dose of the drug:
  - tablets and capsules: tip the required number into the bottle cap, then into a medicine cup; if in foil packaging, check the strip, then push the tablets through the foil into the cup (both methods avoid handling the medication)
  - elixir: invert the bottle several times, hold the bottle with the label to the rear (to avoid obscuring the label with spilt medicine), hold the medicine cup at eye level and pour the liquid into it, ensuring the fluid is accurately on the line. Alternatively insert an oral syringe into the bung, invert the bottle and draw the correct number of millilitres into the syringe, also at eye level.
- Approach the woman by name and confirm her identity.
- Advise the woman on how to take the medication, providing a glass of water if necessary and observe her swallowing the drug (for sublingual preparations, the medication should be placed beneath the tongue; other directions to suck, chew, etc. should be given as indicated).
- Document administration in agreed places.
- Observe for the effects of the medication and take any necessary action.

Precautions

- If the woman is unable to take the medication at the time of administration, it is recorded and the late administration checked before being given. A drug dispensed but not administered should be disposed of safely, rather than left in anticipation or returned to the bottle.
- Compliance is increased if the woman understands the reason for the medication, likely effects and possible side effects. Refusal to take a drug should be recorded, with the reason and the prescribing medical officer informed.
- If the woman vomits soon after administration and only if the tablet is clearly visible, a further stat. dose may be prescribed.
- Controlled drugs may also be prescribed in an oral form; administration should be according to local policy. Tablets are counted; elixir should be measured very carefully using a medicine syringe.

Oral administration to a baby

The baby needs to be awake and able to swallow. The parents should be taught the procedure if they are going to need to repeat it themselves. The prescription is scrutinized as per all prescriptions (see Chapter 18) and local protocols are adhered to. An oral medicine syringe is used (described above).

Patience is needed when administering medication to babies and children; it can be difficult to assess how much the baby has taken if some is seen to dribble down the chin. If this occurs consultation with the paediatrician is necessary regarding the necessity of a further dose.

PROCEDURE: oral administration to a baby

* Wash hands and undertake the thorough checking process described in Chapter 18.
* Confirm the identity of the baby, and where appropriate gain parental consent.
* Draw up the drug accurately in a sterile syringe, see above.
* Place the syringe into the baby's mouth towards the cheek, squeeze a small amount (0.5–1 mL maximum) into the mouth and observe the baby swallowing.
* Administer the next part of the dose, observe the swallow and continue in this way until the drug is fully administered.
* Dispose of syringe into clinical waste, wash hands.
* Document administration.
* If appropriate, observe for the effects of the medication and take any necessary action.

ROLE AND RESPONSIBILITIES OF THE MIDWIFE

These can be summarised as:
* practising within the NMC (2008) guidelines for the safe and effective administration of medicines
* ensuring the drug is dispensed and taken correctly by the woman or baby
* observing the effects and side effects of the drug administered
* education of the woman to aid compliance and effectiveness
* correct record keeping.

Summary

* Oral drug administration involves thorough checking in all parts of the process, as for any other drug administration (see Chapter 18 for details).
* Oral medication may come in different forms; while the majority of oral preparations are swallowed, some are for sucking, chewing, buccal or sublingual use.
* Babies have oral drugs administered in liquid form via a medication syringe where possible.

SELF-ASSESSMENT EXERCISES

The answers to the following questions may be found in the text:

1. Give an example of each of the different types of preparation available for oral administration.
2. What would the midwife do if the drug was dispensed but the woman was not available to take it?
3. Describe how a midwife would administer a sublingual drug to a woman.
4. Describe how drugs are administered orally to a baby.
5. What would the midwife do if the woman vomited her medication shortly after taking it?

Reference

NMC (Nursing & Midwifery Council):
    Standards Medicine Management,
    London, 2008, NMC.

Principles of drug administration: injection technique

20

CHAPTER CONTENTS

Preparations are administered via an injection if they cannot be absorbed, or are absorbed too slowly, when given via other routes. In this chapter the safe administration of drugs via intramuscular (I.M.), subcutaneous (S.C.) and intradermal (I.D.) injection will be reviewed. Intravenous injection is reviewed in Chapter 23. Suitable injection sites in the adult and baby are highlighted and there is discussion about appropriate equipment to use. It is important that this chapter is read in conjunction with Chapter 18.

LEARNING OUTCOMES

Having read this chapter the reader should be able to:

- list the situations in which a midwife is likely to administer medication by injection
- describe, with a rationale for choice, the suitable sites for I.M., S.C. and I.D. injections in the adult and I.M. in the baby
- demonstrate an injection, giving a rationale for each stage
- summarise the role and responsibilities of the midwife.

Indications

The midwife administers drugs by injection on a number of occasions; the following is an indicative, but not exhaustive list:

- oxytocic agent (active third stage of labour or postpartum haemorrhage)
- analgesia or antidote, e.g. pethidine, morphine
- anti-D immunoglobulin
- rubella vaccine
- vitamin K (babies)
- subcutaneous heparin (thromboembolic prophylaxis)
- iron therapy (Z technique indicated)
- steroids (fetal lung maturity in preterm labour)
- intradermal local anaesthetics.

As for all medications, the midwife should be competent to diagnose and manage any unforeseen emergencies, e.g. anaphylaxis or cardiac arrest. Medication given via an injectable route cannot be withdrawn.

Safety

Giving an injection exposes midwives to potential needlestick injury and contact with blood. Used needles must *never* be resheathed, sharps must be disposed of immediately and correctly into a sharps box. A variety of safety devices are becoming increasingly available to reduce the dangers of percutaneous injury; the reader is encouraged to be aware of their availability and use. Disposable gloves are indicated to protect the midwife from potential contact with blood.

Intramuscular injection

Choice of site in the adult

As suggested, intramuscular (I.M.) injection is into muscle. This is considered to be less painful (due to the nature of the pain sensing nerve fibres) than injecting into subcutaneous tissue; deeper muscles can also accommodate irritant substances that subcutaneous tissue can't. A good blood supply ensures that the drug is absorbed quickly and the effects are maximised. Choice of site is important. It may depend on:

- the number of millilitres to be injected
- the nature of the drug
- the mobility of the woman
- the anatomical relation of other structures (nerves, bones, blood vessels)
- the skin and general condition of the woman (presence/absence of fat and subcutaneous tissue, good muscle presence, adequate circulation, any signs of bruising, infection, swelling, inflammation, abscess, frequent or over use of the site)
- the manufacturer's guidelines.

Recommended sites (adults)

There are five recommended sites for I.M. injection (Workman 1999). However, despite Rodger & King's recommendations (based on a literature search of all available evidence) in 2000 to use the ventrogluteal site for preference, it is still rarely seen in UK practice. The five sites are:

1. Deltoid muscle of upper arm (maximum 1 mL) (Fig. 20.1A): the site is approximately 2.5 cm below the acromial process on the lateral surface of the arm. Often the choice of site for vaccinations.

2. Quadriceps muscle (vastus lateralis, maximum 5 mL): this is found by measuring a hand's breadth down from the greater trochanter, and one up from the knee. The remaining middle third of the lateral aspect of the thigh is the correct muscle (Fig. 20.1B).

3. The rectus femoris is adjacent on the anterior aspect of the thigh; it is used less often and is not appropriate in children (Fig. 20.1B).

4. Gluteus maximus muscle (maximum 5 mL): found on the upper outer quadrant of the buttock (Fig. 20.1C). Despite being a popular site injury to the sciatic nerve is a real possibility unless great care is taken with the technique. Dougherty et al (2008) point out that without correct assessment of the muscle position and an appropriately long needle, many medications are placed into gluteal fat. Zaybak et al (2007) agree, suggesting that the deltoid, rectus femoris or vastus lateralis should all be considered as sites of preference for an obese woman, there being less fat and subcutaneous tissue on these sites than on the buttocks.

5. Ventrogluteal site (maximum 2.5 mL): the palm of the midwife's right hand is placed on the greater trochanter of the woman's left hip (or vice versa). The index finger is extended to touch the anterior superior iliac crest while the middle finger stretches as far along the iliac crest as possible. The site is in the 'V' between the index and middle fingers (Fig. 20.1D).

The muscle should be relaxed for minimal discomfort, the site may be supported by the non-injecting hand and some commentators recommend a slight stretching of the skin prior to needle insertion (Hunter 2008). 'Bunching up' the muscle in a thin woman may sometimes be necessary (Workman 1999).

Z-track technique

A Z-track technique (Fig. 20.2) ensures the solution does not leak back to the skin and so irritate the subcutaneous tissue or stain the skin. The skin and subcutaneous tissue are moved sideways or downwards

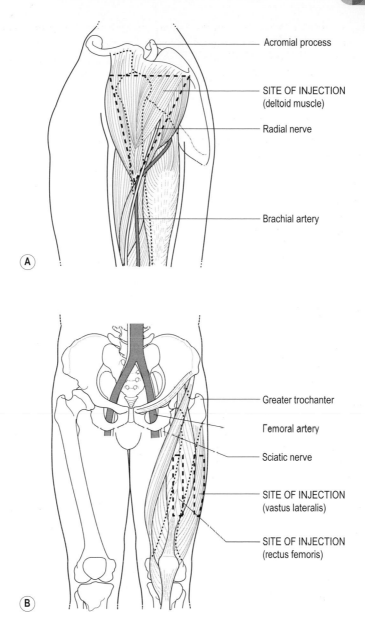

Acromial process

SITE OF INJECTION
(deltoid muscle)

Radial nerve

Brachial artery

Greater trochanter

Femoral artery

Sciatic nerve

SITE OF INJECTION
(vastus lateralis)

SITE OF INJECTION
(rectus femoris)

Figure 20.1 • Sites for adult intramuscular injection. A Deltoid muscle. B Rectus femoris and vastus lateralis (vastus lateralis is the one suitable site for I.M. injection in neonates also).

continued

2–3 cm, the needle is inserted into the original site chosen, the solution is injected and after 10 seconds the needle is removed. The skin is then released (Workman 1999). There are advocates in the literature of Z track being the technique of choice for all I.M. injections (Rodger & King 2000). The reader will need to consult their local protocol.

Choice of equipment

In an average sized woman a 21-g (green) needle is used at a 90° angle (Fig. 20.3). This assessment is individualised, and the needle chosen should reach the muscle with approximately 1 cm of it still visible externally. The needle and syringe should be

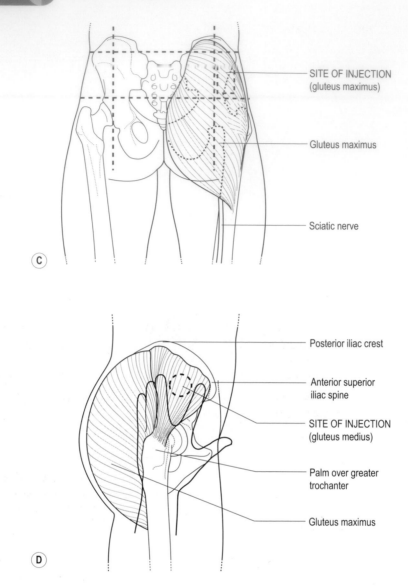

SITE OF INJECTION
(gluteus maximus)

Gluteus maximus

Sciatic nerve

(C)

Posterior iliac crest

Anterior superior
iliac spine

SITE OF INJECTION
(gluteus medius)

Palm over greater
trochanter

Gluteus maximus

(D)

Figure 20.1—cont'd C Gluteus maximus. D Ventrogluteal (Adapted with kind permission from Jamieson et al 1997)
D Ventrogluteal

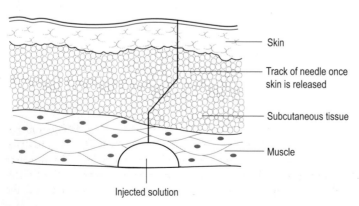

Skin

Track of needle once
skin is released

Subcutaneous tissue

Muscle

Injected solution

Figure 20.2 • Z-track injection. The skin and subcutaneous tissue are moved downwards or sideways for 2–3 cm prior to insertion of the needle and then released once the needle has been removed. The solution is prevented from back tracking to the skin

Figure 20.3 • Intramuscular, subcutaneous and intradermal injections

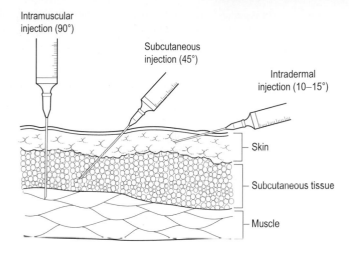

sterile, the syringe being an appropriate size for the amount of fluid to be injected.

It would appear that skin cleansing is not required for I.M. or S.C. injections (Cocoman & Murray 2007) but only if the woman's general hygiene is good. If an alcohol swab is used, it should be used for 30 seconds and the area must be left at least 30 seconds to air dry before injecting. Post-injection, a cotton wool ball or gauze swab is used to cover the puncture site and a plaster applied if necessary.

Ampoules and vials

Ampoules may be glass or, increasingly, plastic, with a top that 'snaps off'. Vials tend to be glass with a rubber bung beneath the metal top. This needs cleaning with an alcohol impregnated wipe before use to reduce the cross infection risk. Ampoules and vials may be completely inverted (without leaking) so that the substance can be removed completely and the scale on the syringe read correctly. Preparations may come as solutions or powder for reconstitution. In the event of needing to reconstitute a drug (e.g. diamorphine) a dilutant, e.g. sterile water, will be required. It is recommended that a new needle is used for the injection, the one used for preparation may have been blunted or be contaminated by glass shards.

Intramuscular injection for a baby

There is one main site for I.M. injection in the baby: quadriceps muscle (vastus lateralis), lateral mid-third of the thigh (see Fig. 20.1B). The deltoid muscle may be used for vaccinations only.

Other sites (e.g. gluteus maximus and ventrogluteal) may be used in older babies, but Hemsworth (2000) suggests that muscular development in these sites is insufficient in neonates. The maximum dose that can be injected is 1 mL. The baby should be in a safe place (e.g. held or in a cot). A 25-g (orange) or 23-g (blue) needle is inserted at a 90° angle (Anonymous 2007).

Subcutaneous injection

A subcutaneous (S.C.) injection places the medication into the connective tissue and fat beneath the skin. These tissues have a reduced blood supply in comparison to muscle, so drug absorption is slow and steady. Common preparations for S.C. use include insulin and heparin. As a single injection only 1–2 mL can be accommodated, but S.C. infusions can also be established and can add up to 3 L of fluid into the circulation over 24 hours.

Generally, a 25-g (orange) needle is used at an angle of 45° (see Fig. 20.3) but studies show that S.C. injections can be inadvertently placed into muscle and so it is necessary to grasp the skin and lift the subcutaneous tissue away from the muscle before injecting (Peragallo-Dittko 1997, Workman 1999). The actual angle chosen will be dependent upon the amount of subcutaneous tissue available. Where the medication is prepacked with a shorter needle (1.2 cm or less; Hayes 1998), a 90° angle is used. Heparin is an example of this: one of the manufacturers suggests that absorption is greater if administered into the abdominal subcutaneous tissue at 90°. Rubbing the site afterwards may cause bruising. A prepacked preparation may also have an air bubble incorporated into the syringe, this air is not to be excluded from the syringe but is the mechanism by which all the medication is delivered. It is also unnecessary to aspirate the plunger back when injecting subcutaneously, it is highly unlikely to be in a vein. S.C. injections are more comfortable for the woman if delivered slowly.

The preferred sites for an adult are:

- outer surface of the upper arm
- lateral upper third of the thigh
- umbilical region of the abdomen
- on the back, beneath the scapulae, either side of the spine.

The site should be examined prior to injection for inflammation, infection, scarring or hardness, which may all indicate poor absorption and increase the level of pain. For repeated injections, the site is rotated. Safety, skin preparation and sterility issues apply as discussed above.

Intradermal injection

A small amount of solution (up to 0.5 mL) is injected locally into the skin using a 25-g (orange) needle at a 10–15° angle (Workman 1999) (see Fig. 20.3). The bevel of the needle is inserted upwards so that a small weal forms and is seen on the skin. The same sites as S.C. injection may be used, but frequently midwives inject intradermally prior to cannulation (see Chapter 47) and therefore inject over the site of the vein to be cannulated. Local anaesthetic is also injected intradermally when infiltrating for perineal repair (see Chapter 34).

PROCEDURE: I.M. and S.C. injections in the adult

- Undertake the thorough checking procedures as for any medication administration (see Chapter 18).
- Gain informed consent and wash hands.
- Gather equipment:
  - two sterile needles and one sterile syringe (correct sizes, in date, undamaged and confirmed to be sterile)
  - portable sharps box
  - disposable tray
  - non-sterile gloves
  - cotton wool or gauze
  - ampoule (already checked thoroughly)
  - medicine administration chart.
- Assemble the needle and syringe by placing them firmly together, protecting their sterility by not touching the needle or syringe hub.
- Loosen the protective sheath over the needle and draw back on the plunger to prepare the syringe.
- Ensure all of the solution is in the ampoule (not retained in the top); snap off the top (protect the fingers with a tissue if a glass ampoule).
- Draw up the required amount of solution, inverting the ampoule if necessary.
- Replace the sheath on the needle: insert it back into the sheath (in the tray) using only one hand and without it touching anything else.
- Invert the syringe and examine it for air. If necessary tap it gently to encourage the air up to the top of the syringe; push the plunger to exclude the air from the syringe and needle, ensuring none of the solution is lost and the dosage in the syringe is correct.
- Replace the needle; discard the old one directly into the sharps box. Take the medicine administration chart, sharps box and tray to the woman.
- Confirm her identity, ensure privacy and expose the injection site.
- Apply gloves.
- For S.C. injection: identify the site, grasp a fold of skin with the non-injecting hand, decisively inject at the correct angle (see above), release the grasp, administer the injection slowly, remove the needle quickly and apply gentle pressure with cotton wool or gauze.
- For I.M. injection: identify the specific site for puncture ensuring the muscle is relaxed. Consider whether a Z-track technique is needed (see above). If not, support the area with the non-injecting hand, then decisively inject at a 90° angle, inserting the needle with approximately 1 cm still visible. Draw back on the plunger (wait for at least 5 seconds to ensure that a vein has not been entered); if 'nothing' is seen, push on the plunger smoothly at a rate of 10 seconds per millilitre to inject the solution. This makes the injection more

comfortable and allows the muscle fibres to expand and absorb the medication. Wait 10 seconds. This allows the medication to diffuse, then remove the needle smoothly. Press gently on the puncture site with the gauze or cotton wool; avoid massage which may cause irritation.

- For all injections: place the syringe and needle directly into the sharps box without resheathing the needle.
- Assist the woman to a comfortable position, remove gloves and wash hands.
- Dispose of equipment correctly.
- Document administration and act accordingly; examine the site 2 hours later for any possible reactions.

Precautions

If blood is seen in the syringe when drawing the plunger back, the needle has punctured a blood vessel and the injection would be intravenous, not intramuscular. The needle and syringe should be withdrawn and discarded. A second injection is prepared and administered.

ROLE AND RESPONSIBILITIES OF THE MIDWIFE

These can be summarised as:

- correct use of equipment and choice of site to facilitate a correct injection technique
- knowledge and application of evidence based best practice
- support of the woman, particularly if anxious
- correct disposal of sharps
- correct record keeping.

Summary

- Injecting into muscle requires selective use of site and equipment to ensure that the technique chosen is correct, particularly if the woman is clinically obese.
- The midwife needs to complete the injection decisively, but ensuring that a vein has not been punctured.
- Subcutaneous injections inject the medication into the tissue beneath the skin and so use a shorter needle and a smaller angle.
- Intradermal injections inject a small amount of solution just beneath the skin.
- Used needles should not be resheathed and sharps should be disposed of correctly at the point of use.

SELF-ASSESSMENT EXERCISES

The answers to the following questions may be found in the text:

1. Cite examples of when injections may be necessary for a childbearing woman.
2. List the sites suitable for intramuscular injection for both the woman and the baby.
3. What would the midwife do if blood appeared in the syringe while drawing back?
4. Demonstrate an I.M. injection for a baby.
5. Compare and contrast the similarities and differences between an I.M. and a S.C. injection in the adult, in relation to the equipment, technique and site.
6. Describe how a Z-track injection is completed.
7. Summarise the role and responsibilities of the midwife when administering an injection.

References

Anonymous: Intramuscular injection technique, *Paediatr Nurs* 19(2):37, 2007.

Cocoman A, Murray J: To swab or not to swab, *World Ir Nurs* 15(8):26–27, 2007.

Dougherty L, Farley A, Hopwood L, Sarpal N: Drug Administration: general principles. In Dougherty L, Lister S, editors: *The Royal Marsden Hospital Manual of Clinical Nursing Procedures*, ed 7, Oxford, 2008, Blackwell Publishing, ch. 8.

Hayes C: Injection technique: subcutaneous, *Nurs Times* 94(41):85–86, 1998.

Hemsworth S: Intramuscular injection technique, *Paediatr Nurs* 12(9):17–20, 2000.

Hunter J: Intramuscular injection techniques, *Nurs Stand* 22(24):35–40, 2008.

Jamieson EM, McCall JM, Blythe R, et al: *Clinical nursing practices*, ed 3, Edinburgh, 1997, Churchill Livingstone.

Peragallo Dittko V: Rethinking subcutaneous injection technique, *Am J Nurs* 97(5):71–72, 1997.

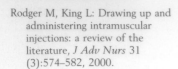

Rodger M, King L: Drawing up and administering intramuscular injections: a review of the literature, *J Adv Nurs* 31 (3):574–582, 2000.

Workman B: Safe injection techniques, *Nurs Stand* 13(39):47–53, 1999.

Zaybak A, Yapucu U, Tamsel S, et al: Does obesity prevent the needle from reaching muscle in intramuscular injections?*J Adv Nurs* 58(6):552–556, 2007.

Principles of drug administration: administration of medicines *per vaginam*

21

The midwife is actively involved in the administration of medicines *per vaginam* (P.V.), largely with prostaglandin for the induction of labour. Placing a drug into the vagina is a means of ensuring that the action of the drug can work directly (locally) to produce the desired effect. Other drugs may also be administered P.V. (e.g. antifungal preparations). This chapter considers the midwife's role and responsibilities and the procedure for administration P.V., focusing largely on the administration of prostaglandin E_2 (PGE_2).

LEARNING OUTCOMES

Having read this chapter the reader should be able to:

- describe how a drug is administered P.V.
- discuss the role and responsibilities of the midwife before, during and after administration
- list the factors that are pertinent to the administration of prostaglandin P.V.

Per vaginam administration

This is generally an embarrassing route for medication administration. Care should be taken that informed consent has been granted and that efforts are made to protect dignity and privacy. Some P.V. medications could often be administered by the woman herself. If the need arose, it is sometimes possible to remove a vaginal tablet or pessary but this is an unreliable action and so should not be factored in as a possibility. The midwife should maintain asepsis, particularly if the membranes have ruptured, and use personal protective equipment as indicated.

Using prostaglandin

In its *Induction of Labour* (IOL) guideline, the National Institute for Health and Clinical Excellence (NICE 2008) is clear about the following points:

- Care should be woman-centred with the woman able to make an informed decision, being particularly aware of the risk of uterine hyperstimulation.
- The wellbeing of the fetus should be confirmed prior to PGE_2 administration.
- The venue and timing of the administration should permit electronic fetal assessment. The morning is often the best time. If prostaglandin is given as an outpatient, instruction *must* accompany the woman as to the need to when to contact the maternity services: after 6 hours if no

signs of labour or earlier if contractions begin. The Bishop's score should be reassessed 6 hours after the PGE$_2$ administration.

- PGE$_2$ tablets or gel should be prescribed. A second dose may be given after 6 hours if labour has not commenced. A controlled release pessary (1 in 24 hours) may be an alternative prescription. The correct place to administer the tablet, gel or pessary is into the posterior vaginal fornix. The woman should remain in a supine position for at least 30 minutes following the administration. The prescription is determined according to the presence or otherwise of intact membranes and the favourability of the cervix (determined by Bishop's scoring).

- A continuous cardiotocogram (CTG; see Chapter 1) should be commenced once contractions have been reported or detected. This may be discontinued once fetal wellbeing is confirmed. Intermittent monitoring is then permitted for healthy women with no other pregnancy complications.

PROCEDURE: administration of medicines P.V.

- Gain informed consent and ensure privacy.
- Wash hands.
- Gather equipment:
  - ○ sterile gloves and hand rub
  - ○ disposable sheet
  - ○ sterile single use lubricant, e.g. KY Jelly®
  - ○ disposable wipes
  - ○ the drug and medicine administration chart.
- Ask the woman to adopt an almost recumbent position (use a wedge to avoid aortocaval occlusion if necessary), with her knees bent, ankles together and knees parted, placing a disposable sheet beneath her buttocks.
- Remove any sanitary towels or underwear, keeping the genital area covered.
- Open the gloves, open the pessary, place it and a blob of the lubricant onto the sterile side of the paper (a sterile vaginal examination pack may be used).
- Apply hand rub and then gloves.
- Ask the woman to remove the covers.

- For PGE$_2$ administration, part the labia with the thumb and forefinger of the non-examining hand:
  - ○ lubricate the two fingers of the examining hand and gently insert into the vagina, in a downwards and backwards direction along the anterior vaginal wall to locate the cervix, ensuring the thumb does not come into contact with the woman's clitoris or anus. Slide the gel applicator between the vaginal wall and the examining hand, until it has been guided into the posterior vaginal fornix by the examining hand. The plunger is then depressed by the other hand and the gel administered. Lubricant may be applied to the tip to aid insertion
  - ○ for the application of a tablet or pessary, either insert the examining hand with the pessary secured between the fingers, guiding it into the fornix as above, or insert the examining hand into the vagina, slide the pessary in using the non-examining hand, and guide it into place using the examining hand. Lubricant may be applied to the pessary to aid insertion.
- Remove fingers, wipe the vulva with the wipes.
- For administration of a pessary with its own applicator, part the labia with the thumb and forefinger of the non-examining hand (a vaginal examination is unnecessary if the positioning of the pessary is not crucial, i.e. antifungal preparations):
  - ○ slide the applicator along the posterior vaginal wall until the pessary is high in the vagina
  - ○ depress the plunger and withdraw the applicator.
- Remove gloves, use hand rub and assist the woman to resume a comfortable semi-recumbent position.
- Dispose of equipment correctly and wash hands.
- Document administration and findings and act accordingly.

ROLE AND RESPONSIBILITIES OF THE MIDWIFE

These can be summarised as:

- assessment prior to administration: the midwife must be familiar with the local protocols for the administration of PGE$_2$, most of which are discussed above
- appropriate checking and dispensing of the drug (as for any prescription): the lubricant used with vaginal

drugs should be appropriate (e.g. KY Jelly®), and sterile for single use. Interaction can occur with some preparations, e.g. obstetric cream and PGE$_2$

- understanding the action and side effects of the drug, and therefore education and support of the woman to prepare her for the effect: as well as hyperstimulation of the uterus, PGE$_2$ can cause fetal distress and uncomfortable uterine contractions. It may also take time for induction of labour to occur, something that the woman and her family need to appreciate. Antifungal preparations may be self-administered, for which the midwife can have a significant role in educating the woman in infection prevention and drug administration

- maintenance of dignity and privacy during an embarrassing procedure: survivors of sexual abuse will find the administration of medicine P.V. a traumatic experience. The midwife is well placed to recognise some of the signs and to obtain appropriate help for the woman

- observations made while undertaking the drug administration: e.g. repeated Bishop's scoring, angle of pubic arch, nature of presenting part, other factors that may affect care

- correct administration technique, placing the medication in the correct place: the preparations for vaginal drugs vary, e.g. tablet, pessary (with or without applicator) or gel (similar to a syringe in appearance). The midwife must be competent with vaginal examination before administering PGE$_2$ P.V., as it does need to be placed accurately

- appreciation of care following administration: in all instances the woman will need to adopt a semi-recumbent position following administration, so that the medicine does not dislodge. Assessment of the fetus must be undertaken if the labour is being induced. Antifungal preparations are often

administered last thing at night. Observations are made both for the expected action and to exclude deviations from the norm

- adherence to national and local protocols with regard to infection control, personal protection, the administration of medicines and aspects of maternity care. NICE (2008) are clear that much of the research around IOL is limited and so will evolve in the near future

- contemporaneous record keeping of the care given before, during and after the administration.

Summary

- Medicines administered P.V. act locally, but the procedure can be embarrassing for the woman.
- The midwife should ensure that PGE$_2$ is administered correctly, following the local protocol.
- A semi-recumbent position should be adopted following the procedure.

SELF-ASSESSMENT EXERCISES

The answers to the following questions may be found in the text:

1. Describe how the midwife prepares the woman for administration of a P.V. medication.
2. Describe how a drug is administered P.V.
3. Discuss the role and responsibilities of the midwife after the administration of a medicine P.V.
4. List the specific considerations when administering PGE$_2$ P.V.

Reference

NICE (National Institute for Health and Clinical Excellence): *Induction of labour,* London, 2008, RCOG Press.

Principles of drug administration: administration of medicines per rectum

22

Medicines inserted into the rectum have two predominant actions:

1. for laxative purposes
2. systemic treatment (sometimes called retention suppositories), e.g. analgesia, antiemetic.

The rectum has a good blood supply and drugs can be absorbed quickly. It is a useful route for the administration of some medicines if the woman is nil by mouth, unconscious or vomiting. This chapter reviews the correct procedure and discusses the role and responsibilities of the midwife.

LEARNING OUTCOMES

Having read this chapter the reader should be able to:

• describe the safe administration of suppositories and enemas, making differentiations accordingly

• discuss the role and responsibilities of the midwife in relation to per rectum (P.R.) administration.

Suppositories

The medication is contained within the pellet that dissolves in the rectum. Suppositories for laxative use vary in their action; widely used glycerin suppositories are designed to melt in the faeces and so soften them. Other types of suppository (e.g. bisacodyl, a stimulant laxative) need to be placed between the faeces and rectal wall. The instructions should be checked prior to administration. Suppositories for systemic use are often firm in texture. Their absorption is enhanced if the rectum is empty and the suppository is placed against the rectal wall.

Which way are they inserted?

The shaping of suppositories has traditionally suggested to practitioners that they should be inserted tapered end first. There is, however, a debate about this. Abd-el-Maeboud et al (1991) considered the anatomy and physiology of the rectum and believed that inserting a suppository blunt end first would facilitate its retention better than if inserted tapered end first. This caused a change in practice (Moppett 2000), but Kyle (2009) has questioned this change. Kyle (2009) considers that Abd-el-Maeboud's trial had a dubious methodology; it particularly failed to differentiate between systemic and laxative suppositories. Abd-el-Maeboud et al (1991) suggest that if inserted blunt end first the anatomy of the rectum 'sucks' the suppository in as the sphincter closes. This means that it is not necessary to insert the administering finger further than pushing the suppository in. Kyle (2009) points out that the necessity for some laxative suppositories to sit against the rectum wall means that it is necessary to insert them 2–4 cm into the rectum. Abd-el-Maeboud et al (1991) believe that inserting a suppository tapered end first prevents the anal sphincter from closing properly. The manufacturers continue to suggest that tapered end first is correct in line with their product licence (Bradshaw & Price 2007). Johnson & Taylor (2000 & 2005) supported the idea that suppositories for systemic use should be inserted blunt end first while laxative ones should be inserted tapered end first. As Kyle (2009) suggests, if this issue is of considerable significance then further rigorous research is needed promptly. The reader should be aware of the devolving argument, any future studies and their locally agreed protocol.

Enemas

Enemas for systemic use are often small (microenemas), whereas laxative ones generally contain more fluid. Both have a nozzle that extends into the sigmoid colon (beyond the rectum), often about 10 cm in length. If a large fluid enema is to be used it should be warmed (40.5–43.3°C) to prevent shock.

General principles

The prescription is scrutinized as for any other administration of medicines. The woman needs to have given informed consent and if the medications are being used for laxative purposes she will need to know what to expect in advance. Both suppositories and enemas require lubrication (e.g. KY Jelly®) on the inserting end so that anal trauma is reduced. Care is always taken not to stimulate the vagus nerve, which may cause bradycardia. The midwife wears non-sterile gloves; an apron is only necessary later if needing to assist with defecation.

Positioning of the woman

It is easier to insert laxative suppositories and all types of enemas if the woman adopts a left lateral position with one or both of her knees flexed (Fig. 22.1).

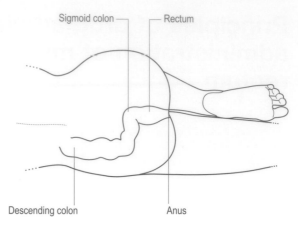

Figure 22.1 • Correct positioning for insertion of P.R. medication (Adapted with kind permission from Jamieson et al 2002)

Insertion then follows the natural anatomy of the colon, flexed knees reduce the discomfort of the anus as the suppository is passed through the sphincter. However, because of the action of only pushing it through the sphincter, the insertion of a blunt end first systemic suppository can be administered in any position, for example while the woman is still in lithotomy after something such as perineal repair.

PROCEDURE: administration of medicines per rectum

- Gain informed consent and ensure privacy. Wash hands. (If the medication is for systemic use the woman should be encouraged to open her bowels before its administration.)
- Gather equipment:
  ○ suppository(ies) or (warmed) enema
  ○ disposable gloves and alcohol hand rub
  ○ disposable sheet
  ○ compatible lubricant, usually KY Jelly®
  ○ gauze swabs
  ○ a trolley or tray with which to work from.
- After removing underwear, the woman is asked to lie in a left lateral position with one or both of her knees flexed. Place the disposable sheet beneath her buttocks.
- Apply hand rub and put on gloves.
- Laxative suppository: lubricate the tapered end, systemic suppository(ies): lubricate the blunt end, enema tubing: the tip, from lubricant on the

gauze swab. Expel the air from the enema tubing by pushing the solution through to the tip.

- Ask the woman to take a deep breath (this relaxes the anal sphincter).
- Lift the woman's right buttock with the non-dominant hand:
  - laxative suppository: insert the suppository tapered end first, 2-4 cm into the rectum using the right index finger. Position according to the manufacturer's instructions (see above). Insert a second suppository in the same way if required
  - systemic suppository: gently push the blunt end first through the anal sphincter. The finger does not need to enter the rectum.
- Insert the enema tubing, advancing it slowly 10–12 cm to ensure that it is in the sigmoid colon. The fluid is gradually squeezed in by rolling up the pack. Withdraw the tubing carefully once completed, maintaining pressure on the pack to prevent the fluid flowing back into it.
- Wipe the perineum with the gauze, remove gloves, apply hand rub and assist the woman into a comfortable position. Wash hands.
- Encourage her to retain the medication for as long as possible. Aim for laxatives to be retained for at least 10–20 minutes.
- Assist later, if needed, to the toilet.
- Dispose of equipment correctly and wash hands.
- Document administration and effect and act accordingly.

ROLE AND RESPONSIBILITIES OF THE MIDWIFE

These can be summarised as:

- appropriate checking and dispensing of the drug (as for any prescription)
- understanding the action and possible side effects of the drug: the effect/side effect should always be reported and recorded. If given for laxative purposes the quantity, colour and consistency of the faeces should be recorded according to the Bristol stool classifications (p 132)
- education and support of the woman: she may associate P.R. drugs specifically with laxatives, not appreciating that systemic suppositories have no laxative effect. The effect of all P.R. medications will be enhanced if the drug is retained by the woman for the required length of time, often around 20 minutes
- maintenance of dignity and privacy during an embarrassing procedure
- correct administration technique, placing the medication in the correct place, upholding the infection control and personal protective equipment protocols
- appreciation of care following administration: toilet facilities should be readily available following administration of medicine P.R. for laxative purposes
- contemporaneous record keeping of the care given before, during and after the administration.

Summary

- Administration of medicines P.R. may be for laxative or systemic purposes. The debate continues as to which end of the suppository should be inserted first.
- The midwife should be familiar with the effect of the drug and how to administer it correctly.

SELF-ASSESSMENT EXERCISES

The answers to the following questions may be found in the text:

1. Describe how a laxative enema is administered.
2. Discuss the responsibilities of the midwife when administering a systemic suppository.
3. Discuss why the woman is positioned in a left lateral position.

References

Abd-el-Maeboud KH, El-Naggar T, El-Hawi E, et al: Rectal suppository: commonsense and the mode of insertion, *The Lancet* 338 (8770):798–800, 1991.

Bradshaw A, Price L: Rectal suppository insertion: the reliability of the evidence as a basis for nursing practice, *J Clin Nurs* 16(1):98–103, 2007.

Jamieson EM, McCall J, Whyte L: *Clinical nursing practices*, ed 4, Edinburgh, 2002, Churchill Livingstone.

Johnson R, Taylor W: *Skills for midwifery practice*, 2005, ed 2, Edinburgh, 2000, Churchill Livingstone.

Kyle G: Practice questions, *Nurs Times* 105(2):16, 2009.

Moppett S: Which way is up for a suppository? *Nurs Times* 96(19): NT Plus Supplement, 12–13, 2000.

Principles of drug administration: intravenous drug administration

23

CHAPTER CONTENTS

The midwife should be trained properly to administer drugs intravenously (I.V.), recognising that in some areas it is an extended role. Updating is often required (according to local protocol) to maintain competence. Antibiotics are the most common drugs administered I.V., but many preparations can be administered in this way. This chapter considers the administration of medicines intravenously, as bolus or 'push' administration, or intermittent infusion, concluding with continuous administration of drugs using a syringe driver and patient-controlled analgesia. Maximum understanding will be gained from this chapter if it is read in conjunction with Chapters 18, 47 and 48.

LEARNING OUTCOMES

Having read this chapter the reader should be able to:

- describe each of the different ways that drugs can be administered intravenously

- discuss the role and responsibilities of the midwife when undertaking intravenous drug administration
- calculate the infusion rate when using a syringe driver.

Drugs given intravenously act quickly: an advantage if a rapid response is required; a disadvantage if allergy occurs. The potential for medication errors, especially drug incompatibility, should be considered particularly when multiple drug infusions are required at the same time and drugs are mixed (Nemec et al 2008). This includes bacterial or particulate contamination as well as physicochemical incompatibilities of intravenous solutions, and steps should be taken to reduce the risk of these occurring (Bertsche et al 2008). Cousins et al (2005) found that errors with drug administration centred around four areas: (1) unlabelled prepared drugs that were left for short periods were being administered to the wrong patient; (2) using the wrong diluent to prepare the drug, resulting in the powder not dissolving properly or being inactivated; (3) bolus drug administration being undertaken too quickly, which can cause phlebitis; and (4) loss of cannula patency and inadherence to aseptic procedures.

As for the administration of all medicines, the woman's details are thoroughly checked, as are the medicine administration chart and drug (and diluent if required) to be administered. Note that the use of medical devices, particularly syringe drivers, features highly in the reported work of the Medicines and Healthcare Products Regulatory Agency (MHRA). It is essential that midwives have a thorough working knowledge of the equipment that they use and its correct maintenance (Murray & Glenister 2001).

The cannulation site should always be checked for patency prior to the administration of intravenous drugs. Signs of infiltration (and, if indicated, extravasation) should be looked for (see Chapter 47) and if present the cannula will require re-siting. Infiltration occurs when the cannula is no longer in the vein or only the tip remains and any drugs injected will therefore infiltrate the surrounding subcutaneous tissues (Dougherty 2008). The site should be flushed with 2–5 mL of normal saline before and after the administration of drugs; if more than one drug is given, the cannula should be flushed between drugs to avoid drug incompatibilities (RCN 2007).

The procedure follows the principles of asepsis as the risk of introducing microorganisms directly into the circulation is real (see Chapter 10). The midwife must also protect her hands from contact with the drug constituents, thus gloves should be worn whilst drawing up and administering the drug. These do not need to be sterile (unless the situation requires this), but should be well fitting and the midwife should use a non-touch technique.

Bolus administration

A bolus administration of a drug produces a high drug concentration without fluid overload but the high concentration can also cause a chemical phlebitis (Scales 2008).

PROCEDURE: bolus or 'push' administration

- A patent cannula should be available with an injection port.
- Gather equipment:
  - the drug, including correct solution (often water for injection) if it is to be diluted, and the woman's medicine administration chart
  - appropriately sized sterile syringe and needles
  - hand rub
  - non-sterile gloves
  - 10 mL sodium chloride 0.9%, needle and syringe for flushing (or locally approved flushing solution)
  - clean injection tray

  - 70% alcohol-impregnated swab
  - disposable sheet
  - portable sharps bin
- Wash hands and put on non-sterile gloves.
- Prepare and draw up the drug according to the manufacturer's instructions, with a second midwife checking the dosages and expiry dates.
- Gently resheath the needle using a non-touch technique and place the prepared syringe on the tray, retaining the ampoule (if not using a needle free port the needle should be changed).
- Draw up the normal saline (if unable to differentiate between the syringes, place on a separate tray and label).
- Confirm the woman's identity then place her arm on the disposable sheet.
- Inspect the cannulation site and, if present, check the infusion for its smooth running.
- Stop the infusion.
- Clean the portal for the I.V. drugs with the alcohol-impregnated swab and allow to dry.
- Flush the cannula using half of the normal saline, the remainder being kept sterile using a non-touch technique.
- Insert the syringe (or needle, if needle port) (Fig. 23.1) using a non-touch technique and inject the first 1 mL of the drug according to the manufacturer's recommendations, observing the woman's condition throughout (Hayes & Williamson 1998). Restart the infusion. If no problems are noticed, stop the infusion, and continue to administer the rest of the drug at the correct rate.
- Repeat the flushing with the remaining normal saline, using pulsation and positive pressure as described on page 326.
- Recommence the infusion at the appropriate rate.
- Dispose of equipment correctly.
- Wash hands.
- Document administration and effect and act accordingly.

Intermittent infusion

Some drugs may be administered as an infusion over 20 minutes to 1 hour. This is done by:

- adding drugs to a burette giving set of an existing infusion, with the existing infusion being stopped until the drugs have been administered, or

Figure 23.1 • A bolus or 'push' administration of intravenous (I.V.) medication

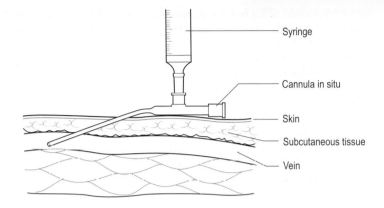

Syringe

Cannula in situ

Skin

Subcutaneous tissue

Vein

- if the drug is already in a prepared infusion (without an existing infusion) it is attached to the cannula with a giving set, *or*
- if there is an existing infusion, it is 'piggy backed' using a Y giving set, with the existing infusion being stopped until the drugs have been administered, to prevent back-tracking of fluid (MHRA 2007).

If the I.V. drugs are the only infusion then the cannula will require flushing before and after administration, as described above. The administration set is often retained for the next dose, but should be renewed after 48 hours. Hand hygiene is essential at each stage of the procedure and it is important that care is taken not to introduce microorganisms into the closed system.

If it is necessary to add drugs to a bag of fluid, it is important that:

- care is taken not to puncture the bag with the needle
- an additive label must be applied with the drug, dose, name and number of the woman, and date and time commenced recorded on it
- the drug and fluid are thoroughly mixed
- the flow rate is correct.

Record keeping should indicate precisely what drug has been administered, over what time and by which method. It should also include whether flushing the cannula was necessary and, if so, with what and should account for any delay of an existing infusion.

Administration using a syringe driver

Syringe drivers (Fig. 23.2) are powered devices that administer controlled doses of medications/fluids by driving the plunger of a syringe at an accurately controlled rate. Kain et al (2006) note that errors involving their use occur in a number of areas: incorrect drug calculation, drug incompatibility and instability, equipment failure, incorrect infusion rate, inadequate user training, inadequate documentation and poor servicing of equipment. It is imperative that the midwife is able to use the syringe driver correctly, having received instruction in its use and ensure that it has been serviced according to manufacturer's instructions.

To calculate the administration rate, the essential information for the midwife is whether it is a 12- or

Figure 23.2 • Syringe driver

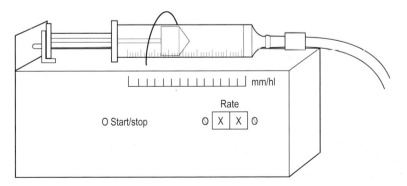

mm/hl

Rate

O Start/stop   O X X O

24-hour pump. The rate is determined by the distance, that is, the length of fluid, measured on the ruler, rather than the number of millilitres. The drug is diluted so that the total length is divisible by 12. Instruction booklets will be provided with each driver, but the general rule is:

$$\frac{\text{Length of fluid (mm)}}{\text{Delivery time (hours)}} = \text{rate setting (mm/hour)}$$

For example, if 36 mm of fluid is to be infused over 12 hours then the rate would be 3 mm/hour. The setting up of the pump relies on several standard principles:

- calculation of the amount of drug that is required over the given period of time with appropriate solution for dilution
- use of sterile syringe, correct size to fit the driver and inserted so that the plunger is secure
- sterile preparation and dilution of the drug
- use of sterile tubing that will fit the cannula used; the tubing must be primed and attached aseptically, after measurement and calculation of the rate
- the syringe must be labelled correctly
- the driver should be maintained and in full working order; alarms for 'occlusion' and 'infusion complete' must be working and the midwife must make regular observations of the pump to ensure it is running to time.

Patient-controlled analgesia

Syringe drivers sometimes have the facility for the woman to increase the analgesia that she is receiving by use of a 'boost' button. They are valuable for postoperative analgesia because there is control over the overall dosage, but the woman can exercise the boost to receive the analgesia when she needs an increase. The woman has control, improving her pain relief and reducing midwifery staff time in administering analgesia. Side effects of I.V. patient-controlled analgesia (PCA) use include nausea, vomiting, pruritus, respiratory depression, sedation, confusion and urinary retention (Momeni et al 2006) but do depend on the drug being infused. Epidural PCA is commonly used during labour.

A mechanism exists to administer a given dose over a set time period – usually 1 or 4 hours – but the machine also has a facility to 'lock out', that is, once a dose has been administered a second dose cannot be given within a predetermined time period

to ensure that the effect of the first dose is felt before the next one is given. The midwife setting up the infusion must set:

- the lockout interval
- a 1- or a 4-hour dose limit
- limit of the drug that the woman can receive with each boost.

A tamper-proof mechanism is also built in to avoid the woman, visitors or others changing the dose.

ROLE AND RESPONSIBILITIES OF THE MIDWIFE

These can be summarised as:

- adherence to local protocols for training and updating of skills
- correct administration procedure, as per the Nursing and Midwifery Council (NMC 2008) and local protocols
- observation of the woman for any unexpected responses
- contemporaneous record keeping.

Summary

- I.V. drugs have a swift effect.
- The midwife needs to be properly trained in their administration and in the correct use of all devices.
- I.V. drugs may be given in the following ways:
  - bolus or 'push'
  - intermittent infusion
  - additives to an infusion
  - syringe driver 12- or 24-hour infusion
  - syringe driver with patient control.
- Sterility must be maintained and flushing is necessary before and after the drug has been administered.

SELF-ASSESSMENT EXERCISES

The answers to the following questions may be found in the text:

1. Describe how a midwife would administer a bolus dose of I.V. antibiotics.
2. Discuss the other ways in which I.V. drugs can be administered.
3. Calculate the rate for a syringe driver: 48 mm of fluid is to be infused over 24 hours.
4. Discuss the advantages of patient-controlled analgesia.
5. Summarise the role and responsibilities of the midwife when administering drugs intravenously.

References

Bertsche T, Mayer Y, Stahl R, et al: Prevention of intravenous drug incompatibilities in an intensive care unit, *Am J Health Syst Pharm* 65(19):1834–1840, 2008.

Cousins DH, Sabatier B, Begue D, et al: Medication errors in intravenous drug preparation and administration: a multicentre audit in the UK, Germany and France, *Qual Saf Health Care* 14(3):190–195, 2005.

Dougherty L: IV therapy: recognizing the differences between infiltration and extravasation, *Br J Nurs* 17(14): 896–900, 2008.

Hayes C, Williamson E: Injection technique: intravenous 2, *Nurs Times* 94(46):40ff, 1998.

Kain VJ, Yates PM, Barrett L, et al: Developing guidelines for syringe driver management, *Int J Palliat Nurs* 12(2):60–67, 2006.

MHRA (Medicines and Healthcare products Regulatory Agency): MDA/2007/089 – Intravenous (IV) infusion lines: all brands, 2007, Online. Available: www.mhra.gov.uk/Publications/Safetywarnings/MedicalDeviceAlerts/CON2033225 16 February 2009.

Momeni M, Crucitti M, De Kock M: Patient-controlled analgesia in the management of postoperative pain, *Drugs* 66(18):2321–2337, 2006.

Murray W, Glenister H: How to use medical devices safely, *Nurs Times* 97(43):36–38, 2001.

Nemec K, Kopelent-Frank H, Greif R: Standardization of infusion solutions to reduce the risk of incompatibility, *Am J Health Syst Pharm* 65(17): 1648–1654, 2008.

NMC (Nursing and Midwifery Council): *Standards for medicine management*, London, 2008, NMC.

RCN (Royal College of Nursing): *Standards for infusion therapy*, London, 2007, RCN.

Scales K: Intravenous therapy: a guide to good practice, *Br J Nurs* 17(19): S4–12, 2008.

Principles of drug administration: inhalational analgesia (Entonox®)

24

CHAPTER CONTENTS

Entonox® (one of its trade names) is 50% oxygen and 50% nitrous oxide. In this concentration it acts as an effective analgesic when inhaled. Its use in the maternity setting is, potentially, for all stages of labour, where the analgesic effect has some value with only minimal side effects for the mother and fetus. This chapter reviews its use and the role and responsibilities of the midwife.

LEARNING OUTCOMES

Having read this chapter the reader should be able to:

- describe the safe and effective use of oxygen and nitrous oxide (50/50)
- discuss briefly its value as an analgesic in labour
- detail the role and responsibilities of the midwife when administering it.

Principles of Entonox® use

Entonox® is a colourless, odourless gas, supplied piped or in cylinders, the cylinder colouring always being blue with blue and white shoulders. Portable cylinders and administration equipment are available. Care should be taken to store the cylinder horizontally above 10 °C; the gases will separate at −6 °C and this may pose a problem to community midwives in the winter until the cylinder is brought back to room temperature.

Entonox® is self-administered by the woman using a mouthpiece or mask to which an expiratory valve is attached. The mask is held over the nose and mouth with an airtight seal or the mouthpiece is placed in the mouth. As the woman breathes, the Entonox® is heard to be released; the apparatus should remain in place during expiration. In this way the woman may breathe through the contraction at a rate that suits her.

Only the woman should hold the apparatus to prevent overdosing; if the woman becomes drowsy she is unable to hold the apparatus to her face. Other side effects may include poor memory of labour, hyperventilation, tingling in hands, nausea and vomiting, dry mouth.

Taken correctly, Entonox® is fully effective within 40 seconds to 1 minute; the effect begins after five deep breaths (approximately 20 seconds; Street 2000). It is excreted from the body within 2–5 minutes.

The skill for the midwife is to support and assist the woman to gain maximum effectiveness from its use. In the first stage of labour, Entonox® needs to be breathed at the onset of the contraction if it is to be effective at the height of the contraction when the pain is at its peak. The midwife needs to palpate the contractions abdominally (see Chapter 1) and encourage the woman to begin breathing before the woman perceives the contraction pain.

Education prior to labour may help the woman to have realistic expectations of the effects of Entonox®. The National Institute for Health and Clinical Excellence (NICE 2007) suggests that it should be available in all birth settings although it is acknowledged that its effectiveness isn't proven. Green (1993) indicates that women have good levels of satisfaction with Entonox® use in labour. From their observations in practice many midwives will agree that one of the benefits of inhalational analgesia is that the woman focuses acutely on breathing regularly, has something to grip on to and therefore has a certain level of distraction that may help her through each contraction.

In the second stage of labour, breathing the analgesia may help the woman if her urge to push is significant, but the presenting part remains high, to encourage descent prior to commencing active pushing, e.g. occipitoposterior position. It can be used effectively for examining the perineum and for suturing at the end of the third stage of labour. Without uterine contractions the woman is able to breathe the gases for a minute or more before any part of the procedure is undertaken.

Entonox® may be contraindicated where a respiratory disease exists. Such women may be reviewed individually by an obstetrician if necessary.

Smoking should not occur in the vicinity of any compressed gas; care should be taken in the woman's home environment (Sealey 2002).

Entonox® is believed to be safe for the fetus but researched evidence is very limited.

Robertson (2006) reiterates the need for occupational awareness of health and safety. Maternity units should have effective ventilation and scavenger systems, staff should also consider wearing personal exposure monitors, particularly if working consistently on labour wards. Vitamin B_{12} can be inhibited with exposure to nitrous oxide, fertility and fetal normality may be affected. Robertson (2006) urges midwives who are planning to become pregnant to consider working in non-nitrous oxide environments.

ROLE AND RESPONSIBILITIES OF THE MIDWIFE

These can be summarised as:

- if appropriately trained in its use, the midwife may, under a patient group direction, administer Entonox® to labouring women – all stages of labour are permitted

- all approved apparatus/equipment should be available for inspection when required (NMC 2004)
- the apparatus should be properly stored, maintained and used correctly on each occasion: cylinders have a batch label and a seal on the valve. The midwife should be fully conversant with fitting the head to the cylinder, ensuring that there is no oil or grease present. The tubing should be cleaned on completion of care
- as a drug, it may only be administered to labouring women, and not to any other group or person 'to try'
- Entonox® is only ever self-administered
- the effect and side effects of the drug are observed; other types of analgesia may be used in conjunction with Entonox® if appropriate, e.g. transcutaneous electrical nerve stimulation (TENS) (see Chapter 26), narcotics, massage
- contemporaneous records are kept
- health and safety at work regulations should be upheld with regard to nitrous oxide use.

Summary

- Due to the nature of its administration its effect in labour is questionable, but it is appreciated by many women. The side effects for the women are transitory and there are no documented effects at this time for the fetus.
- The midwife has responsibilities to ensure that it is stored, serviced and used correctly.
- Working in environments of extensive nitrous oxide use may pose health threats to employees. Health and safety regulations should be upheld.

SELF-ASSESSMENT EXERCISES

The answers to the following questions may be found in the text:

1. Describe how a midwife should support a woman to use Entonox® effectively in the first and second stages of labour.
2. Discuss the advantages and disadvantages of Entonox® as a labour analgesic.
3. Summarise the role and responsibilities of the midwife when caring for a woman using Entonox® in labour.
4. Under which regulations can a midwife administer Entonox® and to whom?

References

Green J: Expectations and experiences of pain in labour: findings from a large prospective study, *Birth* 20(2):65–72, 1993.

NICE (National Institute for Health and Clinical excellence): *Intrapartum care: care of healthy women and their babies during childbirth*, London, 2007, NICE.

NMC (Nursing and Midwifery Council): *Midwives rules and standards*, London, 2004, NMC.

Robertson A: Nitrous oxide – no laughing matter, *MIDIRS Midwifery Digest* 16(1):123–128, 2006.

Sealey L: Nurse administration of Entonox to manage pain in ward settings, *Nursing Times* 98(46): 28–29, 2002.

Street D: A practical guide to giving Entonox, *Nursing Times* 96(34): 47–48, 2000.

Principles of drug administration: epidural analgesia

25

CHAPTER CONTENTS

Epidural analgesia generally provides effective analgesia for women in labour compared to other forms of analgesia or no analgesia (Amin-Somuah et al 2005). A 24-hour epidural service is offered in most consultant delivery units using skilled obstetric anaesthetists and midwives who are competent in epidural management (OAA & AAGBI 2005). The epidural rate in the UK is around 25%, although Odibo (2007) suggests the demand is closer to 70–90%; rates in the USA are much higher than the UK at 58% (Simmons et al 2007). This chapter clarifies the terminology and details the procedures for epidural insertion, top-up and removal. The indications, contraindications, side effects and midwife's role and responsibilities are all highlighted. The reader is encouraged to be aware that the debates surrounding epidural use and normal birth are greater than this text can examine.

LEARNING OUTCOMES

Having read this chapter the reader should be able to:

- discuss the differences between epidural, spinal and combined spinal epidural analgesia
- list the indications, contraindications and possible side effects from epidural analgesia
- describe how an epidural is sited and a top-up administered
- discuss the role and responsibilities of the midwife throughout the procedures
- describe how to remove an epidural catheter.

Epidural analgesia

Epidural analgesia involves the introduction of a local anaesthetic, often combined with an opioid, into the epidural space (Fig. 25.1). The drugs are able to cross the dura and arachnoid membrane and enter the cerebrospinal fluid (CSF). This allows some of the drug to pass into the spinal cord and bind with opioid receptors, some passes into the systemic circulation

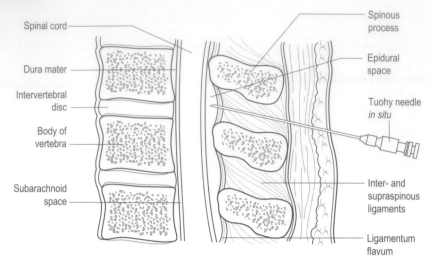

Figure 25.1 • Sagittal section of the lumbar spine with Tuohy needle in the epidural space

whilst the rest attaches to epidural fat (with no analgesic effect) (Chapman 2008).

To achieve this, a Tuohy needle is inserted through the lumbar intervertebral space (between L1 and L4) into the epidural space; a fine catheter is threaded through into the epidural space where it is secured in place to allow administration of the drug either as bolus/intermittent doses or as a continuous infusion.

Spinal analgesia

Spinal analgesia is achieved by injecting the drug through the epidural space, dura and arachnoid membrane, into the intrathecal (subarachnoid) space. Lower doses of the drug can be used as it is placed directly into the CSF where the entire drug can bind to the opioid receptor sites in the spinal cord and it is considered to be 10 times more potent than when placed in the epidural space (Chapman 2008). Onset of analgesia is rapid but not as long lasting as an epidural; it is often the analgesia/anaesthesia of choice for emergency caesarean section where rapid anaesthesia is required or for an elective caesarean section.

Combined spinal epidural analgesia

Combined spinal epidural (CSE) analgesia involves injection of the drug into the intrathecal space immediately before or after the placement of the epidural catheter. Often, it is achieved by using the epidural needle to locate the epidural space at the level of L3 then passing a smaller-diameter long spinal needle through the epidural needle lumen to pierce the dura and arachnoid membrane. The drug can then be injected into the CSF and the spinal needle removed to allow the epidural catheter to be inserted into the epidural space and drugs injected into there (Simmons et al 2007). Amin-Somuah & Smyth (2005) suggest CSE combines the advantages of the faster onset and more reliable analgesia achieved with the spinal with the continuing pain relief of the epidural whilst allowing the woman to remain alert.

Drugs

Local anaesthetics (e.g. bupivacaine, ropivacaine) cross the dura and arachnoid membranes, where they are in contact with the nerve roots and spinal cord. Once there, they inhibit nerve conduction by blocking the sodium ion channels that pass the impulses along the nerve fibres, stopping transmission of the painful impulses to the higher centres. The drug dosage determines which nerve fibres are affected; low doses exert a concentration specific effect and can partially selectively block nerve fibres with the smallest diameter (pain) without blocking the larger motor fibres, reducing the amount of leg weakness and immobility experienced (Amin-Somuah & Smyth 2005, Chapman 2008). CSE is able to achieve a good level of analgesia with lower doses of local anaesthesia.

High doses of local anaesthetics result in numbness from the waist down associated with limited/no mobility. There has traditionally been more difficulty with giving birth with an increased risk of instrumental delivery, increased perineal bruising and pain and postpartum incontinence (Simmons et al 2007). As a consequence low dose local anaesthetics are now combined with opioids to limit these effects. Combining lower doses of local anaesthetics with opioids produces better analgesia than higher doses of the individual drugs (Chapman 2008); the risk of instrumental deliveries has decreased and the woman is more likely to have increased mobility during labour (Simmons et al 2007)

Opioid drugs (e.g. fentanyl, diamorphine) combine with the opioid receptor sites to produce an analgesic effect. Fentanyl is lipid soluble and so passes more readily into the CSF, thus is faster acting compared to diamorphine. However, it has a shorter duration (1–4 hours) compared with diamorphine (6–12 hours) (Chapman 2008).

Indications for epidural analgesia

- Pain relief/maternal request.
- Useful where there is likelihood of instrumental or operative delivery, e.g. malposition, malpresentation, multiple pregnancy, prolonged labour.
- Hypertension, where the potential side effects of hypotension can be helpful.
- Preterm labour, where there may be an early desire to push.
- Postoperative analgesia.

Contraindications

There are contraindications for epidural/spinal analgesia, some of which are absolute whilst others are relative:

- coagulation defects due to the increased risk of haematoma formation
- local sepsis
- some neurological disorders, e.g. multiple sclerosis

- known allergy to drugs used
- raised intracranial pressure
- unavailability of appropriately trained staff in setting up and ongoing care of epidurals
- insufficient midwifery staff to provide 1:1 care for duration of epidural
- spinal deformity.

Whilst an increased BMI is not a contraindication, it is recognised that there is a higher failure rate when the woman's BMI is >30 requiring resiting of the epidural (Dresner et al 2006).

Side effects of epidural and spinal analgesia

The side effects associated with epidural and spinal analgesia result from the effects of the drugs used or complications from the procedure itself:

- Opioid side effects: respiration depression (can occur early, within the first 2 hours of administration or later (6–12 hours) and are more likely to occur with diamorphine than fentanyl); sedation; nausea and vomiting; pruritus (itching); urinary retention.
- Local anaesthetic side effects vary depending on the drug and dosage used: peripheral vasodilatation and resulting hypotension (if severe will also cause loss of consciousness); leg weakness; urinary retention, temperature changes (particularly with the vasodilatory effect of bupivacaine which can cause the woman's feet to be warm, her temperature to rise but her body to shiver).
- Drug toxicity: restlessness, dizziness, tinnitus, metallic taste, drowsiness.
- Anaphylactic drug reaction (see Chapter 18).
- Partial block ('breakthrough' pain): contractions are still felt over one area of the abdomen due to non-uniform spread of local anaesthetic (Amin-Somuah & Smyth 2005).
- Dural puncture: the epidural needle or catheter accidentally punctures the dura mater resulting in reduced intracranial pressure with potential severe headache in the following few days (postdural puncture headache, PDPH).
- Catheter migration: extremely rare complication where the catheter migrates into the CSF (can paralyse the respiratory muscles resulting in apnoea, profound hypotension and respiratory

arrest) or a blood vessel (resulting in sedation from excess opioids or local anaesthetic toxicity noticed by tingling, numbness, twitching, convulsions, apnoea, loss of consciousness).

- Abscess formation which manifests as back pain and tenderness, erythema, purulent discharge from insertion site.
- Haematoma due to trauma to the epidural blood vessels during catheter insertion or removal which presents with back pain and tenderness accompanied by sensory and/or motor weakness.
- Meningitis: an extremely rare complication manifesting as fever, headache, neck stiffness, photophobia, nausea and vomiting.

There is little consensus as to the incidence of risks occurring in practice as many of the studies are too small to be reliable (Middle & Wee 2009) although the majority of risks are rare. However, Ruppen et al (2006) advise that the risks for transient nerve injury are 1:6700, for haematoma formation 1:168 000 and for deep epidural infection 1:240 000. Risks for intrathecal injection are 1:2900, intravascular injection 1:5008 and high/total spinal block 1:16 200 according to Jenkins (2005). The risks determined by the Obstetric Anaesthetists Association for Great Britain and Ireland, which should be given to the woman, are:

- epidural not working effectively and requiring additional pain relief 1:8
- epidural not working effectively at caesarean section necessitating a general anaesthetic 1:20
- severe headache with epidural 1:100, with spinal 1:500
- nerve damage (numb patch on leg or foot, weakness) 1:1000 (temporary), lasting beyond 6 months 1:13 000
- abscess formation 1:50 000
- meningitis 1:10 000
- haematoma 1:170 000
- accidental unconsciousness 1:100 000
- severe injury including paralysis 1:250 000 (OAA 2008).

Effect on labour

Epidural use during labour has traditionally been associated with an increased risk of instrumental delivery, caesarean section, oxytocin augmentation, lower Apgar scores. Odibo (2007) proposes the local anaesthetic drugs are the reason behind many of these risks suggesting they affect the pelvic autonomic and parasympathetic nerves, thus inhibiting oxytocin release, which reduces the frequency and strength of contractions. In the second stage, this affects the expulsive nature of contractions with the urge to push being lost as a result of the sensory blockade. Odibo further states that the pelvic floor muscle tone is reduced, which hampers rotation of the presenting part. However, many of these risks were seen when epidurals were first introduced for obstetric use and high doses of local anaesthetics were used. Over the years, different drugs and dosages have been used to reduce the adverse effects on labour. Even with this, epidural analgesia still impacts on labour. Although women are likely to have a longer second stage, reduced mobility, hypotension, urinary retention, fever and an increased need for oxytocin augmentation and instrumental delivery, Amin-Souah & Smyth (2005) found no significant adverse impact on maternal satisfaction, long-term backache, Apgar scores or the risk of caesarean section.

Changes in practice are also helping to overcome the risks (e.g. delayed pushing; see Chapter 31). Torvaldsen et al (2004) reviewed the evidence concerning the practice of discontinuing the epidural analgesia late in labour to decrease the risk of instrumental deliveries and conclude that there is insufficient evidence to support or refute the practice. Ban Leong et al (2008) are undertaking a Cochrane review to determine whether the timing of the epidural related to the stage of labour makes a difference in respect of labour, maternal and neonatal outcomes, as observational data suggest that early epidural use, particularly during the latent phase of labour, is associated with an increased risk of caesarean section. The reader is advised to review their results when published as this may impact on epidural use in labour.

Simmons et al (2007) suggest the risk of urinary retention increases significantly with combined spinal epidural compared to epidural use. They found no difference in the ability to mobilise or headaches.

PROCEDURE: siting an epidural catheter and analgesia

When a woman requests or requires epidural analgesia, the anaesthetist should be informed, who should attend within 30 minutes unless there are exceptional circumstances (OAA & AAGBI 2005). It is important to consider the staffing levels on the delivery suite to ensure there is a competent midwife able to undertake the ongoing care of the epidural and enough staff for the midwife to provide 1:1 care (OAA & AAGBI 2005). It is the anaesthetist's responsibility to obtain informed consent prior to siting the epidural, and this will include a discussion of the risks involved (Middle & Wee 2009). Written information can be provided by the midwife prior to the anaesthetist's arrival to assist with this (a two-sided epidural information card is available by download from the Obstetric Anaesthetists Association of Great Britain and Ireland website (OAA 2008)).

- Call the anaesthetist, gather the equipment:
  - equipment for cannulation and intravenous infusion (crystalloid fluid)
  - cardiotocograph (CTG) monitor
  - dressings trolley
  - sterile gown and gloves
  - sterile dressing pack, with fenestrated drape and gauze
  - antiseptic lotion, usually chlorhexidine in 70% isopropyl alcohol
  - epidural pack, usually containing a Tuohy needle with stylet, syringe, tubing (catheter) and antibacterial filter
  - local anaesthetics for the skin and epidural, e.g. lidocaine (lignocaine) and bupivacaine
  - opiate analgesia, if required (administered according to controlled drug administration; see Chapter 18)
  - sterile syringes and needles
  - tape/plastic skin dressing.
- Encourage the woman to empty her bladder.
- Cannulate and commence an intravenous infusion: the use of crystalloids to increase effective blood volume is recommended although its efficacy is not clearly evaluated (Delgado & Rodriguez Malagon 2004).
- Record baseline observations of blood pressure, pulse, respirations, pain and sedation score, fetal heart rate assessment.
- Position the woman according to her comfort and the anaesthetist's wishes (usually one of two ways), to promote curvature of the spine so that access can be gained between the vertebrae:

  - in left lateral with knees flexed and chin on chest but with her back very close to the edge of the bed
  - sitting on the edge of the bed with feet supported on a chair, arms resting upon a bed table and head resting on her arms.
- Assist the anaesthetist to 'glove and gown' and to establish a strict aseptic field; pour the lotion, open the needles and syringes, hold ampoules of local anaesthetic for drawing up, etc. (see Chapter 10).
- Encourage the woman to remain still while the epidural is sited by the anaesthetist; all of the activity occurs behind her back, so support and reassurance are needed:
  - the woman's back will be cleansed, the drapes put in place and the local anaesthetic inserted into the skin
  - the Tuohy needle will be inserted when the woman is contraction free and very still (to avoid advancing too far and causing a dural puncture)
  - the stylet will be removed and an epidural syringe will be used (injecting air or saline to assess the resistance) to ensure that the Tuohy needle is in the correct place
  - the catheter tubing is then threaded into place and the Tuohy needle removed.
- If appropriate, spray plastic skin around the puncture site and secure the catheter with tape when the anaesthetist is ready; secure the filter in an accessible place.
- A small test dose is given, the first complete dose is given, or a syringe driver/infusion pump attached when the anaesthetist is satisfied that the catheter is correctly inserted.
- Assist the woman into the position that the anaesthetist suggests for the initial 20 minutes after administration (often semi-recumbent).
- Assess and record blood pressure and pulse after each 5 minutes for the next 20 minutes, and each 30 minutes thereafter.
- Observe the woman's condition, including her level of pain/block, respiratory rate, her warmth, safety, intravenous infusion, colour and signs of nausea.
- Call the anaesthetist if any observations give cause for concern (hypotension may be corrected by increasing the rate of the intravenous infusion, but the anaesthetist should always be called).

- Ensure the anaesthetist has disposed of the equipment correctly, including sharps.
- Monitor the fetal condition and uterine activity, recording the epidural on the CTG tracing.
- If after 20 minutes all observations are within normal limits and the level of analgesia has been achieved, reposition the woman according to her choice (avoiding aortocaval compression) or assist to mobilise.
- Continue all labour care, including care of the bladder: catheterisation may be necessary as urinary retention is a common problem (see Chapter 14), pressure-area care (see Chapter 53) and numb legs, maintaining contemporaneous records.
- If not using a continuous infusion, observe for signs of recurring sensation usually after 2–8 hours; administer a top-up before the woman becomes uncomfortable.
- Administration of patient-controlled analgesia (PCA) allows the woman to administer her own top-ups with or without a low-dose background continuous infusion and will require assessment of the woman's blood pressure and pulse as described above.

Checking the level of the block

The level of the epidural block should be assessed at least once an hour to ensure the level is correct (this will have been previously determined by the anaesthetist). The level can be checked using either an ice cube (wrapped in gauze or tissue to protect the midwife's fingers) or a cold solution (e.g. ethyl chloride spray). Either gently rub the ice cube or spray the cold solution at the top of the woman's chest, moving downwards one side at a time. The woman will be able to feel the coldness of the ice cube/spray in areas where the block is not present but when placed against an area where the block is effective, will not feel it as cold. This should be compared against a dermatome chart (Fig 25.2) and the level recorded. Generally, the level is kept at no higher than T4; if it rises above this, the anaesthetist should be informed. If the level is too low, the woman is likely to be feeling pain and require a top-up or bolus. If the woman is receiving a continuous infusion and the block is too low to be

beneficial, the midwife should check that the catheter is still *in situ* and connected to the bacterial filter with no leaks in the tubing before calling the anaesthetist, who may need to resite the catheter.

Epidural top-ups

Epidural top-ups are given if the administration is not continuous. Midwives who have been properly trained and supervised may undertake top-ups, being familiar with local protocol. The anaesthetist prescribes the dose (concentration and volume), the frequency and the position of the woman. Administering the dose in two halves with 5 minutes between them is often prescribed in case the catheter has migrated into the cerebrospinal fluid. The observations recorded following a top-up also apply to a bolus administered via a PCA pump by the woman.

PROCEDURE: epidural top-up

- Establish the need for the top-up, check the intravenous infusion and gather equipment:
  - the prescribed drug(s)
  - the medicine administration chart and epidural chart
  - sterile needle and syringe
  - alcohol-impregnated swab.
- Position the woman according to the anaesthetist's request, usually lateral during the first stage of labour, sitting for the second.
- Wash hands, check the drugs with another midwife and draw up the correct dose.
- Confirm the woman's identity on the medicine administration chart both verbally with the woman and against her name band.
- When the woman is free from contraction, remove the cap from the filter, clean the port with the swab and inject the local anaesthetic at a rate of 5 mL per 30 seconds (half or whole dose according to prescription).
- Observe the woman throughout for adverse reactions such as tinnitus, drowsiness and slurred speech.
- Reapply the cap.
- Repeat the procedure in 5 minutes (if prescribed in two halves).

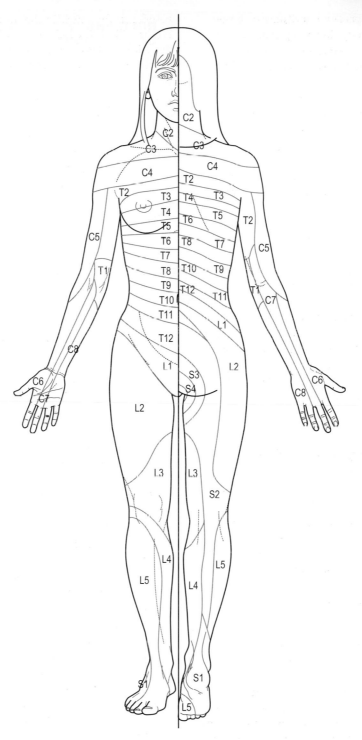

Figure 25.2 • Dermatome levels (Adapted with kind permission from Walsh 1997)

- Pulse and blood pressure are taken as before: every 5 minutes for at least 20 minutes, every 30 minutes thereafter.
- Reposition the woman if necessary.
- Dispose of equipment correctly.
- Document administration and effect and act accordingly.
- Continue to observe for the effects or side effects of the block; summon the anaesthetist if required.

PROCEDURE: removing an epidural cannula

The cannula is removed once the epidural is no longer required, usually once labour is over. If there is any concern about the coagulation status of the woman, coagulation studies should be undertaken and the catheter is removed only when agreed by the anaesthetist.

- Gain informed consent and ensure privacy throughout.
- Wash and dry hands.
- Remove the tape and pull the catheter out carefully, but swiftly in one movement.
- Clean around the site with skin cleansing agent, e.g. chlorhexidine in 70% alcohol swab.
- Apply occlusive dressing for 24 hours.
- Examine the tubing for completeness by assessing the gradations and the rounded appearance of the blue catheter tip; checking with a second person may be required.
- Document removal and act accordingly.

Postnatal care

In the immediate postnatal period the woman may still be numb and may therefore require assistance to care for her baby, to breast feed and help to become mobile again. She will also need observing for signs of urinary retention and headache, two of the most common short-term side effects. Observations for backache may be needed in the longer term.

ROLE AND RESPONSIBILITIES OF THE MIDWIFE

These can be summarised as:

- education and preparation of the woman
- assessing the suitability of the woman, e.g. progress in labour
- consideration of the delivery suite workload and whether the woman can be given 'one-to-one' care following its insertion
- correct positioning and support of the woman during the siting of the epidural
- assistance of the anaesthetist during preparation and siting
- ongoing care and observations of the woman and fetus
- recognising deviations from the norm, responding and summoning the anaesthetist
- training and competence for the provision of top-ups or care of continuous infusion
- correct removal of epidural catheter
- appropriate postnatal care
- contemporaneous record keeping throughout.

Summary

- Epidural, of whichever sort or dose, is generally a very effective form of labour analgesia.
- The midwife has a responsible role at the time of siting the epidural, with the ongoing care and with the management of infusion or top-ups, both during labour and postnatally.
- The midwife works in conjunction with a skilled obstetric anaesthetist.

SELF-ASSESSMENT EXERCISES

The answers to the following questions may be found in the text:

1. Discuss the differences between epidural, spinal and combined spinal epidural analgesia.
2. List the indications, contraindications and possible side effects for epidural analgesia.
3. Describe the midwife's role during epidural siting.
4. How can a midwife assess the level of the block?
5. Describe how an epidural top-up is safely administered by a midwife.
6. Describe how an epidural catheter is correctly removed.

References

Amin-Somuah M, Smyth RMD, Howell CJ: Epidural versus non-epidural or no analgesia in labour, *Cochrane Database Syst Rev* 4: CD000331. DOI: 10.1002/14651858.CD000331.pub2, 2005.

Ban Leong S, Lim Y, Sia YT: Early versus late initiation of epidural analgesia for labour, *Cochrane Database Syst Rev* 3: CD007238. DOI: 10.1002/14651858.CD007238, 2008.

Chapman S: Pain management: epidural and intrathecal analgesia. In Dougherty L, Lister S, editors: *The Royal Marsden Hospital Manual of Clinical Nursing Procedures*, ed 7, Oxford, 2008, Wiley Blackwell, pp 585–604

Delgado M, Rodriguez Malagon N: Interventions for preventing hypotension in adults receiving spinal anaesthesia, *Cochrane Database Syst Rev* 3: CD005057. DOI: 10.1002/14651858.CD005057, 2004.

Dresner M, Brocklesby J, Bamber J: Audit of the influence of body mass index on the performance of epidural analgesia in labour and the subsequent mode of delivery, *Br J Obstet Gynaecol* 113 (10):1178–1181, 2006.

Jenkins JG: Some immediate serious complications of obstetric epidural analgesia and anaesthesia: a prospective study of 145000 epidurals, *Int J Obstet Anesth* 14: 37–42, 2005.

Middle JV, Wee MYK: Informed consent for epidural analgesia in labour: a survey of UK practice, *Anaesthesia* 64(2):161–164, 2009.

OAA: Epidural information card, 2008. Online. Available: www.oaa-anaes.ac.uk/assets/-managed/editor/File/Info%20for%20Mothers/2008_eic_english.pdf 4 April 2009

OAA, AAGBI: Guidelines for Obstetric Anaesthetic Services, revised edition, 2005. *Obstetric Anaesthetists' Association/The Association of Anaesthetists of Great Britain and Ireland*, London. Online. Available: www.oaa-anaes.ac.uk/assets/-managed/editor/File/PDF/Publications/obstetric-guidelines.pdf 4 April 2009.

Odibo L: Does epidural analgesia affect the second stage of labour? *Br J Midwifery* 15(7):429–435, 2007.

Ruppen W, Derry S, McQuay H, et al: Incidence of epidural haematoma, infection and neurologic injury in obstetric patients with epidural analgesia/anaesthesia, *Anesthesiology* 105:394–399, 2006.

Simmons SW, Cyna AM, Dennis AT, et al: Combined spinal-epidural versus epidural analgesia in labour, *Cochrane Database Syst Rev* 3: CD003401. DOI: 10.1002/14651858.CD003401.pub2, 2007.

Torvaldsen S, Roberts CL, Bell JC, et al: Discontinuation of epidural analgesia late in labour for reducing the adverse delivery outcomes associated with epidural analgesia, *Cochrane Database Syst Rev* 4: CD004457. DOI: 10.1002/14651858.CD004457.pub2, 2004

Walsh D: *TENS: Clinical Applications and Related Theory*, Edinburgh, 1997, Churchill Livingstone.

Principles of drug administration: transcutaneous electrical nerve stimulation

26

CHAPTER CONTENTS

This chapter considers the midwife's role in the application and use of transcutaneous electrical nerve stimulation (TENS) for the purposes of pain relief in labour and postoperatively. TENS is not a pharmaceutical drug, but it is widely used for analgesia in labour.

LEARNING OUTCOMES

Having read this chapter the reader should be able to:

- discuss the principles by which TENS is considered to be effective when in labour
- describe how it is applied and used
- summarise the role and responsibilities of the midwife.

How does TENS work?

The 'gate control' theory of pain suggests that stimulation of larger peripheral nerve fibres inhibits pain signals entering the central pain pathway, reducing the perception of pain – TENS provides this stimulation. Additionally, it is believed that the electrical stimulation also activates the release of the body's own endorphins.

TENS is available as a handheld battery operated unit. Electrodes are placed onto the skin over specific spinal nerves. The electrodes need to be the correct size to stimulate the nerve fibres at the correct rate and density (Coates 1998). A water-based electrode gel is required to facilitate the current. Tape is used to keep the electrodes securely in the correct place if self-adhesive electrodes are unavailable.

TENS machines are adjusted according to the pulse frequency (the number per second), pulse duration and amplitude (strength of the current). The constant background tingling closes the gate on the pain and promotes endorphin production. With the boost facility the duration, amplitude and frequency are all increased, enhancing the pain relieving action yet further. The woman experiences the sensation as tingling on the skin; this should be through both electrodes and be at a comfortable level. If supplied with indicator lights, these are seen to flash intermittently, or to remain on continuously, according to the frequency. TENS should not be used in water, it may interfere with a cardiac pacemaker, damaged or sore skin should be avoided and it should not be used in the first trimester (Poole 2007a) or on the abdomen at any stage of pregnancy.

Suitability as a labour analgesic

Studies conflict when considering the effect of TENS, so much so that NICE (2007) state that TENS should not be offered to women in established labour. However, levels of consumer satisfaction are good (Carroll et al 1997). As a non-pharmacological analgesic it has no known ill effects for the mother (so long as it is used according to the manufacturer's instructions) or fetus. It allows the woman to mobilise, to utilise other analgesics as well and to have some control – aiding both her physiological and psychological equilibrium. Application in early labour is indicated to promote an increase in the woman's natural endorphin level. Poole (2007b) suggests that it may take 20–30 minutes for the effects of TENS to be felt. Women often hire and apply their TENS machines in labour before meeting with a midwife. The woman may need guidance on how to use it correctly; the midwife may not be familiar with the actual machine but should be able to apply the correct principles.

Positioning of TENS

Hawkins (1994) suggests that correct positioning of the electrodes is essential. Bryant and Yerby (2004), Coates (1998) and Hamilton (2009) all indicate (when labouring) the need to place the electrodes over the spinal nerves that supply the uterus and pelvic floor: T10–L1 and S2–S4.

Coates (1998) suggests that if the woman's arms are relaxed and hanging loosely by her sides, then the lower tip of her scapula is at T7. Three spinal vertebrae can then be counted down to locate T10. The top of the upper pad is placed level with T10. S2 is located by identifying the iliac crests and placing the top of the lower electrode one vertebra below this. The pads should be placed centrally either side of the spinal column, with 3 cm between them (Fig. 26.1).

PROCEDURE: applying a TENS unit for a labouring woman

- Clarify that this is the woman's choice of analgesia; discuss what to expect.
- Position the woman so that access can be gained to her back.
- Ensure the unit is switched off, but fully charged with the electrodes connected and all the controls on the lowest possible setting.

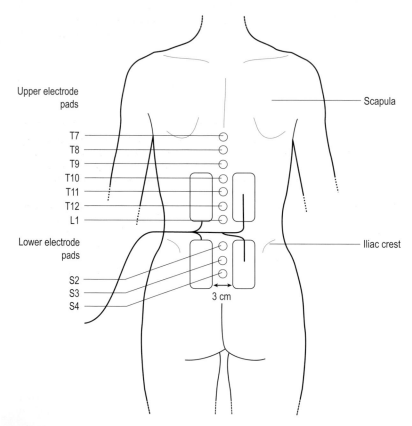

Figure 26.1 • Positioning of the electrodes for transcutaneous electrical nerve stimulation (TENS) (Adapted with kind permission from Coates 1998)

- Identify the correct positions for the electrodes (see Fig. 26.1) and apply them using tape and electrode gel if required.
- Switch the unit on, demonstrate the boost and how to increase the intensities according to need.
- Ensure that the woman is comfortable.
- Replace clothing, securing the unit in a pocket if appropriate, leaving the boost button accessible.
- Document application and effect, ensure that there is no electrical interference with any other items being used.
- Discontinue the use of TENS at the end of labour or according to the woman's wishes (switch the unit off, remove electrodes, clean reusable electrodes, service and maintain the unit according to the manufacturer's instructions).

ROLE AND RESPONSIBILITIES OF THE MIDWIFE

These can be summarised as:

- education and empowerment of the woman in her choice of analgesia, but cautiously if national guidelines suggest otherwise
- appropriate training, updating and application of TENS
- care and maintenance of the TENS unit
- observation of the effectiveness
- contemporaneous record keeping.

Summary

- TENS works on the 'gate control' theory of pain: electrical impulses of differing frequencies close the gate and encourage the body to release endorphins.
- Many women view TENS as being a good non-pharmacological analgesic for labour; research questions its validity.
- It has minimal side effects and allows both mobility and control.
- The midwife has a role in ensuring that it is applied, used and maintained correctly.

SELF-ASSESSMENT EXERCISES

The answers to the following questions may be found in the text:

1. How are the effects of TENS achieved?
2. How does a midwife decide where to place the electrodes?
3. Which signs indicate to the woman and the midwife that the TENS unit is working effectively?
4. When should TENS not be used?
5. Summarise the role and responsibilities of the midwife in relation to the use of TENS in labour.

References

Bryant H, Yerby M: Relief of pain during labour. In Henderson C, Macdonald S, editors: *Mayes' midwifery: a textbook for midwives*, ed 13, Edinburgh, 2004, Baillière Tindall, pp 458–475.

Carroll D, Tramer M, McQuay H, et al: Transcutaneous electrical nerve stimulation in labour pain: a systematic review, *Br J Obstet Gynaecol* 104(2):169–175, 1997.

Coates T: Transcutaneous electrical nerve stimulation: TENS, *Pract Midwife* 1(11):12–14, 1998.

Hamilton A: Comfort and support in labour. In Fraser DM, Cooper MA, editors: *Myles textbook for midwives*, ed 15, Edinburgh, 2009, Churchill Livingstone, pp 493–507.

Hawkins J: The use of TENS for pain relief in labour, *Br J Midwifery* 2 (10):487–490, 1994.

NICE (National Institute for Health and Clinical Excellence): *Intrapartum care: care of healthy women and their babies during childbirth*, London, 2007, NICE.

Poole D: Use of TENS in pain management Part One: how TENS works, *Nurs Times* 103(7):28–29, 2007a.

Poole D: Use of TENS in pain management Part Two: how to use TENS, *Nurs Times* 103(8):28–29, 2007b.

Facilitation of related childbearing skills: optimal fetal positioning

27

Malposition and malpresentation in labour are associated with an increased risk of intervention during labour, instrumental and/or operative delivery and increased morbidity to the woman and baby. Reducing the incidence of malposition and malpresentation prior to labour could minimise the risks to both the woman and the baby. This chapter focuses on the use of different positions and alternative therapies used by the woman during pregnancy to encourage the fetus into an optimal fetal position.

LEARNING OUTCOMES

Having read this chapter the reader should be able to:

- discuss the evidence surrounding the use of optimum fetal positioning
- discuss the different positions and postures a woman can use during pregnancy to encourage the fetal occiput to rotate from a posterior to an anterior position
- discuss the different methods that may change the presentation from breech to cephalic
- identify some of the hazards associated with malpositions and malpresentations for the woman and baby.

Malposition of the occiput: occipitoposterior position

Approximately 10% of labours at term occur with an occipitoposterior (OP) position. Whereas many of these undergo a long rotation to become an occipitoanterior position during labour, a small number will persist in the posterior position. OP labour and deliveries are associated with a number of possible complications:

- higher presenting part with wider diameters that will take longer to negotiate the pelvis
- early rupture of membranes, increasing the risk of ascending infection
- cord prolapse
- uncoordinated uterine action leading to prolonged labour
- urinary retention
- premature urge to push
- increased risk of trauma to vagina and pelvic floor
- increased risk of instrumental and/or operative delivery, which may be associated with an increased blood loss
- abnormal moulding which may result in an unsettled baby and increase the risk of intracranial haemorrhage

- lower Apgar scores
- increased perinatal mortality and morbidity.

(Adapted from Lewis 2004)

Sutton & Scott (1996) strongly advocate using different positions and postures to encourage the fetus to rotate to a lateral or anterior position and so facilitate engagement from 34 weeks gestation onwards. They do caution women to discuss this with the health professional overseeing their pregnancy to ensure there are no contraindications to this.

The assumption behind their recommendations is to provide the fetus with room to rotate within the uterus and adopt a position that is more comfortable and better for delivery. The fetus will be able to adopt a more flexed position if in a lateral or anterior position; as the head flexes the engaging diameters will reduce and hence engagement is likely to occur earlier rather than later. Their advice centres on using upright and forward leaning postures regularly, particularly during Braxton Hicks contractions, as this is believed to assist the fetus to manoeuvre into the optimum position.

Favourable positions to adopt

- Use upright and forward leaning postures regularly (to create more space for the fetus to turn).
- To read, sit on a dining chair with elbows resting on the table, lean slightly forward and keep the knees apart.
- Sit on a dining chair facing the back, stretching and resting arms over the back of the chair.
- When sitting generally, make sure the knees are lower than the hips and keep the back straight by placing a small cushion over the small of the back for support.
- While watching television, kneel on the floor and lean over a large bean bag or cushion
- When driving, place a wedge cushion under the bottom.
- When swimming try to keep the abdomen forward; breast stroke is better for this than back stroke.
- When lying on one side, place a pillow between the legs with the top knee resting on the bed.

Positions to avoid

- Avoid relaxing in semi-reclining positions that cause the knees to be higher than the hips.
- If driving using bucket seats, have regular stops to change position and use a wedge cushion under the bottom.
- Do not sit with crossed legs or legs up.
- Do not squat in late pregnancy unless the fetus is no longer in the OP position as the head may be forced into the pelvis in the OP position.

Sutton & Scott's (1996) work is not research based but they have strong anecdotal evidence to support their claims. This is an area that needs researching but at present does not appear to have any disadvantages for suitable women.

Another method that has been proposed since the 1950s is for the woman to adopt an 'all-fours' position, using knees and hands for support, used in conjunction with pelvic rocking. This method has been recommended over the years and used by many women without being researched as to its effectiveness. Hunter et al (2007) following a systematic review of the studies evaluating this intervention conclude that whilst adopting this position for 10 minutes twice a day resulted in a change in the position of the baby at the time, it had no effect on the position of the fetus at term, and thus do not recommend the hands–knees position as an intervention; however, use of this position during labour reduced the incidence of backache. Kariminia et al's (2004) small study compared this intervention (for 10 minutes twice daily) with a control group who had to undertake walking each day from 37 weeks. They concluded that although the hands–knees posture combined with pelvic rocking exercises is a practice commonly used within midwifery to encourage rotation from the posterior to the anterior position, their results did not support this practice and recommended that in the absence of any beneficial effects, the practice should be discontinued. Encouraging rotation of the occiput from a posterior to an anterior position remains an area for further research.

Malpresentation: breech presentation

The fetus will present by the breech in approximately 3–4% of pregnancies at term; this figure is higher earlier in pregnancy and the majority of breech presentations that turn spontaneously do so by 34 weeks. Midwives need to maintain their skills in undertaking a vaginal breech delivery through simulation, as the number of vaginal breech births is low. Many women with a breech presentation deliver by caesarean section as this is considered to decrease the perinatal morbidity and mortality (RCOG 2006a).

Breech labour and delivery is associated with a number of complications:

- early rupture of membranes, with increased risk of ascending infection
- uncoordinated contractions leading to prolonged labour
- increased risk of cord compression during first and second stage
- cord, foot, leg and arm prolapse
- early urge to push
- increased risk of operative delivery
- no moulding; head undergoes compression and decompression increasing the risk of intracranial haemorrhage during vaginal birth
- increased risk of trauma to vagina and pelvic floor
- increased risk of birth asphyxia
- increased perinatal morbidity and mortality.

A variety of methods can be used to encourage the fetus to turn from the breech to a cephalic presentation, including external cephalic version, adopting a knees chest position and acupuncture.

External cephalic version

External cephalic version (ECV) is undertaken by experienced personnel, usually obstetricians but could include midwives who have undergone further training. It should be offered to all women at or after 37 weeks who have an uncomplicated pregnancy and breech presentation to reduce caesarean section rates and the incidence of breech presentation at term (Hofmeyr & Kulier 2002a, Hutton & Hofmeyer 2006). The Royal College of Obstetricians and Gynaecologists (RCOG 2006b) suggests that nulliparous women should be offered ECV from 36 weeks. The National Institute for Health and Clinical Excellence (NICE 2008) agrees that all women with breech presentation should be offered ECV at 37 weeks; if this is not possible it should be at 36 weeks. Hutton & Hofmeyer (2006) found that ECV undertaken at 32–34 weeks

does not affect presentation at term or the caesarean section rate but concluded that there is insufficient evidence as to whether ECV between 34–36 weeks significantly affects either presentation or caesarean section rates and advise further research. Steen & Kingdon (2008) and the RCOG (2006b) suggest that ECV has a 50% success rate and is thus an important intervention in reducing the caesarean section rate undertaken routinely for breech presentation. Contraindications include:

- ruptured membranes
- oligohydramnios
- multiple pregnancy
- hydrocephalus
- placenta praevia
- antepartum haemorrhage within the previous 7 days
- abnormal cardiotocography
- major uterine abnormality
- maternal hypertension.

ECV should be undertaken during daylight hours in a unit where emergency facilities are available. Very occasionally, the fetus can become compromised during the procedure necessitating immediate delivery as a result of placental abruption or knotting of the umbilical cord.

It is important to ensure the following points are adhered to; the midwife can undertake many of these:

- the location of the placenta should be determined by ultrasonography because placenta praevia is a contraindication
- an abdominal palpation should be undertaken before the procedure to ensure there has been no spontaneous version and that the breech has not engaged
- cardiotocography should be undertaken before and after the procedure and should be reassurring
- the woman should have an empty bladder
- the uterus should not be contracting
- if pain is felt the procedure should be stopped
- anti-D immunoglobulin should be administered to Rhesus negative women within 72 hours of the procedure
- if the membranes rupture during the procedure, exclude cord prolapse
- the procedure is abandoned if the fetus does not turn easily (it can be reattempted after several days).

ECV encourages the fetus to rotate 180° by moving the breech away from the pelvic brim and then with one hand over each fetal pole, the fetal head is turned downwards while the breech is rotated upwards. The fetus is usually rotated face downwards to maintain flexion. However, if this is unsuccessful, an attempt can be made to turn the fetus backwards but it is important to maintain flexion of the head.

Knees–chest posture

This has been advocated by many health professionals over the years without being properly evaluated. Woman with breech presentations have been encouraged to assume a knees–chest posture for varying amounts of time, either every day or for a set number of days. There are variations in the frequency and duration of the posture; for example, the Elkins procedure requires women to adopt the position for 15 minutes every 2 hours when awake for 5 days (Smith et al 1999). Smith et al (1999) evaluated a modified Elkins procedure (knees–chest position for 15 minutes, three times a day) and found this did not reduce the incidence of breech presentation in labour or increase the success rate of ECV. They conclude that postural management is not an effective management option that should be offered routinely.

Dover (1999) suggests there are unanswered issues resulting from this study and suggests that postural management does not harm and may have some positive effects in relation to maternal emotional wellbeing. Hofmeyr & Kulier's (2002b) systematic review of the studies found the controlled studies were too small to provide any support or refute the use of postural management with breech presentation. Due to the ease with which postural management could be undertaken they suggest larger randomised trials should be performed to evaluate this further.

Acupuncture

Acupuncture is a form of traditional Chinese medicine that uses the energy (meridian) lines and acupuncture points believed to run throughout the body. The belief is that a difficulty within one of the energy lines will disrupt the body–mind–spirit relationship, thus correction and rebalancing the energy levels is at the centre of this treatment.

Acupuncture can only be administered by a trained acupuncturist who may use conventional acupuncture (insertion of needles into the skin at acupuncture sites), electroacupuncture (passing a small electric current through the needles inserted into the skin at acupuncture points) and moxibustion (applying moxa sticks to an acupuncture point on both feet (the lateral corner of the fifth toenail bed) for 15 minutes up to 10 times each day for a set number of days; the sticks are lit and allowed to smoke which applies heat to the acupuncture points).

Several studies report on the efficacy of acupuncture although the study numbers are generally small. One small study of 67 women demonstrated a highly significant effect of acupuncture in altering the presentation (78.7% of the intervention group versus 21.2% of the control group, $p < 0.001$) when undertaken twice a week from 34 to 37 weeks (Habek et al 2003).

Moxibustion has received favourable reports that it increases fetal activity that in turn encourages the fetus to move from a breech to a cephalic presentation (Budd 2000, Steen & Kingdon 2008) although Coyle et al (2005) caution that whilst moxibustion may reduce the number of ECVs undertaken and the use of oxytocin, the studies so far have been small and they recommend further research is undertaken.

Budd (2000) suggests that the treatment is cheap, with most women requiring only two moxa sticks, and that with further research to demonstrate the efficacy of moxibustion, midwives could be trained to undertake this, who in turn could instruct women or their partners in its use. Grabowska (2006) recommends using moxibustion twice a day for 15–20 minutes until the presentation changes to cephalic. Neri et al's (2007) small study found that the presentation changed following three treatments.

This is an area of growing interest and the reader is advised to keep abreast of the developments within acupuncture.

ROLE AND RESPONSIBILITIES OF THE MIDWIFE

These can be summarised as:

- keeping abreast with current changes in optimal fetal positioning to provide good evidence-based care
- education and support of the woman
- assisting at ECV unless trained to undertake the procedure.

Summary

- Postural management for rotating the occiput from a posterior to an anterior position is mainly anecdotal, with little support for undertaking the hands–knees position during pregnancy.
- Postural management for breech appears to bring no benefit but is not considered harmful.
- ECV in uncomplicated pregnancies has a high success rate although complications can arise during the procedure.
- Acupuncture, particularly moxibustion, increases fetal activity to encourage the breech to change to a cephalic presentation.
- Postural intervention requires further research to evaluate its efficacy.

SELF-ASSESSMENT EXERCISES

The answers to the following questions may be found in the text:

1. What advice can the midwife offer the woman regarding her posture and positioning that may assist the fetal occiput to rotate from a posterior to an anterior position?
2. What procedures can be used to change the presentation from breech to cephalic?
3. What are the role and responsibilities of the midwife in relation to optimal fetal positioning?
4. List the hazards associated with malpositions and malpresentations for the woman and the baby.

References

Budd S: Acupuncture. In Tiran D, Mack S, editors: *Complementary therapies*, ed 2, Edinburgh, 2000, Baillière Tindall, pp 79–104.

Coyle ME, Smith CA, Peat B: Cephalic version by moxibustion for breech presentation, *Cochrane Database Syst Rev* 2: CD003928 DOI: 10.1002/14651858.CD003928.pub2, 2005.

Dover S: Abstract writers' comments, *MIDIRS Midwifery Dig* 9(4):450, 1999

Grabowska C: Turning the breech using moxibustion, *Midwives* 9(12): 484–485, 2006.

Habek D, Habek JC, Jagust M: Acupuncture conversion of fetal breech presentation, *Fetal Diagn Ther* 18(6):418–421, 2003.

Hofmeyr GJ, Kulier R: External cephalic version for breech presentation at term, *Cochrane Library* 2: Update Software, Oxford, 2002a.

Hofmeyr GJ, Kulier R: Cephalic version by postural management for breech presentation, *Cochrane Library* 2: Update Software, Oxford, 2002b.

Hunter S, Hofmeyr GJ, Kulier R: Hands and knees posture in late pregnancy or labour for fetal malposition

(lateral or posterior), *Cochrane Database Syst Rev* 4: CD001063 DOI: 10.1002/14651858. CD001063.pub3, 2007.

Hutton EK, Hofmeyr GJ: External cephalic version for breech presentation before term, *Cochrane Database Syst Rev* 1: CD000084 DOI: 10.1002/14651858. CD000084.pub2, 2006.

Kariminia A, Chamberlain ME, Keogh J, et al: Randomised controlled trial of effect of hands and knees posturing on incidence of occiput posterior position at birth, *Br Med J* 328 (7438):490, 2004.

Lewis P: Malpositions and malpresentations. In Henderson C, MacDonald S, editors: *Mayes midwifery: a textbook for midwives*, ed 13, Edinburgh, 2004, Baillière Tindall.

Neri I, De Pace V, Venturini P, Facchinetti F: Effects of three different stimulations (acupuncture, moxibustion, acupuncture plus moxibustion) of BL.67 acupoint at small toe on fetal behavior of breech presentation, *Am J Chin Med* 35(1): 27–33, 2007.

NICE (National Institute for Health and Clinical Excellence): *Antenatal care: routine care for the healthy pregnant woman*, London, 2008, NICE.

RCOG (Royal College of Obstetricians and Gynaecologists): *The management of breech presentation Green Top Guideline 20b*, London, 2006a, RCOG.

RCOG (Royal College of Obstetricians and Gynaecologists): *External cephalic version and reducing the incidence of breech presentation Green Top Guideline 20a*, London, 2006b, RCOG.

Smith C, Crowther C, Wilkinson C, et al: Knee–chest postural management for breech at term: a randomised controlled trial, *Birth* 26(2):71–75, 1999.

Steen M, Kingdon C: Breech birth: Reviewing the evidence for external cephalic version and moxibustion, *Evidence Based Midwifery* 6(4): 126–129, 2008.

Sutton J, Scott P: *Understanding and teaching optimal foetal positioning*, ed 2, Tauranga, New Zealand, 1996, Bay Print.

Facilitation of related childbearing skills: speculum use

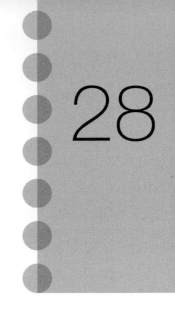

28

CHAPTER CONTENTS

A speculum is an instrument that is inserted into the vagina to open the vaginal walls and allow access to the top of the vagina and cervix. It can be an uncomfortable and embarrassing procedure for the woman and it is important it is undertaken correctly and sensitively. This chapter focuses on the use of the Cusco speculum.

LEARNING OUTCOMES

Having read this chapter the reader should be able to:

- discuss the indications for using a Cusco speculum
- describe how to insert the speculum
- discuss the role and responsibilities of the midwife in relation to speculum use.

Indications

The midwife may need to use a speculum:

- during preterm labour to assess the cervix

- to inspect around the top of the vagina and cervix for the presence of amniotic fluid when prelabour rupture of membranes is suspected
- to obtain a high vaginal swab
- to obtain a cervical smear.

Cusco speculum

The speculum is made of either metal (reusable) or plastic (disposable). It has two short blades that are curved across their width (Fig. 28.1). When the speculum is closed the blades close together, but when it is opened they separate to press against the vaginal walls. At one end there is a circular opening through which the vagina and cervix can be visualised and swabs inserted when required. Attached to this end are the handles that open and close the speculum by means of a screw mechanism. When the handles are apart the blades are closer together. To open the blades, bring the handles together. When inserting the speculum, ensure it has been introduced far enough into the vagina otherwise it will be difficult to visualise the cervix and take a swab (Hardy 2007).

Although insertion of the speculum is not usually painful, it may cause discomfort to the woman, particularly if she has sustained vaginal lacerations. A cold speculum may heighten the discomfort felt. The procedure may also be a source of embarrassment for the woman, provoking anxiety. Wright et al (2005) found that discomfort and anxiety were reduced when women were offered the opportunity for self-insertion of the speculum; however, these

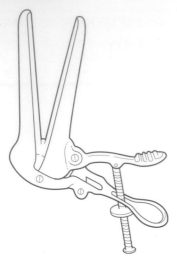

Figure 28.1 • Cusco speculum (Adapted with kind permission from Chilman & Thomas 1987)

were non-pregnant women, there have been no studies looking at the effects of self-insertion of speculums during pregnancy.

Asepsis

The speculum should be sterile and asepsis maintained throughout as ascending infection can result in uterine and neonatal sepsis; single-use disposable speculums are recommended (Tattersall 2006) and should not be reused (Wilkinson 2006). Sterile gloves should be worn if the membranes have ruptured; however, when obtaining a high vaginal swab or cervical smear, non-sterile gloves may be worn. A sterile vaginal examination (VE) pack and warm water can be used to clean the area and create a sterile field.

PROCEDURE: using a speculum

- Gain informed consent and privacy.
- Gather equipment:
  - sterile or non-sterile gloves (depending on the reason for speculum use)
  - speculum and lubricating jelly, e.g. KY Jelly®
  - disposable sheet
  - sterile VE pack containing swabs and a bowl
  - warm water
  - light source.
- Encourage the woman to empty her bladder.

- Ask the woman to adopt an almost recumbent position (a wedge can be used to avoid aortocaval occlusion if necessary), with her knees bent, ankles together and knees parted.
- Position the disposable sheet under the woman.
- Remove any sanitary towels or underwear, keeping the genital area covered.
- Wash hands and apply gloves.
- Clean the genital area by swabbing the perineum from front to back using cotton-wool balls or gauze soaked with the warm water, passing the swabs from the examining (clean) hand to the non-examining (dirty) hand; use each swab once and dispose of it (see Chapter 10).
- Lubricate the outer aspect of the blades of the speculum with a water-soluble lubricant, keeping the blades closed.
- Part the labia with the non-dominant hand and use the dominant hand to insert the speculum into the vagina in a downwards direction (with the width of the blades in the anterior–posterior diameter).
- When in place, turn the speculum 90° so that the handles are uppermost.
- Open the blades by unscrewing the handles and bringing them closer together, informing the woman that she may feel pressure as the blades stretch the vagina.
- Inspect the vagina and cervix if indicated, using a good light source to obtain the high vaginal swab (see Chapter 11) or cervical smear.
- To remove the speculum, close the blades taking care not to trap any maternal tissue, rotate the speculum back to its insertion position and withdraw the speculum.
- Remove the disposable sheet and assist the woman to replace her sanitary towel and knickers.
- Remove and dispose of gloves and equipment.
- Assist the woman into a comfortable position.
- Wash hands.
- Document findings and act accordingly.

ROLE AND RESPONSIBILITIES OF THE MIDWIFE

These can be summarised as:

- recognising the need for using a Cusco speculum
- ensuring the procedure is undertaken correctly, with minimal discomfort
- correct documentation.

Summary

- Speculum use can be an embarrassing and uncomfortable procedure for the woman.
- Undertaking the procedure correctly can reduce the discomfort experienced.
- Maintenance of asepsis is important to reduce the risk of uterine and neonatal infection.

SELF-ASSESSMENT EXERCISES

The answers to the following questions may be found in the text:

1. When might a midwife need to use a Cusco speculum?
2. What are the role and responsibilities of the midwife when using a speculum?

References

Chilman A, Thomas M: *Understanding nursing care*, ed 3, Edinburgh, 1987, Churchill Livingstone.

Hardy J: How to take a sample for cervical screening... art & science clinical skills: 13, *Nurs Stand* 21 (50):40–44, 2007.

Tattersall S: The use of vaginal specula in improving infection control, *Nurs Times* 102(9):53–55, 2006.

Wilkinson E: The implications of reusing single-use medical devices, *Nurs Times* 102(45):23, 2006.

Wright D, Fenwick J, Stephenson P, Monterosso L: Speculum 'self-insertion': a pilot study, *J Clin Nurs* 14(9):1098–1111, 2005.

Facilitation of related childbearing skills: membrane sweep

29

CHAPTER CONTENTS

This chapter considers the skill of sweeping or 'stripping' the membranes. As the cervical os is gently dilated (stretch) and the amnion is digitally separated from the lower uterine segment (sweep), intrauterine prostaglandin synthesis commences and so labour may be induced (Boulvain et al 2005). It is generally used prior to formal induction of labour (Enkin et al 2000). However, while the woman may appreciate assistance to commence labour without further intervention, sweeping the membranes is an uncomfortable procedure that may induce bleeding *per vaginam* and discomfort. Informed consent should include these aspects as well as expected outcome (see Chapter 30 for supporting information).

LEARNING OUTCOMES

Having read this chapter the reader should be able to:

- discuss the indications for membrane sweeping
- discuss the current evidence available
- describe how the procedure is performed
- summarise the role and responsibilities of the midwife.

The evidence

The Royal College of Obstetricians and Gynaecologists (RCOG 2001) indicates that sweeping the membranes increases the likelihood of spontaneous birth within 48 hours and birth within 1 week. It does, therefore, reduce the incidence of birth after term and formal methods of induction, e.g. prostaglandin (PGE_2), both of which have associated risks. The woman and baby do not appear to be at an increased risk of infection (Boulvain et al 2005). Although some studies suggest prelabour rupture of membranes is more likely to occur with membrane sweeping, de Miranda et al (2006) found this not to be so. Operative delivery figures are unchanged with the use of membrane sweeping. It is noted above that the woman may experience pain and bleeding with and after the procedure and some intermittent uterine activity in the hours and days following. The recommendation is that membrane sweeping should be offered to all women (except placenta praevia and any situation where labour or vaginal birth is not indicated) over 40 weeks gestation, prior to formal induction of labour. Nulliparous women should be offered the opportunity of a membrane sweep at 40 and 41 weeks; for parous women this should be offered at 41 weeks and both groups may be offered additional sweeps if labour does not begin spontaneously (NICE 2008).

De Miranda et al (2006) found membrane sweeping to be effective when repeated every 48 hours (three times a week) until labour commenced or the pregnancy reached 42 weeks' gestation and undertook three 360° sweeps on each occasion; however, the frequency at which membrane sweeping should be undertaken is still subject to debate. It is considered that prostaglandin synthesis directly correlates with the surface area of membrane detached. NICE (2008) and Enkin et al (2000) suggest that where the cervix is closed (and therefore the membranes inaccessible) cervical massage is undertaken; De Miranda et al (2006) suggest this is achieved by using the fore and middle fingers to make circular pushing and massaging movements on the cervix for 15 seconds duration. Whilst MacKenzie (1999) suggests that the cervix should be favourable, i.e. a Bishop score >8, for a membrane sweep to take place, it can be undertaken with lower Bishop scores in order to assist with ripening of the cervix.

The procedure should be completed according to local protocols, but it is likely that the woman already comes into the category of requiring induction of labour, that is, >40 weeks or a pregnancy complication that requires delivery. Care should be taken to avoid membrane rupture when the presenting part is not a well-engaged cephalic presentation, due to the dangers of cord prolapse. The procedure can be carried out in an outpatient setting, the home or hospital; asepsis should be maintained. The woman must be fully informed of what to expect following the procedure. The midwife needs to be trained in this aspect of care before undertaking the procedure. Contemporaneous record keeping should document the findings as well as the action taken.

PROCEDURE: stretch and sweep of the membranes

* Prepare for and undertake the examination *per vaginam* (as detailed on p 206 as far as 'Locate the cervix …') expecting to find a posterior, largely uneffaced, almost closed cervix (do not rupture the membranes).
* Undertake a Bishop's scoring (or similar) assessment of the cervix.
* Insert one or two fingers into the cervix and gently dilate the os. If the cervix is closed, undertake cervical massage for 15 seconds.

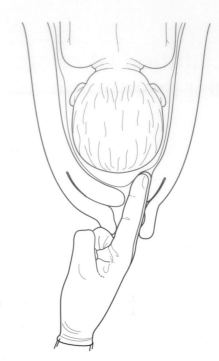

Figure 29.1 ● Sweeping the membranes

* Insert one or two fingers between the lower uterine segment and the fetal membranes and move the finger(s) with a sweeping circular action through 360° with some inward pressure (Fig. 29.1). Do this fairly decisively as the woman will be uncomfortable and this will be increased if the procedure is unnecessarily prolonged.
* Remove the examining hand gently, remove gloves.
* Auscultate the fetal heart.
* Assist the woman to dress and resume a comfortable position; discuss the findings.
* Dispose of equipment appropriately and wash hands.
* Document the findings and act accordingly.

ROLE AND RESPONSIBILITIES OF THE MIDWIFE

These can be summarised as:
* undertaking evidence-based care with knowledge and professionalism
* correct contemporaneous documentation.

Summary

- Sweeping the membranes involves dilating the cervical os and separating the membranes from the lower uterine segment prior to induction of labour for women who are to be formally induced.
- It is an uncomfortable procedure for the woman but may assist labour to begin naturally.

SELF-ASSESSMENT EXERCISES

The answers to the following questions may be found in the text:

1. Discuss the indications for membrane sweeping, citing the supporting evidence.
2. What clinical information does the midwife require prior to undertaking the procedure?
3. Describe how a midwife prepares for and carries out a membrane sweep.
4. Summarise the role and responsibilities of the midwife in relation to this procedure.

References

Boulvain M, Stan CM, Irion O: Membrane sweeping for induction of labour, *Cochrane Database Syst Rev* 1: CD000451. DOI: 10.1002/14651858.CD000451, pub2, 2005.

De Miranda E, van der Bom JG, Bonsel GJ, Bleker OP, Rosendaal FR: Membrane sweeping and prevention of post-term pregnancy in low-risk pregnancies: a randomised controlled trial, *Br J Obstet Gynaecol* 113(4): 402–408, 2006.

Enkin M, Keirse MJNC, Neilson J, et al: *A guide to effective care in pregnancy and childbirth*, Oxford, 2000, Oxford University Press.

MacKenzie I: Labor induction including pregnancy termination for fetal anomaly. In James D, Steer P, Weiner C, et al, editors: *High risk pregnancy*, London, 1999, W B Saunders, ch 62.

NICE (National Institute for Clinical Excellence): *Induction of labour*, London, 2008, NICE.

RCOG (Royal College of Obstetricians and Gynaecologists): *Induction of labour*, London, 2001, RCOG.

Principles of intrapartum skills: first-stage issues

30

CHAPTER CONTENTS

The first stage of labour is divided into two phases: latent and established. The National Institute for Health and Clinical Excellence (NICE 2007) defines the latent phase as the time when painful contractions occur with some cervical change, including effacement and dilatation up to 4 cm. Labour is established when the contractions are regular and painful and are accompanied by progressive cervical dilatation.

This chapter focuses on a selection of the skills used when caring for a woman during the first stage of labour; it is acknowledged that these skills may also be employed during the second stage of labour. In particular, this chapter addresses the skills of examination *per vaginam* during labour, commonly referred to as a vaginal examination (VE). This is an essential skill for the midwife when caring for a labouring woman, one that should be undertaken sensitively due to the intimate nature of the examination, but efficiently as the information gained will help assess progress and inform care. The procedure is invasive and considered a medical intervention, thus it should only be undertaken when necessary (Mandaza & Nolan 2001). The procedures for performing amniotomy and applying a fetal scalp electrode are also described. The chapter concludes with a discussion on different positions that may be adopted by the woman during the first stage of labour.

Having read this chapter the reader should be able to:

- list the indications for undertaking a VE during labour
- discuss the information that may be obtained from a VE and how this assesses progress
- discuss the role and responsibilities of the midwife when undertaking a VE
- describe the procedures for VE, amniotomy and the application of a fetal scalp electrode
- discuss the different positions that a woman may adopt during the first stage of labour and when each of these may be recommended.

Examination *per vaginam*

Indications

An examination *per vaginam* is an intimate procedure that should be undertaken only when there is a clear clinical indication. Levin et al (2005) found that women experience an average of three VEs during labour; some women will have more than this. NICE (2007) advise that the midwife (and doctor) should be sure that it is absolutely necessary and that the findings will provide important information to the decision making process; they advise that for women in normal labour the frequency of the examination should be every 4 hours, although this may be considered as too frequent by some women and midwives who will undertake the examination only when clinically indicated.

Women can find this procedure very distressing and it is important that the procedure is discussed with the woman prior to undertaking the procedure. This discussion should include: the rationale for the procedure, what will happen, what is expected of the woman and confirmation that the procedure can be stopped at any point if requested by the woman. This discussion should be undertaken in a manner that allows the woman to ask questions and also to refuse the examination. During the examination itself, it is important to maintain both verbal and non-verbal communication with the woman, recognising when she is experiencing discomfort/pain and requires the procedure to end and providing her with information (Stewart 2005). Levin et al (2005) found that only 70% of women recalled having the subject of VE discussed

with them before the procedure although 95% considered they were well informed of the findings. Only 40% felt they could refuse the examination and sadly 22.2% considered that their permission was not sought.

During labour, the midwife may undertake a VE to:

- confirm the onset of labour
- assess progress during labour
- identify the presentation and position
- perform an artificial rupture of membranes
- apply a fetal scalp electrode
- exclude cord prolapse following spontaneous rupture of the membranes where there is an ill-fitting presenting part
- confirm the onset of the second stage of labour, especially with a breech presentation and multiple pregnancy.

Contraindications

The midwife should not undertake a VE when there is:

- bleeding
- placenta praevia
- preterm rupture of the membranes
- preterm labour (the initial VE should be undertaken by the obstetrician; the midwife may perform subsequent examinations)
- no consent from the woman.

Information gained from undertaking an examination *per vaginam*

External genitalia

Any abnormalities such as varicosities, oedema, warts or signs of infection should be noted, as should scarring, particularly if indicative of previous perineal or labial trauma or female genital mutilation; NICE (2007) warns that a VE may be very difficult in the presence of fibulated genital mutilation. The colour, consistency, amount and odour of any discharge or bleeding from the vagina should be recorded; amniotic fluid may be seen if the membranes have ruptured.

Vagina

The vagina should feel warm and moist, with soft distensible walls. A hot, dry vagina could be indicative of dehydration, infection or obstructed labour. A vagina that feels tense may be associated with fear or previous scarring. The presence of varicosities, a cystocoele or rectocoele should be noted. A full rectum may be felt through the posterior vaginal wall.

Cervix

The cervix is assessed for position, consistency, effacement, dilatation and application to the presenting part. Prior to labour, the cervix is usually in a central or posterior position, firm, non-effaced with the os closed (unripe). In the latter weeks of pregnancy and early labour, the structure and position of the cervix alters as the cervix ripens, resulting in a cervix that feels less rigid and in an anterior position. A ripe cervix that feels soft and stretchy is associated with good dilatation of the os uteri, whereas a tight unyielding unripe cervix at term is more likely to be associated with prolonged labour. An unripe cervix requires three to four times more uterine effort than a ripe cervix (Burnhill et al 1962).

A cervix that is well applied to the presenting part is associated with good uterine activity (Blackburn 2007). The reverse may be true, that a poorly applied cervix is associated with less efficient uterine activity and slower progress. For example, when the fetus is in an occipitoposterior position, the head is not pushed directly onto the cervix; rather it is directed downwards and forwards against the back of the symphysis pubis, leading to a decrease in the effectiveness of uterine contractility, slower cervical dilatation and prolonged labour (Chamberlain 1993). The application of the cervix to the presenting part can be assessed by feeling between them.

Effacement usually precedes dilatation with the primigravida; these may appear to occur simultaneously with the multigravida. Effacement is assessed by the length of the cervix and the degree to which it protrudes into the vagina. A non-effaced cervix feels long and tubular, with the os closed or partly dilated. As effacement occurs, the cervix thins out and feels shorter, as the lower uterine segment takes it up (Fig. 30.1). A fully effaced cervix feels continuous with the lower uterine segment and does not protrude into the vagina.

Dilatation of the os uteri is measured in centimetres and is assessed by inserting one or both fingers through the external os and parting the fingers to assess the diameter. In early labour, when the cervix is less than 2 cm dilated, usually only one finger can be inserted. Towards the end of the first stage it may be easier to feel around the remaining rim of cervix to estimate dilatation; for example, a rim of 1 cm equates to a dilatation of 8 cm, as there is 2 cm of cervix remaining. When the cervix can no longer be felt, full dilatation has occurred, equal to 10 cm. This is the point at which the fetal head can pass through the cervix although for the preterm fetus, this may be less than 10 cm. If the presentation is breech, it is possible for the foot and leg to protrude through the cervix before it is fully dilated (footling breech). Dilatation of the os uteri should occur progressively throughout the first

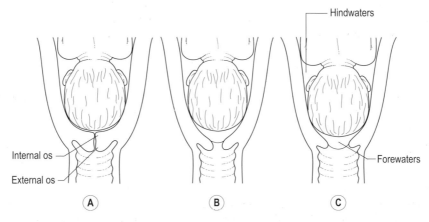

Figure 30.1 • Effacement of the cervix

stage of labour and is one factor in determining progress (NICE 2007 suggest this to be 0.5 cm or more per hour).

The os uteri is usually closed in the primigravida until labour begins, but the os of the multigravida may allow one or two fingers through before labour, commonly referred to as a 'multips os'.

The membranes

Intact membranes may be felt as a shiny surface over the presenting part. This can be difficult to feel, particularly in early labour or if the forewaters are shallow and the membranes tightly pressed against the presenting part. If the membranes are difficult to feel, it may be mistaken for ruptured membranes. When the presenting part is poorly applied to the cervix, the membranes contain a greater amount of fluid and may bulge through the cervix. As the pressure increases in the forewaters during contractions, the membranes can become tense and may rupture spontaneously. This usually occurs earlier when the presenting part is ill-fitting or poorly applied; for example, with a malposition such as an occipitoposterior position, malpresentation such as face presentation or a high presenting part. If the membranes are felt intact but amniotic fluid is leaking, a hindwater rupture is the likely cause. Pulsation felt beneath the membranes may be indicative of cord presentation or vasa praevia.

Presentation

In conjunction with information gained from the abdominal examination, the identification of landmarks on the presenting part help to confirm the presentation:

- A cephalic presentation is smooth, round and firm, and sutures or fontanelles may be felt. Moulding can be assessed by the degree of overlapping of the bones of the vault. Caput succedaneum may also be felt as a soft or firm mass on the presenting part, which can make the identification of sutures and fontanelles more difficult.
- Both the breech and face presentation feel soft and irregular. The sacrum may be palpable as a hard bone, with the anus close by and the landmarks are felt in a straight line. If a finger is inadvertently inserted into the anus, it will be gripped. Fresh meconium is also likely to be present.

- With the face presentation, the orbital ridges may be felt and a finger inserted into the mouth may be sucked, the landmarks are located in a triangular position. If a face presentation is suspected or confirmed, care should be taken to avoid damaging the eyes; application of a fetal scalp electrode is not recommended and obstetric cream should not be used as it could initiate a chemical conjunctivitis.
- If the cord presents, the pulsations can be palpated through the membranes – the membranes should not be ruptured due to the danger of cord prolapse. If a cord is felt without membranes the emergency procedure for managing cord prolapse should be instigated whilst the examining midwife keeps her fingers in the vagina in an attempt to push the presenting part off the cord.

Level of the presenting part

This is determined by assessing the distance between the presenting part and the ischial spines in centimetres (Fig. 30.2). The ischial spines are referred to as zero station, with the presenting part being above (− cm) or below (+ cm) this. The ischial spines may be difficult to palpate; this becomes a subjective measurement. It is important for the midwife to ensure it is the level of the presenting part being assessed and not caput succedaneum. Descent of the presenting part is one indicator of progress during labour and the assessment should correlate with the findings from the degree of engagement determined during the abdominal examination.

Position

With a cephalic presentation, identification of sutures and fontanelles will confirm the position and attitude:

- The sagittal suture is easily identified as a long straight suture; its position is taken in relation to the maternal pelvis, moving from back to front.
- A sagittal suture in the right oblique is felt moving from the posterior right quadrant of the maternal pelvis obliquely forwards to the left anterior quadrant (Fig. 30.3) and is indicative of left occipitoanterior position or right occipitoposterior position.
- The posterior fontanelle is felt as a small triangular area, with three sutures running

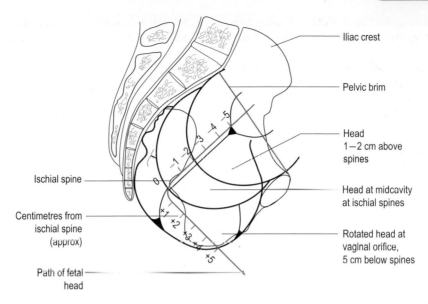

Figure 30.2 • Level of presenting part in relation to the ischial spines

Figure 30.3 • Rotation of a cephalic presentation felt on examination *per vaginam*

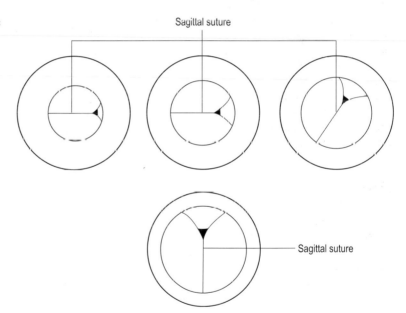

from it; it is indicative of a well-flexed cephalic presentation, usually occipitoanterior position.

- The anterior fontanelle is felt as a larger, diamond-shaped area, with four sutures running from it and is associated with a deflexed head, usually with an occipitoposterior position.

Progress is indicated where there is progressive flexion (or extension if a face presentation) and

rotation. Comparing the position of the landmarks from all previous VEs should demonstrate this.

Pelvic outlet

This is assessed by feeling for the ischial spines; if prominent, the transverse diameter of the outlet is reduced and could affect progress, particularly in the second stage of labour. The subpubic angle is assessed by moving the top part of the two examining fingers towards the pubic arch. Two fingers should fit snugly under the pubic arch, indicating an angle of 90° or greater. A reduced subpubic angle is often found with prominent ischial spines and may be associated with an android pelvis. This can result in more pressure being placed on the perineum and increased perineal trauma as well as delay in the second stage of labour. Care should be taken when assessing the subpubic angle to avoid the clitoris; pressure on this structure can be painful.

PROCEDURE: examination
per vaginam

The procedure should be carried out using an aseptic technique. Although sterile VE packs and lotions to wash the genital area are used in many labour wards, McCormick (2001) has demonstrated that the infection rate is unaffected by their use. She proposes that stringent hand hygiene and using sterile gloves (and avoiding their contamination) is as effective in minimising the risk of infection and more cost effective than using VE packs and lotions. NICE (2007) advise that tap water is sufficient for perineal cleansing where it is required. The midwife should refer to the hospital policy for local requirements on perineal cleansing. The procedure for perineal cleansing follows this procedure. If an assistant is present, she can open packs and equipment for the midwife.

- Discuss the procedure fully with the woman and gain informed consent.
- Ensure privacy.
- Gather equipment:
  ○ apron
  ○ sterile gloves
  ○ lubricant, e.g. water-soluble lubricant, obstetric cream (the latter should not be used with a face presentation)
  ○ disposable sheet
  ○ other equipment as necessary, e.g. amnihook, fetal scalp electrode
  ○ Pinard stethoscope or sonicaid.
- Encourage the woman to empty her bladder.
- Undertake an abdominal palpation to ascertain the lie, presentation, position, degree of engagement and auscultate the fetal heart.

- Ask the woman to adopt an almost recumbent position (use a wedge to avoid aortocaval occlusion if necessary), with her knees bent, ankles together and knees parted, placing the disposable sheet beneath her buttocks (be aware of the difficulty experienced by women with pelvic girdle pain when opening their legs).
- Remove any sanitary towels or underwear, keeping the genital area covered.
- Apply apron; wash and dry hands.
- Open the equipment to be used including the lubricating gel.
- Apply hand gel, allow to dry then put on gloves.
- Ask the woman to lift up the cover to allow access to the genital area.
- Lubricate the first two fingers of the dominant hand with antiseptic cream.
- With the thumb and forefinger of the non-examining hand, part the labia, observing the condition of the vulva.
- Inform the woman of what you are about to do and then, if no contraction present, gently insert the first two fingers of the examining hand into the vagina, in a downwards and backwards direction along the anterior vaginal wall, ensuring the thumb does not come into contact with the woman's clitoris or anus.
- Locate the cervix and determine the position, tone, degree of effacement and dilatation and application to the presenting part.
- Move the fingers through the cervical os to ascertain the presence of the forewaters and the presentation, position, degree of flexion and level of the presenting part; the presence of caput succedaneum and degree of moulding should be noted.
- If necessary and consent has been gained prior to the examination, rupture the membranes and/or apply a fetal scalp electrode (pp 207–209).
- Withdraw the fingers gently, assessing the pelvic outlet.
- Auscultate the fetal heart.
- Assist the woman into a comfortable position, reapply sanitary pad if required and discuss the findings.
- Dispose of equipment appropriately and wash hands.
- Document the findings and act accordingly.

PROCEDURE: perineal cleansing

A VE pack and water for cleansing will be required. The midwife should follow the procedure for examination *per vaginam* up to asking the woman to lift the cover up. The midwife is then required to:

- Swab the perineum from front to back using cotton-wool balls or gauze soaked with the warm water, passing the swabs from the examining (clean) hand to the non-examining (dirty) hand (see Chapter 10); use each swab once and dispose of it.
- The procedure then continues as described above in the section 'PROCEDURE: examination *per vaginam*' from the point 'Lubricate the first two fingers of the dominant hand . . .'.

Amniotomy (artificial rupture of membranes)

Intact membranes provide a cushion that fits appropriately into the cervix during labour, helping to apply an even pressure and giving some protection to the presenting part from compression and infection. Many midwives would not rupture membranes unless specifically indicated, believing that spontaneous rupture follows a more natural labour. Romano (2008) suggests that over two-thirds of women reach full dilatation prior to spontaneous rupture of the membranes occurs.

Amniotomy disrupts the normal process of labour and may lead to other interventions occurring (Andrees & Rankin 2007, Svardby et al 2007). NICE (2007) and Smyth et al (2007) caution that amniotomy should not be undertaken with normal progressing labour. When the membranes are not present the presenting part presses more directly onto the cervix; pain is often greater as more prostaglandin is released and so contractions increase in strength and frequency. Svardby et al (2007) advise that amniotomy is commonly undertaken where labour progress is slow or absent; based on cervical dilatation only, this occurs when the cervix dilates at less than 0.5 cm per hour (NICE 2007). NICE (2007) concurs with this, advising amniotomy will shorten the labour length by 1 hour but may increase the strength of the contractions and therefore increase the amount of pain felt. Smyth et al (2007), however, disagree with this view and recommend that amniotomy is not undertaken routinely in labours that are prolonged.

Variations of the fetal heart (namely, early decelerations) can be seen after artificial rupture of membranes (ARM). These may lead to further intervention; there is an increased risk of caesarean delivery and cord prolapse (Smyth et al 2007). Amniotic fluid embolism (anaphylactoid syndrome of pregnancy) is known to be a rare side effect associated with ARM (Mato 2008).

The use of standard precautions is indicated and the sharpness of the amnihook means that the midwife must take care to avoid personal injury and must dispose of the hook into a sharps box.

Indications

- Induction of labour.
- Augmentation of labour.
- Application of fetal scalp electrode and/or assessment of liquor colour.
- Maternal request.
- Often prior to birth of second twin.

Contraindications

- High presenting part (risk of cord prolapse).
- Preterm labour.
- Known vaginal infection.
- Maternal HIV-positive status.
- Caution is taken with polyhydramnios or any malposition or malpresentation.
- Placenta praevia.
- Vasa praevia.

A controlled ARM is sometimes performed when the presenting part is high. An obstetrician performs the ARM while the midwife applies light pressure to the fundus. This encourages the presenting part to engage in the pelvis as the membranes rupture. The obstetrician ensures that the fluid has drained and no cord has prolapsed before removing the hand.

PROCEDURE: artificial rupture of the membranes

- Discuss the indication with the woman and gain her informed consent.
- Gather equipment:
  - equipment as for vaginal examination
  - amnihook.

- Undertake a vaginal examination as detailed on page 206, maintaining the sterility of the amnihook.
- Locate the cervix using the examining hand; ensure that all factors are favourable for ARM to be undertaken, e.g. descent of presenting part, keeping fingers in the cervix, no pulsation felt beneath the examining fingers.
- Use the non-examining hand to slide the amnihook carefully, with the hook pointing downwards, between the examining hand and anterior vaginal wall.
- Guide the amnihook into place with the examining hand, placing the hook against the membranes.
- Twist the amnihook slightly using the non-examining hand to tear the membranes.
- Withdraw the amnihook gently, retaining the fingers in the cervix as the amniotic fluid drains out (ensuring the amniotic fluid does not come into contact with the midwife's clothing).
- The examining fingers can then locate the tear and digitally increase the size of the opening.
- Undertake a reassessment of the cervix, fetal descent and position.
- A scalp electrode can be applied if indicated (see below).
- Withdraw the hand, auscultate the fetal heart.
- Assist the woman re: hygiene, comfort and position.
- Discuss the findings with the woman.
- Dispose of equipment correctly and wash hands.
- Document the indications for ARM with the findings and act accordingly.

Rupturing the membranes with an amnihook is sometimes easier to do if a contraction is present and the membranes are bulging under the pressure. This is not an absolute necessity, however. Clearly the membranes do need to be intact; membranes that are tight across the baby's head may be deceptive, causing the midwife to question their presence. Care should be taken to ensure that neither the baby nor the woman is scratched with the hook.

Application of a fetal scalp electrode

When continuous cardiotocograph monitoring is indicated, a fetal scalp electrode (FSE) may be applied to ensure continuity of contact. The electrode transfers fetal heart sounds from conductivity in the fetal scalp to a transducer located on the woman's thigh, attached to the electrocardiograph (ECG) port on the monitor. The sound of the fetal heart is continuous regardless of maternal or fetal position. It is not accompanied or confused by sounds of fetal movement or uterine blood flow. It is an invasive procedure for both the woman and the fetus; the electrode is secured under the fetal scalp, with either a clip or spiral connection. It is assumed that the fetus experiences some pain and the transfer of viruses such as HIV and herpes simplex (Baker 2007) from mother to child is more likely (both are contraindications to FSE use). Skin infection or long-term scarring can occur.

Needs et al (1992) found clip electrodes performed better than other types with regard to attachment. The clip is applied by rotating the end of the electrode: anticlockwise rotation causes the clip to recede into the electrode head; clockwise rotation causes it to emerge from the electrode head and be caught on the scalp. It is often spring loaded and therefore rarely requires an active rotation clockwise. The Copeland FSE is commonly used and is considered to reduce the risk of needlestick injury as it has a protecting penetrating needle; this also controls the depth of penetration reducing the risk of fetal injury to the skull (Cutlan 2006). A spiral electrode is rotated in the direction of the spiral, usually clockwise, until caught under the scalp.

Accuracy of scalp electrodes depends upon their correct application. If membrane is between the electrode and the scalp then the tracing is likely to be unreliable, sometimes known as 'artefact'. Interpretation of the trace is impossible. The electrode should not be near or through a fontanelle or suture line, the cervix or vagina – it should be on the skin folds of the scalp. It can be used on the buttocks of a breech presentation, but causes obvious scarring. It should not be used with a face presentation.

PROCEDURE: application of a fetal scalp electrode

- Discuss the indication with the woman and gain her consent.
- Ensure that the monitor has the ECG facility and correct leads.
- Gather equipment:
  ○ equipment as for vaginal examination with amnihook if membranes are intact
  ○ sterile fetal scalp electrode.

- Undertake a vaginal examination as detailed on page 206.
- Perform ARM (pp 207, 208) if membranes intact.
- Locate the fetal scalp using the examining hand; ensure that sutures and fontanelles are avoided.
- Use the non-examining hand to slide the scalp electrode carefully between the examining hand and vaginal wall.
- Guide the electrode into place with the examining hand, supporting the head of the electrode against the scalp.
- Turn the end of the electrode anticlockwise, then release to attach to the scalp, using the non-examining hand.
- The electrode should be attached to the scalp; a gentle pull will confirm whether it is attached.
- An assistant may attach the leads to the transducer and the transducer to the monitor while the examining hand remains in place; if the electrode is not working reapplication may be tried.
- Check that the electrode is securely placed over an appropriate area of the scalp, withdraw the hand.
- Apply conductive gel to the transducer or the appropriate fastening and attach around the woman's thigh using a small belt or attach to the monitor on the woman's abdomen if appropriate (e.g. EZIplug 3 attaches to either the leg or the abdomen; Cutlan 2006); ensure that monitoring is satisfactorily taking place.
- Assist the woman with regard to hygiene, comfort and position.
- Explain the differences that can be heard.
- Dispose of equipment correctly and wash hands.
- Document the indications for FSE with other aspects of the examination and act accordingly.

Removal of the fetal scalp electrode

An FSE is usually removed at delivery. To do this the electrode head is held against the scalp while the end is rotated anticlockwise. Care should be taken not to create any trauma while removing it. An obvious scar should be noted on the initial birth examination. The electrode should be disposed of as per the disposal of sharps policy.

Maternal positioning

During the first stage of labour women should be encouraged to adopt whichever positions they find comfortable (NICE 2007). Lewis et al (2002) suggest that, given the freedom to do so, women will change position throughout labour and a change in positions should be encouraged to avoid the occurrence of pressure ulcer formation (see Chapter 53). Some women will find changing position more difficult due to constraints such as epidural anaesthesia or continuous fetal heart rate monitoring; the midwife can still enable the woman to make some changes to her position (e.g. side-lying). The Royal College of Midwives (RCM) (2008) suggest that the midwife is in a key position to encourage mobility and position changes for labouring women.

Positions adopted vary from upright (including walking, sitting, kneeling, squatting, all fours) to recumbent (including supine, semi-recumbent, lateral or side-lying); Chapman (2009) suggests that upright positions are more comfortable than sitting positions. Upright positions can also result in a shorter first stage, less severe pain and less narcotic and epidural use (Lamaze 2009, RCM 2008). The National Childbirth Trust (NCT 2009) encourage women to keep moving in labour and also advocate rocking, swaying or hip wiggling, walking around and up and down stairs and the use of a birthing ball to remain upright. Lamaze (2009) support the use of upright positions, suggesting gravity can assist with descent of the presenting part, and moving around during labour can help the pelvic bones accommodate the fetus during its travels through the pelvis, a view supported by Simkin & Ancheta (2005). Midwives advocate the use of stair walking or lifting one leg onto a surface so that the leg is higher than the other knee where labour appears to be slowing or asynclitism is present.

There is a lack of randomised controlled trials evaluating positions used in the first stage of labour; much of the evidence is anecdotal. Lewis et al (2002) are undertaking a systematic review of the randomised controlled trials looking at the effects of different positions in relation to maternal, fetal and labour outcomes for the Cochrane database and the reader is advised to read their review when it is available.

All fours

Stremler et al (2005) found that women who were labouring with fetuses in an occipitoposterior position experienced less backache when adopting an all fours position. This may also be achieved by leaning over a birthing ball to relieve pressure on the woman's arms. It may be more comfortable for the woman if she has support/cushioning under her knees (e.g. pillow, padded mat). Hanson (2009) suggests an open knee–chest position can help to reduce the premature urge to push whilst a closed knee–chest position is useful if the cervix is oedematous.

Lateral (side-lying)

To encourage fetal rotation from an occipitoposterior to an occipitoanterior position, Ridley (2007) suggests that women should lie on their side, ensuring it is the same side as the position of the fetal spine (e.g. lie on right side for right occipito-posterior position), as this was found to increase the incidence of spontaneous vaginal delivery, decrease the length of labour and the risk of caesarean section compared with lying on the opposite side or any other position. For women with restricted mobility, such as those with an epidural *in situ*, side-lying may be a way of alternating position and relieving pressure from the buttocks and sacral area.

Supine

When the woman lies flat, the weight of the pregnant uterus can compress the major blood vessels (aortocaval compression) which can compromise maternal cardiac function and uterine blood flow. This in turn can affect the fetus and cause alterations in the fetal acid-base status (Lewis et al 2002). Contractions can appear to be less strong in the supine position compared to upright or lateral positions (Lewis et al 2002). Thus if a woman wishes to lie supine, it is advisable to place a wedge under her right side to relieve the pressure off the aorta.

Semi-recumbent

This is often the position adopted by women in labour and is convenient for the midwife when certain procedures are required (e.g. abdominal palpation, examination *per vaginam*). Kerrigan (2006) suggests there is little evidence to support use of

this position; however, some women may need to rest and adopt this position periodically during labour.

These can be summarised as:

- undertaking a competent examination in which all of the information is gained
- undertaking an amniotomy correctly, if indicated
- appropriate application of a fetal scalp electrode, if indicated
- encouraging the use of appropriate alternative positions to enhance the comfort of the woman and labour progress
- recognising deviations from the norm and instigating referral
- education, explanations and support of the woman
- appropriate record keeping.

Summary

- An examination *per vaginam* is an invasive procedure but one that can yield valuable information in relation to the assessment of progress in labour.
- Amniotomy may be undertaken for induction or augmentation of labour.
- Fetal scalp electrodes offer continuity of contact if continuous fetal monitoring is indicated.
- The risk of ascending infection is high; an aseptic technique should be used throughout.
- Women should be encouraged to change position during the first stage of labour and use those which are most comfortable.
- There is a need for more evidence regarding the advantages and disadvantages of the different positions used.

SELF-ASSESSMENT EXERCISES

The answers to the following questions may be found in the text:

1. For what reasons would the midwife undertake an examination *per vaginam* during labour?
2. What is the procedure for performing an examination *per vaginam*?
3. How could the midwife identify a flexed cephalic presentation?
4. How does the information gained from an examination *per vaginam* help to assess progress?

5. Describe how to perform an amniotomy and application of a fetal scalp electrode.

6. What are the role and responsibilities of the midwife in relation to an examination *per vaginam*, artificial rupture of the membranes and application of a fetal scalp electrode?

7. What advice can the midwife give to a woman regarding positioning during the first stage of labour?

References

Andrees M, Rankin J: Amniotomy in spontaneous, uncomplicated labour at term, *Br J Midwifery* 15(10): 612–616, 2007.

Baker DA: Consequences of herpes simplex virus in pregnancy and their prevention, *Curr Opin Infect Dis* 20(1):73–76, 2007.

Blackburn ST: *Maternal, fetal and neonatal physiology: a clinical perspective*, ed 3, St Louis, 2007, Saunders.

Burnhill MS, Donezis J, Cohen J: Uterine contractility during labour studied by intra-amniotic fluid pressure recordings, *Am J Obstet Gynaecol* 83:561–571, 1962.

Chamberlain GVP: *Obstetrics by ten teachers*, ed 16, London, 1993, Arnold.

Chapman V: Slow progress and malpresentations/malpositions in labour. In Chapman V, Charles C, editors: *The midwife's labour and birth handbook*, ed 2, Chichester, 2009, Wiley-Blackwell, pp 106–134.

Cutlan C: Electronic fetal monitoring and infection control, *Br J Midwifery* 14(10):584–585, 2006.

Hanson L: Second stage labour: challenges in spontaneous bearing down, *J Perinat Neonatal Nurs* 23(1):31–39, 2009.

Kerrigan A: The mother-midwife partnership: A critical analysis of intrapartum care, *Br J Midwifery* 14(6):346–350, 2006.

Lamaze : The six cares that support normal birth, 2009: *Care Practice #2:*

Freedom of Movement Throughout Labour. Online. Available: http://www.lamaze.org/carepractices/CarePractice2.pdf 26 March 2009.

Levin D, Fearon B, Hemmings V, et al: Informing women during vaginal examination, *Br J Midwifery* 13(1):26–29, 2005.

Lewis L, Webster J, Carter A, et al: Maternal positions and mobility during first stage of labour, *Cochrane Database Syst Rev* 4: CD003934. DOI.:10.1002/14651858. CD003934, 2002.

Mandaza P, Nolan M: Clinical file. Case study. Vaginal examinations in labour, *Pract Midwife* 4(6):22, 2001.

Mato J: Suspected fluid embolism following amniotomy: a case report, *AANA* 76(1):53–59, 2008.

McCormick C: Vulval preparations in labour: use of lotions or tap water, *Br J Midwifery* 9(7):453–455, 2001.

National Childbirth Trust: NCT information sheet: Straightforward birth. Online. Available: www.nct.org.uk/info-centre/publications/view/45 26 March 2009, 2009.

Needs L, Grant A, Sleep J, et al: A randomised controlled trial to compare three types of fetal scalp electrode, *Br J Obstet Gynaecol* 99 (4):302–306, 1992.

NICE (National Institute for Health and Clinical Excellence): Intrapartum care: Care of healthy women and their babies during childbirth, London, 2007, NICE.

RCM (Royal College of Midwives): Positions for labour and birth, *Midwifery Pract Guide*. Online Available: http://www.rcm.org.uk/college/standards-and-practice/practice-guidelines/ 26 March 2009, 2008.

Ridley RT: Diagnosis and intervention for occiput posterior malposition, *J Obstet, Gynaecol Neonatal Nurs* 36(2):135–143, 2007.

Romano AM: Research summaries for normal birth, *J Perinat Educ* 17 (1):48–52, 2008.

Simkin P, Ancheta R: *The labor progress handbook: Early interventions to prevent and treat dystocia*, ed 2, Oxford, 2005, Blackwell.

Smyth RMD, Alldred SK, Markham C: Amniotomy for shortening spontaneous labour, *Cochrane Database Syst Rev* 4: CD006167. DOI.:10.1002/14651858. CD006167, pub2, 2007.

Stewart M: 'I'm just going to wash you down': sanitizing the vaginal examination, *J Adv Nurs* 51(6): 587–594, 2005.

Stremler R, Hodnett E, Petryshen P, et al: Randomised controlled trial of hands-and-knees positioning for occipitoposterior position in labour, *Birth: Issues Perinat Care* 32(14): 243–251, 2005.

Svardby K, Nordstrom L, Sellstroni E: Primiparas with or without oxytocin augmentation: A prospective descriptive study, *J Clin Nurs* 16(1):179–184, 2007.

Principles of intrapartum skills: second-stage issues

31

CHAPTER CONTENTS

The second stage of labour lasts from the time the cervix is fully dilated until the birth of the baby, during which time the baby descends and rotates through the pelvis, the contractions change to become expulsive and the perineum stretches and thins out. This chapter will review the current evidence and clinical skills utilised during care in the second stage of labour and will encompass a discussion on the definition and duration of the second stage, the effects of directed and spontaneous pushing, different maternal positions and the management of a nuchal cord. The chapter concludes with a discussion on when and how to undertake an episiotomy.

LEARNING OUTCOMES

Having read this chapter the reader should be able to:

- discuss the evidence and opinions relating to recognition, duration, pushing, positions, nuchal cord and perineal management during the second stage of labour
- discuss the preparation for and conduct of a normal delivery
- describe how to infiltrate the perineum and incise an episiotomy
- discuss the role and responsibilities of the midwife throughout.

Definition

The second stage of labour has traditionally been defined by a very clinical description: from full dilatation of the os uteri to the complete birth of the baby. It is now recognised that this stage of labour has both a passive and an active phase [National Institute for Health and Clinical Excellence (NICE) 2007].

The passive phase is the time from when the cervix is fully dilated but there is no urge to push. This has also been referred to as the 'rest and descent', 'rest and be thankful' or the 'pause for rotation' stage when the fetus descends passively (Brancato et al 2008, Long 2006, Williams 2007). Long (2006) suggests that this follows the transition phase, which occurs at the end of the first stage, and that it is a time when the woman may feel drowsy and relaxed; the presenting part may still be high. Yildirim & Beji (2008) argue that women cannot push effectively if the urge to push is absent and that pushing during the passive phase should be discouraged as this can lead to maternal exhaustion.

The active phase is recognised when the woman experiences expulsive contractions and has a strong urge to push, the cervix is fully dilated and the baby is visible (NICE 2007). The active phase will also commence when the woman begins to push once the cervix is fully dilated even in the absence of expulsive contractions, for example, with epidural anaesthesia (NICE 2007). The urge to push begins with the stimulation of the Ferguson's reflex as the fetus descends onto the pelvic floor.

Delaying pushing until the woman is in the active phase of the second stage has many advantages for both the woman and the baby. These include: less maternal exhaustion, increased confidence in her own ability, less perineal trauma, reduced incidence of bladder and pelvic injury, reduced risk of instrumental delivery, reduced incidence of fetal heart abnormalities, higher Apgar scores at 1 and 5 minutes and higher umbilical cord arterial pH (Allbers & Borders 2007, Brancato et al 2008, Nicholl & Cattell 2006, Roberts & Hanson 2007, Roberts et al 2004, Schaffer et al 2005, Simpson & James 2005, Yildirim & Beji 2008).

Recognition

Recognition of the second stage has been classified by signs such as a change in contraction frequency and nature (expulsive), a heavy blood-stained show (as the operculum descends), pouting of the vulva and anus (as the fetal head descends onto the soft tissues), visible fetus at the introitus (always ensure this is not caput succedaneum) or use of vaginal examination which reveals the absence of a locatable cervix. However, skilled, intuitive, observant midwives will be very familiar with situations in which the urge to push is gradual or arises before full dilatation. Equally, the woman may become particularly vocal or particularly quiet and withdrawn, have a purple line that extends up the anal cleft (Hobbs 1998), display changes in abdominal shape (Burvill 2002) or sacral curve (rhombus of Michaelis; Sutton 2003) or feel that she can't go on, is tired or – in contrast – is renewed with energy. Our researched understanding of these issues remains limited; nevertheless a truly 'tuned

in' midwife will support the woman in her intuitive actions and sounds while maintaining good clinical observation and skill.

Duration

NICE (2007) suggests that the baby should be born within 3 hours (nulliparous women) or 2 hours (multiparous women) from the beginning of the active phase for most women although they suggest referral may be required an hour before the end of these time limits. Cheng et al (2007) found that a second stage lasting longer than 3 hours for multiparous women was associated with increased risk of operative delivery, increased maternal morbidity and lower Apgar scores. The length of the second stage will be affected by factors such as maternal position and epidural anaesthesia and the midwife should continue to observe for signs of normality and progress whilst recognising and managing any deviations from the norm.

Pushing: directed or spontaneous

Spontaneous pushing is likely to occur when the woman reaches the active phase of the second stage of labour due to the strong urge to push that accompanies this stage. Women may not begin to push until the contraction has built up and will often use short pushes lasting 5–7 seconds 3–5 times during a contraction (Di Franco et al 2007, Perez-Botella & Downe 2006). The duration of the second stage is not significantly increased with the use of spontaneous pushing (Sampselle et al 2005), with some studies suggesting the time is reduced (Yildirim & Beji 2008).

Directed pushing occurs when the woman is told how to push – usually this involves breath holding, taking breaths quickly between pushes and 3–4 sustained pushes from when the contraction begins to when it ends. Breath holding increases intrathoracic pressure which can decrease the venous return to the heart, thereby reducing cardiac output and blood pressure. This in turn can reduce uterine blood flow and placental perfusion, and the amount of oxygen available to the fetus, increasing the likelihood of fetal heart rate abnormalities occurring (Perez-Botella & Downes 2006, Roberts & Hanson 2007). Hanson (2009) advises that women should be encouraged to push spontaneously or breathe through a contraction where fetal heart rate abnormalities occur until the fetus recovers. Additionally there is more strain placed on the urinary, pelvic and perineal structures increasing their risk of damage (Roberts & Hanson 2007, Schaffer et al 2005). Breath holding can make women feel dizzy, causing them to gasp; a sudden surge of blood back to the heart may occur, resulting in rebound hypertension (Perez-Botella & Downes 2006).

Women should be encouraged to follow what their bodies are telling them to do and push when they have the urge (NICE 2007). In some situations the woman may not experience the urge to push (e.g. epidural anaesthesia). In this situation women may need some instruction on when and how to push (Young 2005); the principles of spontaneous pushing should be followed, for example, no breath holding, short bursts allowing the contraction to build up first.

Position

De Jonge et al (2007a) propose that the routine use of the supine position should be considered an intervention in normal labour as when given the choice women opt to use a variety of positions during the second stage of labour. They highlight the importance of midwives facilitating choice for women rather than encouraging a semi-recumbent position which is more comfortable for the midwife. Lewis et al (2002) agree suggesting that women who are able to move around have an increased sense of control and require less analgesia. NICE (2007) also recommend women should be encouraged to adopt the position of their choice whilst being discouraged from lying supine or semi-supine.

Gupta et al (2004) found the use of an upright position (standing, squatting, kneeling, all fours, birthing chair or stool, sitting upright) reduced the length of the second stage, the incidence of assisted deliveries, the incidence of abnormal fetal heart rates and reporting of less severe pain. There was also an increased risk of second-degree tears and blood loss greater than 500 mL. However, Allbers & Borders (2007) found that fewer perineal tears and less pain were associated with upright and lateral delivery positions. De Jonge et al (2007b) found the increased blood loss associated with upright positions originated from perineal damage, those women with an intact perineum did not have an increased blood loss when

semi-sitting or sitting. Di Franco et al (2007) consider upright positions make use of gravity and allow the pelvic diameters to increase although they acknowledge they are more tiring than semi-recumbent positions. To combat this, they recommend the use of a supported squat where the woman is supported under her arms allowing her to put less weight on her legs and feet, and her trunk to become longer, which can provide greater space for the fetus to move through the pelvis. Soong & Barnes (2005) found a significant increase in perineal trauma in women adopting the semi-recumbent position compared with the all fours position. These effects were more noticeable with women undergoing their first vaginal birth and where the birth weight was in excess of 3500 g. The use of the all fours position may be more comfortable for women who are labouring with the fetus in an occipito-posterior position.

Ragnar et al (2006) compared the use of kneeling and sitting upright and conclude that they do not differ significantly in their outcomes, although kneeling was associated with more favourable maternal experiences and reduced pain. It was considered that kneeling allowed women the freedom to modify their position more easily, thus allowing women to feel more in control.

Sutton (2003) suggests that pelvic diameters are increased when the woman adopts a lateral position. Soong & Barnes (2005) found that women with epidural anaesthesia were more likely to require suturing when they were in a semi-recumbent rather than a lateral position. Nicholl & Cattell (2006) support the use of a lateral position when delivery is undertaken on the bed as this helps to increase the number of intact perineums and reduce the incidence of fourth-degree tears.

Women should avoid excessive and prolonged knee holding (more likely in supine and semi-recumbent positions or prolonged squatting) as this can cause compressive peroneal neuropathy (functional and/or pathological changes to the peroneal nerve which supplies the calf and foot) which can present as knee tenderness, foot drop, decreased sensation over the dorsum of the foot (Sahai-Srivastava & Amezcua 2007).

Midwives can therefore:

- encourage and support women to adopt the positions of their choice in which they are most comfortable, while remembering the advantages of an upright position (or lateral where an epidural anaesthesia is present)

- consider the suitability of the environment and accessibility of equipment such as beanbags, birthing balls, rocking chairs, birthing chairs/stools, etc.
- teach women and their birthing partners how to utilise upright positions together
- have confidence in their own ability to facilitate safe deliveries in different positions.

Asepsis

It is important that delivery is an aseptic procedure for both the woman and the baby to reduce the incidence of postnatal infection. The midwife will use a sterile delivery pack, establishing a sterile field both on the working surface and in the area of the woman's perineum. Adaptations are necessary according to the environment and the position that the woman has adopted. The midwife must attend to scrupulous hand hygiene and the use of all personal protective equipment including aprons, gowns, sterile gloves and eye protection (eye protection is sometimes interpreted as damaging the relationship with the woman but for certain delivery positions it should be considered). Once the sterile gloves have been applied for delivery they should be kept sterile or changed as needed. An anal pad may be used to cover or remove any faeces that may escape from the anus.

Management of the perineum

The HOOP Trial (McCandlish et al 1998) provides the means of giving women the choice as to how their perineum is managed. The hands-on approach – controlling the speed of delivery of the baby's head, guarding of the perineum (placing the hand next to the perineum to support it) and applying traction to deliver the shoulders – demonstrated less perineal pain for women at 10 days after the birth. All other outcomes (e.g. perineal trauma) were similar, thus allowing women to make an informed choice. It is possible to achieve control of the speed of delivery with verbal guidance, but equally the woman may wish to deliver the baby herself onto her abdomen; both of these methods are modifications of the hands-on technique. NICE (2007) advises either technique can be used. Research into this aspect of care is ongoing and the reader needs to be aware of this.

The umbilical cord

The presence of a nuchal cord (cord around the baby's neck at delivery) occurs in 10–37% of deliveries; it is thought to be more common in males due to their tendency to have longer cords (Reed et al 2009). The evidence of whether to feel for a nuchal cord and how to manage it (looping a loose cord over the baby's head, clamping and cutting a tight cord or attempting to deliver the baby through the cord) is limited and inconclusive (Phillips 2004, Reed et al 2009). Although the option of slipping a loose cord over the baby's head is favoured by many midwives, this requires the woman to stop pushing, which may be very difficult and cause her to panic and handling the cord may stimulate the umbilical arteries to vasoconstrict, reducing blood flow to the baby. Reed (2007) also suggests that feeling around the perineum for the cord can be a painful process for the woman. Clamping and cutting the cord severs the oxygen supply for the baby, which can be detrimental in cases of shoulder dystocia and may be the causative factor behind babies having lower Apgar scores and lower pH levels in studies reviewing the effects of nuchal cords at delivery (Reed et al 2009). In addition, Reed et al (2009) suggest that studies looking at nuchal cord management do not distinguish between loose and tight cords. They suggest that leaving the cord intact and delivering the baby with the cord around his neck can be advantageous as the placental blood flow can be resumed following the birth of the baby. Reed et al (2009) suggest the Somersault technique can be used for this – slowly deliver both shoulders without handling the cord and as the shoulders deliver, flex the baby's head to push his face close to the mother's thigh, then keeping the head next to the perineum, assist the baby to somersault out of the vagina and unwrap the cord. Sadan et al (2007) undertook a small study looking at the management of single nuchal cord and conclude that leaving the nuchal cord intact or cutting it after the delivery of the anterior shoulder has no adverse effects on perinatal outcomes.

The management of nuchal cord at delivery remains a contentious issue with little evidence to support a particular management option. However, with the risk of shoulder dystocia it would appear prudent not to clamp and cut the cord unless the delivery is prevented by a tight short cord and therefore it may be unnecessary to feel for a nuchal cord unless there is a clear clinical indication.

Preparation of the environment

As a continuum of labour care, it is anticipated that the support, communication, physical care, observations and record keeping that have extended through the first stage of labour will continue. NICE (2007) recommends hourly blood pressure and pulse, 4-hourly temperature, ½-hourly recording of the frequency of the contractions and intermittent auscultation of the fetal heart for 1 minute following a contraction every 5 minutes. Specifically for the second stage the environment should:

- contain all that is required for management of an aseptic delivery
- be warm and ready to receive the baby
- be calm and relaxed
- have a midwife present throughout, with an assistant for delivery (depending on local protocol, but ideally a second midwife)
- have a mechanism to call for emergency assistance
- be equipped to begin emergency management for mother or baby. All equipment must have been checked and the midwife must be competent in its use.

PROCEDURE: normal delivery

Adaptations are made according to the birth environment and position of the woman. Note should be taken of the discussions above:

- Prepare the environment and gather equipment:
  ○ delivery trolley or surface to work from
  ○ sterile delivery pack, including warm towels to dry/wrap the baby
  ○ sterile gloves, gown, etc.
  ○ disposable sheets, gloves and sanitary towels
  ○ extras: urinary catheter, amnihook, lidocaine, needles and syringes, oxytocic (ecbolic) agent
  ○ an infectious waste refuse bag should be available, usually a floor bin.
- Ensure that the room temperature is correct (21–24°C) and draughts are excluded.
- Give ongoing reassurance and explanations to the woman, support her in her choice of position and analgesia and maintain maternal and fetal observations.

- Place the disposable sheets strategically in the area of the perineum, while wearing disposable gloves.
- When delivery is imminent, put on apron and eye protection, wash and dry hands and open the outer covering of the delivery pack.
- Place all other sterile items onto the delivery pack using a non-touch technique.
- Apply hand rub, allow to dry and then put on sterile gloves.
- Check the swabs and instruments in the delivery pack.
- Arrange the trolley in a way that suits, having cord clamps and the receiver for the placenta accessible.
- Continue to observe the advancing fetus while carrying out these procedures (some women experience short second stages of labour).
- Place sterile drapes appropriately to provide a sterile field.
- Position the anal pad if being used, have a warm towel on hand, e.g. on woman's abdomen, ready to receive the baby.
- As the fetus reaches the perineum, the perineum is seen to stretch.
- As the head crowns, consider applying gentle pressure to it with one hand to slow the delivery, guard the perineum with the other hand if adopting a hands-on approach.
- Encourage the woman to breathe and give gentle pushes as the head extends and emerges, note the time.
- Restitution will be seen followed by external rotation of the head as the shoulders rotate internally.
- As the next contraction occurs and the woman has urges to push again, apply traction to the anterior shoulder (in a direction away from the symphysis pubis) to deliver it, followed by traction in the opposite direction to deliver the posterior one.
- Deliver the body and limbs of the baby by lateral flexion, following the curve of the birth canal, in an upward direction towards the woman's abdomen; the woman may assist.
- Note the time of delivery.
- The baby is placed ideally skin to skin with his mother and is dried completely; parents or midwife will check the gender.

- Drying acts as stimulation, during which time the baby will take its first breath and cry; complete Apgar score (see Chapter 37) at 1 minute. Act swiftly (before 1 minute) if resuscitation is required (see Chapter 56).
- Clamping and cutting of the cord will be undertaken according to the parents' wishes and chosen management of the third stage of labour. Breastfeeding may be facilitated.
- Share in the joy of the moment, but stay alert to the clinical situation.
- Care moves into management of the third stage of labour; this may have included the administration of an intramuscular or intravenous oxytocic agent following delivery of the anterior shoulder or the birth of the baby.

Episiotomy

Episiotomy is the surgical incision into the perineum to widen the vulval outlet. Rates of episiotomy vary across the world from 9.7% (Sweden) to 100% (Taiwan) with reported rates of 62.5% in the USA and 30% in Europe (Carroli & Mignini 2009). The work of Sleep et al (1984) indicates that a protocol of restricted episiotomy can be safely applied so that it is performed solely for fetal or maternal distress or with lack of progress and instrumental delivery. A restricted policy is associated with less posterior perineal trauma (posterior vaginal wall, perineal muscles and anal sphincter), less suturing and fewer complications compared with the routine use of episiotomy. However, there is an increased risk of anterior perineal trauma (labia, anterior vagina, urethra, clitoris) although there is little associated morbidity (Carroli & Mignini 2009, Fernando et al 2007).

A midwife may perform an episiotomy if it is indicated, with the woman's consent, and if properly trained. The timing of gaining informed consent is a more difficult issue; parenthood education during the antenatal period may assist the woman to understand what it is and why it may be necessary; her birth plan may include her wishes. The urgency of the need to undertake one at the time prevents detailed explanations, but consent is still required.

If required, the episiotomy should be in the right mediolateral position rather than in the midline, as this is less likely to extend to a third-degree tear (Eogan et al 2006). The incision should begin at the posterior fourchette and be undertaken at an angle of 45–60° (Eogan et al 2006, NICE 2007). Thomas & Cameron (2007) found that the angle of the incision could vary between 29–80° from the midline. A small episiotomy angle increases the risk of anal sphincter injury occurring (Eogan et al 2006).

Infiltration of the perineum with an anaesthetic is necessary prior to the incision. The timing of the episiotomy is important; the presenting part needs to descend sufficiently onto the perineum to displace the levator ani (deep muscles). The incision is then only likely to affect the skin, posterior vaginal wall and superficial pelvic floor muscles (see Fig. 34.1, p 242, which indicates the muscles of the pelvic floor). If performed too early, the deep pelvic floor muscles may be incised and haemorrhage is likely to occur from the wound. The delivery of the presenting part usually follows immediately, the midwife being required – almost simultaneously – to remove the scissors from the vulva, control the delivery of the head and support the perineum so that the episiotomy does not extend. The procedure and repair (see Chapter 34) are both aseptic events.

PROCEDURE: infiltration of the perineum and episiotomy

- Gain informed consent.
- Between contractions, draw up the correct dose of anaesthetic agent, e.g. lidocaine using a sterile needle (21-g green) and syringe.
- Insert two fingers into the vagina behind the perineum to protect the presenting part.
- Insert the full depth of the needle centrally at the introitus, draw back; if not in a blood vessel inject one-third of the anaesthetic as the needle is withdrawn. Avoid taking the needle completely out of the tissue, but as the introitus is reached reposition the needle and reinsert it in a mediolateral direction. Instil the anaesthetic as described and then repeat for a third time (Fig. 31.1A) to infiltrate a fan-shaped area of the perineum.
- Allow the agent time to work, two or three contractions if possible.

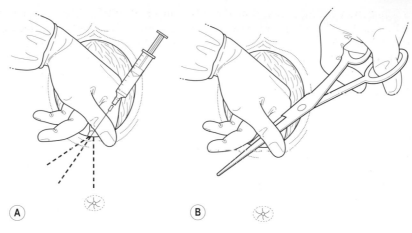

Figure 31.1 • A Infiltration of the perineum. B Incision of episiotomy

- Reinsert two fingers to protect the presenting part again. Using the straight scissors supplied in the delivery pack, make one decisive right mediolateral incision of approximately 4–5 cm long, beginning at the posterior fourchette and at an angle of 45–60 ° from the midline, at the height of the contraction at which the delivery is anticipated (Fig. 31.1B).
- Immediately apply control to the fetal head, removing the scissors onto the trolley; guard the perineum if able and facilitate the slow delivery of the head.
- Continue with the delivery as described above.
- Ensure that after examination of the genital tract (see Chapter 32) the episiotomy is repaired appropriately (see Chapter 34).
- Records should specifically include details of the indication, infiltration and incision.

ROLE AND RESPONSIBILITIES OF THE MIDWIFE

These can be summarised as:

- thorough preparation of the environment and equipment
- care and observations throughout the second stage
- safe, evidence-based management of the birth for woman and baby
- respect and appropriate facilitation of the woman's wishes

- recognition of any deviation from the norm; referral as necessary
- contemporaneous record keeping.

Summary

- Many factors contribute to satisfying, safe and evidence-based care in the second stage of labour.
- Midwives should have confidence to allow women to push spontaneously in whichever is the position of their choice, preferably upright.
- Restricting the length of the second stage is inappropriate providing that there is progress and maternal and fetal wellbeing.
- Delivery is an aseptic procedure in which standard precautions and personal protective equipment are all used.
- Controlling the speed of delivery of the head, support of the perineum and lateral flexion to the shoulders may result in less perineal pain in the short term.
- Episiotomy should be restricted to instances of maternal and fetal distress. It is an aseptic procedure, incising the perineum to increase the vulval outlet. Anaesthetic is used, consent is essential and timing vital.
- The midwife has an autonomous and highly responsible role during the second stage of labour.

SELF-ASSESSMENT EXERCISES

The answers to the following questions may be found in the text:

1. How may the midwife recognise the second stage of labour?
2. Describe how the environment is prepared for birth.
3. Discuss the evidence relating to management of the second stage of labour, including length, pushing and delivery positions.
4. Demonstrate how a normal birth is conducted including management of the equipment and positioning of the hands.
5. Describe how to infiltrate the perineum and incise an episiotomy.
6. Summarise the role and responsibilities of the midwife when providing complete care during the second stage of labour.

References

Allbers LL, Borders N: Minimizing genital tract trauma and related pain following spontaneous vaginal birth, *J Midwifery Womens Health* 52(3): 246–255, 2007.

Brancato RM, Church S, Stone PW: A meta-analysis of passive descent versus immediate pushing in nulliparous women with epidural analgesia in the second stage of labour, *J Obstet, Gynecol Neonatal Nurs* 37(1):4–12, 2008.

Burvill S: Midwifery diagnosis of labour onset, *Br J Midwifery* 10(10): 600–605, 2002.

Carroli G, Mignini L: Episiotomy for vaginal birth, *Cochrane Database Syst Rev* 1: CD000081, DOI:10.1002/14651858. CD000081, pub2, 2009.

Cheng YW, Hopkins LM, Laros RK, et al: Duration of the second stage of labor in multiparous women: Maternal and neonatal outcomes, *Am J Obstet Gynaecol* 196(6):585. e1–e6, 2007.

De Jonge A, Teunissen DAM, van Diem MTh, et al: Women's positions during the second stage of labour: views of primary care midwives, *J Adv Nurs* 63(4):347–356, 2007a.

De Jonge A, van Diem MTh, Scheepers PLH, et al: Increased blood loss in upright birthing positions originates from perineal damage, *Br J Obstet Gynaecol* 114 (3):349–355, 2007b.

Di Franco JT, Romano AM, Keen R: Care Practice #5: Spontaneous pushing in upright or gravity-neutral positions, *J Perinat Educ* 16(3): 35–38, 2007.

Eogan M, Daly L, O'Connell P, et al: Does the angle of episiotomy affect the incidence of anal sphincter injury? *Br J Obstet Gynaecol* 113:190–194, 2006.

Fernando RJ, Williams AA, Adams EJ: The management of third or fourth degree perineal tears, *RCOG Greentop Guidelines No 29*, London, 2007, RCOG.

Gupta JK, Hofmeyr GJ, Smyth RMD: Position in the second stage of labour for women without epidural anaesthesia, *Cochrane Database Syst Rev* 1: CD002006. DOI: 10.1002/14651858.CD002006, pub2, 2004.

Hanson L: Second stage labor care: challenges in spontaneous bearing down, *J Perinat Neonatal Nurs* 23(1):31–39, 2009.

Hobbs L: Assessing cervical dilatation without VEs – watching the purple line, *Pract Midwife* 1(11):34–35, 1998.

Lewis L, Webster J, Carter A, et al: Maternal positions and mobility during the first stage of labour, *Cochrane Database Syst Rev* 4: CD003934, DOI: 10.1002/14651858.CD003934, pub2, 2002.

Long L: Redefining the second stage of labour could help to promote normal birth, *Br J Midwifery* 14(2): 104–107, 2006.

McCandlish R, Bowler U, van Asten H, et al: A randomised controlled trial of care of the perineum during second stage of normal labour, *Br J Obstet Gynaecol* 105(12):1262–1272, 1998.

NICE (National Institute for Health and Clinical Excellence): *CG55 Intrapartum Care*, London, 2007, NICE.

Nicholl MC, Cattell MA: Getting evidence into obstetric and midwifery practice: reducing perineal trauma, *Aust Health Rev* 30(4):462–467, 2006.

Perez-Botella M, Downe S: Stories as evidence: Why do midwives still use directed pushing? *Br J Midwifery* 14(10):596–599, 2006.

Phillips S: To cut or not to cut? *Pract Midwife* 7(7):26–27, 2004.

Ragnar I, Altman D, Tyden T, et al: Comparison of the maternal experience and duration of labour in two upright delivery positions – a randomised controlled trial, *Br J Obstet Gynaecol* 113(2):165–170, 2006.

Reed R: Nuchal cords: think before you check, *Practising Midwife* 10(5): 18–20, 2007.

Reed R, Barnes M, Allan J: Nuchal cords: sharing the evidence with parents, *Br J Midwifery* 17(2): 106–109, 2009.

Roberts CL, Torvaldsen S, Cameron C: Delayed versus early pushing in women with epidural analgesia: A systematic review and meta-analysis, *Br J Obstet Gynaecol* 111:1333–1340, 2004.

Roberts J, Hanson L: Best practices in second stage labor care: Maternal bearing down and positioning, *J Midwifery Womens Health* 52(3):238–247, 2007.

Sadan O, Fleischfarb Z, Everon S, et al: Cord around the neck: should it be severed at delivery? A randomized controlled study, *Am J Perinatol* 24(1):61–64, 2007.

Sahai-Srivastava S, Amezcua L: Compressive neuropathies complicating normal childbirth: Case report and literature review, *Birth: Issues Perinat Care* 34(2):173–175, 2007.

Sampselle CM, Miller JM, Luecha Y, et al: Provider support of spontaneous pushing during the second stage of labor, *J Obstet, Gynecol Neonat Nurs* 34(6): 695–702, 2005.

Schaffer JI, Bloom SL, Casey BM: A randomized trial of the effects of coached versus uncoached maternal pushing during the second stage of labor on postpartum pelvic floor structure and function, *Am J Obstet Gynecol* 192(5):1692–1696, 2005.

Simpson KR, James DC: Effects of immediate versus delayed pushing during second stage of labour on fetal wellbeing: A randomized controlled trial, *Nurs Res* 54(3):149–157, 2005.

Sleep JM, Grant A, Garcia J, et al: West Berkshire perineal management trial, *Br Med J* 289:587–590, 1984.

Soong B, Barnes M: Maternal position at midwife-attended birth and perineal trauma: Is there an association? *Birth: Issues Perinat Care* 32(3): 164–169, 2005.

Sutton J: Birth without active pushing. In Wickham S, editor: *Midwifery best practice*, Edinburgh, 2003, Elsevier Science, pp 90–92.

Thomas E, Cameron H: Midwives' management of episiotomy at a district general hospital, *Br J Midwifery* 15(11):680–683, 2007.

Williams C: Arbitrary time limits for the second stage of labour – do they disempower women from achieving normal birth? *MIDIRS Midwifery Dig* 17(4):527–533, 2007.

Yildirim G, Beji NK: Effects of pushing techniques in birth on mother and fetus: a randomized study, *Birth: Issues Perinat Care* 35(1):25–30, 2008.

Young G: Review: delayed pushing reduces rotational or mid-pelvic instrumental deliveries but increases duration of the second stage of labour in women having epidurals, *Evid Based Med* 10(4):122, 2005.

Principles of intrapartum skills: third-stage issues

32

CHAPTER CONTENTS

The third stage of labour can be a dangerous stage for the woman as primary postpartum haemorrhage (PPH) remains a cause of maternal mortality and mismanagement of the third stage increases the risk. In the UK, the risk of death from haemorrhage is very small (nine women died from PPH during 2003–2005) (Lewis 2007). However, worldwide, particularly in developing countries, the death rate can be much higher, accounting for 11% of maternal deaths (Lewis 2007). Following the delivery of the baby, the midwife has a responsibility to ensure the placenta and membranes are delivered safely and competently. This chapter focuses on the principles of the management of the third stage of labour, discussing both physiological and active management, examination of the genital tract following delivery of the placenta and estimation of blood loss; relevant anatomy and physiology are included.

LEARNING OUTCOMES

Having read this chapter the reader should be able to:

- describe the physiology of the third stage of labour
- discuss the effects of early and delayed cord clamping on the baby
- discuss the different methods of managing the third stage
- discuss how blood loss is estimated
- describe how the genital tract is examined following delivery.

Physiology of the third stage of labour

The third stage is from the birth of the baby to the complete expulsion of the placenta and membranes, involving the separation, descent and expulsion of the placenta and membranes and the control of haemorrhage from the placental site. It also encompasses examination of the genital tract following delivery and, if necessary, perineal repair.

Placental separation has previously been thought to result from the placenta being squeezed following the reduction in the size of the uterus at the beginning of the third stage. This was thought to result in an increased pressure within the blood vessels of the spongy layer of the decidua, causing them to rupture. The escaping blood between the placental surface and the thin septa of the spongy layer resulted in the placenta shearing from the decidua. However, following ultrasound visualisation of placental separation, a different understanding of the physiology has emerged (Herman 2000, Herman et al 2002, Krapp et al 2000) with three phases identified: latent, contraction/detachment and expulsion.

With the delivery of the baby, the intrauterine volume reduces drastically (from 4 L before labour to 0.5 L) as the uterus becomes smaller. Intrauterine pressure increases from 100 mmHg in the second stage to 140 mmHg in the third stage.

Phase 1: latent phase

Contraction and retraction of the myometrium continues as with the first and second stages of labour causing extensive thickening of most of the myometrium. However, the area of myometrium beneath the placental site is unable to thicken to the same extent.

Phase 2: contraction/detachment phase

With further contraction and retraction, the myometrium under the lower pole of the placenta begins to contract with a reduction in the surface area. Consequently, the shearing forces cause the placenta to tear away from the spongy layer of the decidua. With the onset of placental detachment, the wave of separation passes upwards and the remaining placenta

detaches, with the uppermost part of the placenta detaching last. At this point, the maternal sinuses within the decidua are exposed. The oblique muscle fibres surrounding the blood vessels contract, sealing off the torn ends of the maternal vessels, helping to prevent haemorrhage.

Phase 3: expulsion phase

The placenta descends into the lower uterine segment, causing the membranes (which had begun to detach from the uterine wall as the internal cervical os dilated) to peel away from the walls of the uterus. As the uterus contracts, the placenta descends into the vagina, assisted by gravity, with the membranes following.

The placenta and membranes are then expelled by maternal effort. The fetal surface appears first at the vulva, with the membranes behind, and any blood loss is contained within this – the 'Schultze' method of expulsion (Fig. 32.1A). Sometimes the lower edge of the placenta descends first, so that the maternal surface appears at the vulva, sliding out lengthways with membranes (Fig. 32.1B). This is a slower process, with increased blood loss (the mechanisms to control haemorrhage are less effective when the placenta is still partially attached) – also known as the 'Matthews Duncan' method of expulsion.

Brandt (1933) demonstrated by radiographic studies that the placenta usually separates within

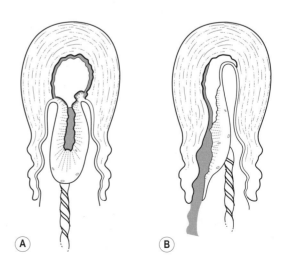

Figure 32.1 • Methods of placental expulsion. A Schultze. B Matthews Duncan

3 minutes of the birth of the baby. Herman (2000) suggests that the duration of the third stage is dependent on the length of the latent phase; however, the time taken for the descent and expulsion of the placenta and membranes can also vary individually, influenced by factors such as posture and whether the third stage is managed actively or expectantly.

Signs of separation and descent

These are not absolute and may occur for other reasons:

- Bleeding: 30–60 mL of blood may trickle from the vagina: this may also occur with a partially separated placenta, although bleeding is often heavier, or from a laceration.
- Lengthening of the cord: this occurs as the placenta descends, but may also occur if the cord is coiled and then straightens out.
- Uterus becomes globular, hard, high, mobile and ballottable: this is assessed by palpating the fundus but should be undertaken with caution as it may cause irregular contractions, resulting in a partially separated placenta and membranes, and excessive bleeding. The fundus is palpable below the umbilicus, and is broad, until placental separation and descent into the lower uterine segment.

The fundal height increases, usually above the umbilicus, with the fundus narrowing (Fig. 32.2).

Control of haemorrhage

Bleeding from the placental site can be profuse and rapid, as the placental circulation is approximately 500–800 mL/minute at term. It is imperative that haemorrhage is controlled. The body attempts to do this in three ways:

1. The middle oblique fibres of the uterus contract and retract, constricting the blood vessels running through them. This causes the vessels to kink, slowing down and stopping the blood flow, allowing for clot formation at the placental site.
2. The walls of the uterus become in apposition to each other, exerting pressure on the placental site.
3. The blood clotting mechanism begins to work at the placental site, within the sinuses and torn vessels. The damaged tissue releases thrombokinase, converting prothrombin to thrombin. This combines with fibrinogen to form fibrin, which then combines with platelets to form a clot. Vitamin K, calcium and the other clotting factors are required for this process to happen efficiently.

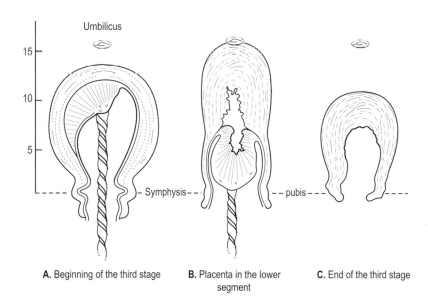

A. Beginning of the third stage   B. Placenta in the lower segment   C. End of the third stage

Figure 32.2 • Position of the uterus before and after placental separation

Clamping of the umbilical cord

The custom of cutting the cord was introduced in the seventeenth century. Its introduction coincided with the practice of giving birth in bed, which resulted in the bedding becoming blood-soaked; the practice of clamping the cord became widespread to reduce this. With active management, the cord is clamped immediately after delivery, usually within 30 seconds; with expectant management, it is not cut until it has stopped pulsating (McDonald & Middleton (2008) suggest this is often within 2 minutes). There is much debate currently regarding the timing of cord clamping for active management as evidence is emerging that delayed clamping (30 seconds to 5 minutes after delivery) has a beneficial effect on the health and wellbeing of the baby (see below). An increasing number of women are opting for a 'lotus birth', which leaves the baby attached to the placenta and cord until the cord shrivels and detaches naturally from the umbilicus (Cook 2007).

Placental separation relies on the ability of the uterus to contract and retract. If the cord is clamped, a counter-resistance is set up in the placenta, preventing the transfer of blood to the baby. The size of the placenta does not reduce as much and this can inhibit contraction and retraction, resulting in a slower separation process. The effect of this is twofold:

1. The delay in complete separation means there is delay in sealing off the torn maternal vessels, resulting in a retroplacental clot and increasing the risk of haemorrhage.
2. The cervix may retract before the placenta is expelled, resulting in a retained placenta, which often necessitates a manual removal of the placenta and membranes under an epidural, spinal or general anaesthetic.

Clamping the cord and Rhesus isoimmunisation

When the cord is clamped, more fetal blood remains in the placenta, increasing the pressure within the placenta. As the uterus contracts, the pressure increases further and the surface placental vessels rupture. Fetal blood cells are released into the uterine cavity and may pass into the maternal circulation. Thus active management can increase the risk of fetomaternal transfusion (Enkin et al

2000). If the baby is Rhesus positive and the woman is Rhesus negative, she will produce antibodies against the Rhesus-positive blood cells. Rhesus iso-immunisation can affect future pregnancies, as the antibodies are small enough to pass through to the placenta and haemolyse fetal cells if the fetus is Rhesus positive. All Rhesus-negative women should receive anti-D immunoglobulin at birth if the baby is Rhesus positive to reduce the risk of isoimmunisation occurring. If antibodies are already present and known to be haemolysing fetal red blood cells, the cord should be clamped immediately at birth to reduce the number of antibodies transferred to the baby at delivery. This may help to reduce the severity of anaemia and jaundice occurring from isoimmunisation.

Clamping the cord: the effect on the baby

Airey et al (2008) suggest delayed cord clamping increases placental transfusion to the baby by 20%, the equivalent of an extra 20–30 mL/kg blood and 20–40 mg/kg of iron for the term baby. This extra blood may be required for the newly established pulmonary circulation. Early cord clamping reduces the amount of blood transferred to the baby, with resulting hypovolaemia, which may be a factor in the development and severity of respiratory distress syndrome and can compromise the baby who is born with low haemoglobin.

There are many benefits associated with delayed cord clamping. For the term baby there is increased tissue oxygenation within the first week of life, increased haematocrit, haemoglobin and blood volume, reduced incidence of anaemia at 2 months and beyond which is thought to improve the baby's resistance to infection and aid neurodevelopment in infancy – for some babies this can be the difference between life and death in infancy (Airey et al 2008, Cook 2007, Weckert & Hancock 2008). With the preterm baby, delayed cord clamping is associated with a reduced need for blood transfusion and ventilation, decreased incidence of hypotension, anaemia, intraventricular haemorrhage, improved cerebral oxygenation, increased blood volume (20–60% increase in red blood cells), haemoglobin levels (at 1 hour, 10 weeks and 6 months) and ferritin levels (Airey et al 2008, Baenziger et al 2007, Chapparo et al 2006, Cook 2007, McDonald & Middleton 2008, Rabe et al 2004, Ultee et al 2006). The increase in early protein and iron levels with a 50% reduction in the number of blood transfusion needs for very low birthweight babies was found even with a delay in clamping of 30 seconds (Rabe et al 2009).

To achieve optimum placental transfusion, Cook (2007) suggests the baby should be delivered onto the woman's abdomen. Airey et al (2009) suggest the earlier studies looking at placental-baby blood flow which suggested the baby should be placed 40 cm below the introitus for 30 seconds were undertaken when ergometrine was the drug used to manage the third stage. However, as the blood flow in the umbilical vein, which transfers placental blood to the baby increases as the uterus contracts, Airey et al (2009) suggest that keeping the baby level with the placental bed, or within 10 cm above or below, has little effect on the size and speed of placental transfusion. They are currently undertaking a review of the studies comparing different positions of the baby relative to placental position prior to cord clamping – the reader is advised to look for their findings on the Cochrane database when they are published.

There is a risk of overtransfusing red blood cells predisposing the baby to jaundice particularly when an oxytocic drug is given; however Airey et al (2008) question whether there is an increased requirement to treat the jaundice. Cernadas et al (2006) found increased levels of polycythaemia although no babies were symptomatic or required treatment; additionally these differences did not persist beyond 24–48 hours and there were no significant differences in bilirubin levels when the cord was clamped immediately or at 1 or 3 minutes. However McDonald & Middleton (2008) found an increase in jaundice requiring treatment with phototherapy.

Cord clamping and maternal outcome

Clamping the cord immediately following the birth of the baby or delaying clamping up to 3 minutes makes no significant difference to PPH rates (McDonald & Middleton 2008). Cernadas et al (2006) also found that delayed cord clamping made no difference to maternal outcomes. Draining the placenta is associated with a shorter third stage and a decreased risk of retained placenta (Soltani et al 2005), although further research into these effects is needed.

Management of the third stage

This is either expectant (physiological, passive) or active.

Expectant management

This is delivery of the placenta without intervention: no oxytocic drug, no cord clamping unless it has stopped pulsating, no controlled traction, no palpation of the abdomen. The placenta is delivered by maternal effort, assisted by gravity and the baby suckling at the breast. Signs of separation and descent are seen.

Women should only be considered for expectant management if they have had a physiological first and second stage as Fry (2007) advises that the physiological process of placental separation and delivery are dependent on a finely tuned balance of hormonal, neurological, physiological and psychological interactions. If any of these have been disturbed, Fry (2007) suggests the safety of the third stage is compromised; this includes the use of syntocinon which desensitizes oxytocin receptors (Gyte 2006). Equally the environment needs to be private and warm, with fear, anxiety and tension dissipated otherwise adrenaline levels increase which can inhibit oxytocin release and interfere with the physiological process of uterine contraction and retraction, and thus placental separation and descent (Blackburn 2008, Buckley 2004). Kanikasamy (2007) suggests that a calm confident midwife who is able to instil confidence and practise non-invasive care will promote the release of oxytocin. Blackburn (2008) agrees, suggesting that the woman should be undisturbed, as this causes catecholamine levels to reduce whilst high levels of oxytocin and prolactin are released. Uninterrupted skin-to-skin contact and suckling should also be encouraged as this promotes a surge in oxytocin release (Blackburn 2008, Page 2007). Expectant management can be undertaken with preterm labour; however, it is acknowledged that this may not be possible if the baby requires active resuscitation.

Expectant management is associated with a higher blood loss (Prendiville et al 2000), partly because blood loss measurement is more accurate. Provided this is not excessive and the woman is not compromised, it may be a physiological loss with which the body can cope. Wickham (1999) suggests that the blood loss in the early postnatal period is less when the third stage is managed expectantly compared with active management. However, it is important to discuss this with the woman, ideally during the antenatal period or early labour, as active management should ensue if the woman begins to haemorrhage. The woman should be aware of the risks and consent to change from expectant to active management in the presence of haemorrhage.

Expectant management can take longer to complete than one that is actively managed – possibly up to 1 hour. Provided the woman's condition remains stable, with no excessive bleeding, there is no cause for concern. This may be a time when breastfeeding is initiated, with the added benefit of increased oxytocin release to promote uterine contraction. The National Institute for Health and Clinical Excellence (NICE 2007) advises that the placenta should be delivered within 1 hour with expectant management. If there is concern that the placenta has not delivered after 1 hour, the midwife should assess whether the placenta has separated by placing the woman on her back and gently pressing her abdominal wall just above the pubic bone (using only fingertips) and observing the cord. If the cord does not move, Odent (1998) advises the placenta has separated.

Principles of expectant management

- Note the time of delivery of the baby.
- Keep the baby on the woman's abdomen skin to skin.
- Maintain a safe, warm and private environment, taking steps to reduce any anxiety in the woman.
- The midwife can continue to wear the gloves worn for delivery of the baby but these will need to be changed prior to examining the genital tract.
- Ensure the woman's bladder is empty.
- Encourage the woman to adopt an upright position.
- Observe the general condition of the woman throughout, particularly any blood loss *per vaginam*, colour, respirations (NICE 2007) and recording the maternal pulse every 15 minutes or more frequently if indicated.
- Do not touch the cord, allowing it to stop pulsating naturally.

- Encourage and assist the woman to breast feed when the baby is ready.
- Do not palpate the uterus unless blood loss becomes excessive.
- Place a bedpan or suitable receptacle under or next to the woman when she is ready to push the placenta out.
- Encourage the woman to deliver the placenta by her own efforts, bearing down to expel the placenta.
- Note the time the placenta and membranes are expelled (usually within 1 hour of the birth).
- The cord can be clamped and cut when it has stopped pulsating (unless the woman has requested a lotus birth), applying the clamp 3–4 cm from the abdominal wall (longer if the baby is preterm, as catherisation of the umbilical vein may be required; this is more successful when the cord is longer).
- Assess the condition of the woman, noting the condition of the uterus, amount of blood loss, pulse and blood pressure following completion of the third stage; the condition of the genital tract should also be determined, suturing can be undertaken when appropriate.
- Assist the woman into a comfortable position, removing any soiled linen; if all her observations are within the expected parameters, leave the woman and her baby together (with her partner or labour supporter), ensuring the call bell is close at hand.
- Examine the placenta (Chapter 33) and record total blood loss.
- Dispose of the placenta and equipment correctly (if the woman is taking the placenta home, it should be double wrapped and placed in a suitable container).
- Document findings and act accordingly.

If the woman wishes to have an expectant third stage but the umbilical cord has been severed, the maternal end of the cord should be cut 2–3 cm above the clamp and the cord placed in a sterile receiver. This will allow a limited amount of blood to drain from the placenta, helping to reduce its overall size. This helps to minimise retroplacental bleeding and decreases the risk of partial separation and isoimmunisation (Lucas 2006). The principles of management are the same. However, this is not as effective and may inhibit the physiological process. In the presence of any signs of haemorrhage, an oxytocic drug may be required and the third stage actively managed. Blood drained from the placenta should not be included in the total estimate of blood loss following delivery, being placental and not maternal blood.

If the woman has requested a lotus birth, the cord remains unclamped and the baby stays attached to the placenta and cord until it detaches naturally usually 3–10 days after birth. Blackburn (2008) suggests that once the placenta has been checked and washed, it should be covered with salt and placed into the woman's chosen wrapping.

Active management

This involves the administration of an oxytocic drug, early cord clamping and delivery of the placenta using controlled cord traction (CCT) (NICE 2007, Pena-Marti & Comunian-Carrasco 2007). It is often quicker than a physiological third stage, with a reduced blood loss; however, the oxytocic drugs can have unpleasant side effects, e.g. raised blood pressure, nausea, vomiting (Maughan et al 2006) and there is a higher incidence of retained placenta (Prendiville et al 2000). Prendiville et al (2000) suggest active management should be the management of choice for deliveries in maternity hospitals; no comment is made about home births. Traditionally, active management does not require signs of separation to be seen prior to undertaking CCT (Spencer 1962); however, Pena-Marti & Comunian-Carrasco (2007) recommend using controlled cord traction only after signs of separation are seen, and an oxytocic drug administered. Fundal pressure should not be used.

The use of oxytocic drugs has been a major contributor in the reduction in maternal deaths from PPH (DH 1996); active management is recommended for women considered to be at high risk of PPH. These include:

- previous PPH
- grande multiparity
- fibroids
- multiple pregnancy
- polyhydramnios
- anaemia
- pre-eclampsia
- antepartum haemorrhage, both placental abruption and placenta praevia

- tocolytic drugs given for preterm labour
- induced labour
- augmented labour
- prolonged labour
- precipitate labour
- general anaesthesia.

Oxytocic (ecbolic) drugs

These are drugs that stimulate the uterus to contract and consist of oxytocin, in the form of syntocinon, ergometrine or a combination of the two. They are administered prophylactically during active management to reduce the risk of PPH or as part of the emergency management of PPH to arrest bleeding. NICE (2007) recommend the use of 10 IU syntocinon for prophylactic use during active management.

Syntocinon

Syntocinon causes the uterus to contract rhythmically and strongly, mainly the upper uterine segment, mimicking the body's actions. Given intravenously (I.V.) it takes effect within 40 seconds; with intramuscular (I.M.) use it takes around 2–3 minutes to take effect. Its main side effect is fluid retention due to its antidiuretic nature although Cotter et al (2001) caution there is insufficient evidence about the adverse effects of syntocinon and suggest further research is needed. They do suggest that syntocinon is associated with a reduction in the incidence of manual removal of placenta and less hypertension compared with ergometrine. The usual dose is 5 or 10 units; however, Cotter et al (2001) suggest this may need to be increased and call for research to determine the optimum dose and route of administration.

Ergometrine

Ergometrine causes a non-physiological continuous spasm of the uterus and cervix, lasting for up to 2 hours; it is therefore a useful drug to give when a PPH is due to uterine atony. It also causes vasospasm, which can increase blood pressure and should not be administered routinely to hypertensive women. Constriction of the smooth muscle of the bronchioles may also occur, which may be problematic for women with asthma. Given I.V. it takes effect within 40 seconds; with I.M. use, it takes around 5–7 minutes.

The usual dose is 0.25–0.5 mg. The side effects are mainly related to the effects of smooth muscle contraction and include tinnitus, headache, chest pain and palpitations, cramp-like pains in the back and legs, nausea and vomiting, a sharp rise in blood pressure, and a decreased prolactin level; if the woman has had a general anaesthetic, ergometrine increases the risk of acute pulmonary or cerebral oedema post-delivery.

Syntometrine

This is composed of ergometrine 0.5 mg and syntocinon 5 units in 1 mL. It combines the effects of the two drugs and is commonly the drug of choice when the third stage is being actively managed; unfortunately, it also combines the side effects of the two drugs. Compared with syntocinon alone, it achieves a small but significant reduction in bleeding when the blood loss is 500–1000 mL but there is no difference between syntometrine and syntocinon when the blood loss is above 1000 mL (McDonald et al 2004). There is a significant increase in the incidence of diastolic hypertension, vomiting and nausea when syntometrine is used compared with syntocinon and McDonald et al (2004) suggest the advantages of reducing the risk of a blood loss of 500–1000 mL be measured against the risk of side effects occurring when deciding whether to use syntocinon or syntometrine.

When an oxytocic drug is to be administered prophylactically, it is usually given I.M. either as the anterior shoulder is being delivered or following the birth of the baby, as this provides sufficient time for the drug to take effect before delivering the placenta. Soltani & Dickinson (2006) are currently undertaking a review for the Cochrane database addressing the timing of prophylactic oxytocic drugs, cord clamping and the effects on maternal and neonatal outcomes; the reader is advised to review this when it is published. Nardin et al (2006) suggest that the use of the umbilical vein could be an alternative way of administering an oxytocic drug as this would direct the drug directly to the placental bed and uterine wall. They propose that this would result in earlier uterine contraction and placental separation with less systemic side effects. However, they acknowledge the need for training for this to be viable. They are currently reviewing the evidence surrounding the use of umbilical vein injections of saline with and without oxytocic drugs versus other routes of administration and expectant management. Their results will be on the Cochrane database and the reader is advised to read this when published.

With multiple births, the oxytocic drug should be administered as the anterior shoulder of the final baby is delivered or as the baby is born depending on the local policy.

Principles of active management

- As the anterior shoulder of the baby is born or the baby is delivered, an intravenous or intramuscular oxytocic drug is given.
- Clamp and cut the cord at birth within 3 minutes unless this is contraindicated (e.g. Rhesus isoimmunisation with antibodies; discussed earlier), ensuring both ends are secure and placing the maternal end (often clamped with artery forceps) in a sterile receiver, positioned close to the vulva.
- Place a sterile towel over the woman's abdomen and place the non-dominant hand over the fundus and await a contraction, keeping the hand still, during which time signs of placental separation and descent may be seen.
- When the uterus is contracted and signs of separation and descent are noted, place the non-dominant hand above the symphysis pubis, with the thumb and fingers stretched across the abdomen and palm facing inwards (Fig. 32.3).
- Grasp the cord with the dominant hand and apply steady downward traction (controlled cord traction); at the same time, push the uterus upwards towards the umbilicus with the non-dominant hand (to reduce the risk of uterine inversion).
- Controlled cord traction is best achieved if the midwife is able to keep the hand applying traction close to the vulva. The grip should be secure by holding the artery forceps on the cord close to the vulva; as the cord lengthens the clamp should be moved up to remain near to the vulva. Alternatively, wrap the cord around the fingers of the dominant hand, moving them nearer the vulva as necessary.
- If resistance is felt, stop, relieve the pressure from the dominant then the non-dominant hand (the placenta may not have separated) and wait for a minute before attempting again, ensuring the uterus is contracted.

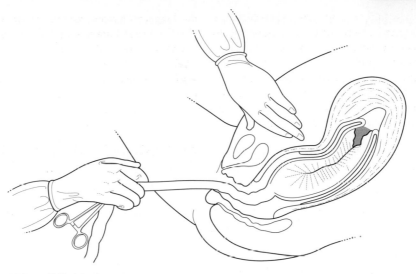

Figure 32.3 • Position of hand to 'guard' the uterus during controlled cord traction

- When the placenta appears at the vulva, traction should be applied in an upward direction to follow the curve of the birth canal.
- The non-dominant hand is moved down to help ease the placenta into the receiver, allowing the membranes to be expelled slowly.
- If there is any difficulty delivering the membranes, they should be 'teased out' either by moving them gently up and down (artery forceps can be positioned on the membranes to help with this) or by twisting the placenta round to make the membranes into a rope-like structure, either way encouraging the membranes to separate and be expelled.
- Observe the condition of the woman throughout, particularly any blood loss *per vaginam*.
- Note the time the placenta and membranes are expelled (often within 5–10 minutes).
- Assess the condition of the woman, noting the condition of the uterus, amount of blood loss, pulse and blood pressure following completion of the third stage; the condition of the genital tract should also be determined, suturing can be undertaken when appropriate.
- Assist the woman into a comfortable position, removing soiled sheets; if all her observations are within the expected parameters, leave the woman and her baby (skin to skin) together (with her partner or labour supporter), ensuring the call bell is close at hand.

- Examine the placenta (see Chapter 33) and record total blood loss.
- Dispose of the placenta and equipment correctly (if the placenta is being taken home by the woman, it should be double wrapped and placed in a suitable container).
- Document findings and act accordingly.

If there is concern that the placenta is not delivering within 30 minutes (NICE 2007), the midwife should determine whether the placenta has separated (pp 225, 228) and refer to an obstetrician if it has not separated, if blood loss is excessive or if a manual removal of placenta is required.

Once third-stage management is complete the delivery records are completed in detail, including the birth notification. The new family are given time together, vital sign observations are checked, as is the woman's uterus and lochial loss. Refreshments are given and the baby care is attended to; infant feeding should begin.

Estimation of blood loss

Estimating blood loss is notoriously inaccurate, with estimates usually lower than the actual amount of blood lost. Brant (1967) demonstrated that although blood loss up to 300 mL was accurately assessed, blood loss in excess of this was generally underestimated. Haswell (1981) used a pouch situated under the woman's buttocks to 'catch' the blood loss and suggested that blood loss over 500 mL was usually underestimated by half. Levy & Moore's (1985) study of midwives' ability to estimate blood loss found that as the actual amount of blood increased, the accuracy of the estimation reduced; for example, 100 mL blood loss was estimated as 111 mL (mean), 300 mL blood loss was estimated as 197 mL (mean), with 500 mL the mean estimate was 307 mL and, when the blood loss was 1200 mL, the mean estimated blood loss was 718 mL. Bose et al (2006) undertook a similar study assessing obstetricians, anaesthetists, midwives, nurses and healthcare assistants' ability to assess blood loss using sanitary pads, gauze swabs, kidney dishes, inco-pads, floor spills and a bed soaked with different amounts of blood. The anaesthetists were most accurate in their assessment but tended to overestimate blood loss, whereas all the other categories of healthcare professional seriously underestimated blood loss. In particular, Bose et al found that there was significant underestimation for large floor spillages, large gauze swabs and where the blood loss was over the bed and onto the floor. They developed guidelines to assist with the visual estimation of blood loss, which include looking at saturated gauze swabs (small 10×10 cm $= 60$ mL, medium 30×30 cm $= 140$ mL, large 45×45 cm $= 350$ mL), saturated sanitary pad (100 mL), floor spillages (50 cm diameter $= 500$ mL, 75 cm $= 1000$ mL, 100 cm $= 1500$ mL) and whether the bleeding with a PPH is restricted to the bed (unlikely to exceed 1000 mL) or spills over the bed and onto the floor (likely to exceed 1000 mL) (Bose et al 2006).

Blood loss should be estimated as accurately as possible as it forewarns of impending haemorrhagic state (Bose et al 2006). This includes blood loss on disposable sheets, linen and collected within receivers during and after the third stage. It is important to retrieve as much blood from the sheets as possible into a container for measurement. Obvious blood loss can be measured in a jug, but when the blood has seeped onto the sheets, it becomes harder to estimate blood loss.

The woman who has an expectant third stage often delivers the placenta into a bedpan, or container, enabling blood loss to be collected more easily. The increased blood loss with an expectant third stage may be due (in some instances) to the more efficient collection and measurement of blood.

The estimated amount of blood loss should be documented appropriately and referral should be made if this is excessive or the woman is compromised. Women are affected differently by blood loss, many women who are in good health with good predelivery haemoglobin levels can tolerate a 500 mL loss (this amount is only slightly more than is removed from the body during a blood donation session) with little or no effect (Begley et al 2008). McDonald & Middleton (2008) agree, suggesting healthy women are able to tolerate a blood loss up to 1000 mL without being compromised.

Examination of the genital tract following delivery

Trauma to the cervix, vagina, labia and perineum can increase blood loss, cause increased pain for the woman or result in infection. The midwife should examine the woman's genital tract following birth to ascertain the degree of trauma and whether suturing is indicated. Bruising and oedema may be evident, which can affect the examination. The area is likely to be extremely tender, and the examination should be undertaken sensitively; the woman should be offered Entonox® (NICE 2007). It is important that there is a good light source to visualise the genital tract clearly.

PROCEDURE: examination of the genital tract

- Explain the procedure to the woman and gain informed consent.
- The midwife continues to wear the gloves that have been used for the delivery of the placenta and membranes if sterility has been maintained, otherwise a new pair of sterile gloves should be worn.
- Ask the woman to adopt an almost recumbent position, with her knees bent, ankles together and knees parted.
- Wash down the external genitalia gently with a sterile swab and warm tap water, wiping from front to back to remove any blood or debris.
- Examine the vulva, noting any trauma, particularly to the labia.
- Wrap a sterile swab around the first two fingers of the examining hand, fingers slightly parted.
- Separate the labia gently with the fingers of the non-examining hand and insert the swabbed fingers carefully into the vagina, directing the fingers in a downwards and backwards direction.

- Gently press down to examine the anterior and side walls of the vagina and cervix (if the cervix cannot be seen, the woman may need to lie flat) for trauma, replacing the gauze as necessary.
- Slowly begin to remove the swabbed fingers from the vagina, examining the posterior vaginal wall.
- When the fingers have been removed, examine the perineum for trauma.
- Assist the woman into a comfortable position, remove gloves, wash hands and discuss the findings.
- Suturing may be undertaken when appropriate (see Chapter 34).
- Dispose of equipment appropriately.
- Document findings and act accordingly.

- The placenta and membranes may be delivered expectantly (by the woman) or actively (by the midwife).
- Delayed cord clamping confers many benefits for the baby and does not appear to compromise the woman.
- Active management decreases the length of the third stage and the blood loss, but is associated with increased side effects from the oxytocic drugs and retained placenta.
- Estimation of blood loss is often inaccurate and under-assessed; as the blood loss increases, this inaccuracy also increases.
- The genital tract should be examined following delivery of the placenta and membranes for signs of trauma.

ROLE AND RESPONSIBILITIES OF THE MIDWIFE

These can be summarised as:

- undertaking the procedures correctly
- recognising deviations from the norm and instigating referral
- appropriate record keeping.

Summary

- The third stage of labour is concerned with the delivery of the placenta and membranes and the control of haemorrhage.
- During this stage, the woman is at increased risk of morbidity and mortality from haemorrhage.

SELF-ASSESSMENT EXERCISES

The answers to the following questions may be found in the text:

1. Describe the physiology of the third stage of labour.
2. What are the advantages for the baby of delayed cord clamping?
3. What is the midwife's role when the third stage is to be expectant?
4. Name the drugs used with active management of labour and discuss their side effects
5. How is controlled cord traction applied?
6. How is blood loss estimated?
7. How does the midwife assess the genital tract for trauma following delivery of the placenta and membranes?

References

Airey R, Farrar D, Duley L: Timing of umbilical cord clamping: Midwives views and practices, *Br J Midwifery* 16(4):236–239, 2008.

Airey R, Farrar D, Duley L: Alternative positions for the baby at birth before clamping the umbilical cord, *Cochrane Database Syst Rev* (1) CD007555, DOI:10.1002/14651858.CD007555, 2009.

Baenziger O, Stolkin F, Keel M, et al: The influence of the timing of cord clamping on postnatal cerebral oxygenation in preterm neonates: a randomised controlled trial, *Pediatrics* 119(3):455–459, 2007.

Begley CM, Devane D, Murphy DJ, et al: Active versus expectant management for women in the third stage of labour, *Cochrane Database Syst Rev* (4) CD007412, DOI:10.1002/14651858.CD007412, 2008.

Blackburn S: Physiological third stage of labour and birth at home. In Edwins J, editor: *Community Midwifery Practice*, Oxford, 2008, Blackwell, pp 66–86.

Bose P, Regan F, Paterson-Brown S: Improving the accuracy of estimated blood loss at obstetric haemorrhage using clinical reconstructions, *Br J Obstet Gynaecol* 113(8):919–924, 2006.

Brandt M: The mechanism and management of the third stage of labour, *Am J Obstet Gynecol* 23:662–667, 1933.

Brant HA: Precise estimation of postpartum haemorrhage: difficulties and importance, *Br Med J* 1:398–400, 1967.

Buckley SJ: Undisturbed birth – nature's hormone blueprint for safety, ease and ecstasy, *MIDIRS Midwifery Dig* 14(2):203–206, 2004.

Cernadas JMC, Carroli G, Pellegrini L, et al: The effect of timing on cord clamping on neonatal venous haematocrit values and clinical outcome at term: A randomized controlled trial, *Pediatrics* 117 (4):779–787, 2006.

Chapparo CM, Neufeld LM, Tena Alvarez G, et al: Effect of timing of umbilical cord clamping on iron status in Mexican infants: a randomized controlled trial, *Lancet* 367:1997–2004, 2006.

Cook EL: Delayed cord clamping or immediate cord clamping? A literature review, *Br J Midwifery* 15 (19):562–571, 2007.

Cotter AM, Ness A, Tolosa JE: Prophylactic oxytocin for the third stage of labour, *Cochrane Database Syst Rev* (4) CD001808. DOI: 10.1002/14651858.CD001808, 2001.

DH (Department of Health): Report on confidential enquiries into maternal deaths in the United Kingdom 1991–1993, London, 1996, HMSO.

Enkin M, Keirse MJNC, Neilson J, et al, editors: The third stage of labour. In *A guide to effective care in pregnancy and childbirth*, ed 3, Oxford, 2000, Oxford University Press, ch 33.

Fry J: Physiological third stage of labour: support it or lose it, *Br J Midwifery* 15(11):693–695, 2007.

Gyte G: *NCT Evidence Based Briefing Third Stage of Labour*, 2006.

Haswell JN: Measured blood loss at delivery, *J Indiana State Med Assoc* 74(1):34–36, 1981.

Herman A: Complicated third stage of labor: time to switch on the scanner, *Ultrasound Obstet Gynecol* 15:89–95, 2000.

Herman A, Zimerman A, Arieli S, et al: Down–up sequential separation of the placenta, *Ultrasound Obstet Gynecol* 19:278–281, 2002.

Kanikasamy F: Third stage: the 'why' of physiological practice, *Midwives* 10 (9):422–425, 2007.

Krapp M, Baschat AA, Hankeln M, et al: Greyscale and color Doppler

sonography in the third stage of labor for early detection of failed placental separation, *Ultrasound Obstet Gynecol* 15(2):138–142, 2000.

Levy V, Moore J: The midwife's management of the third stage of labour, *Nurs Times* 1(5):47–50, 1985.

Lewis G, editor: The Confidential Enquiry into Maternal and Child Health (CEMACH). Saving Mothers' Lives: reviewing maternal deaths to make motherhood safer – 2003–2005, *The Seventh Report on Confidential Enquiries into Maternal Deaths in the United Kingdom*, London, 2007, CEMACH.

Lucas M: Reflections on the third stage, *Pract Midwife* 9(6):30–31, 2006.

Maughan KL, Heim SW, Galazka SS: Preventing postpartum haemorrhage: Managing the third stage of labor, *Am Fam Physician* 73(6):1025–1028, 2006.

McDonald S, Middleton P: Effect of timing of umbilical cord clamping of term infants on maternal and neonatal outcomes, *Cochrane Database Syst Rev* (2) CD004074. DOI:10.1002/14651858.CD004074, pub2, 2008.

McDonald SJ, Abbott JM, Higgins SP: Prophylactic ergometrine-oxytocin versus oxytocin for the third stage of labour, *Cochrane Database Syst Rev* (1) CD000201. DOI:10.1002/14651858.CD000201, pub2, 2004.

Nardin JM, Carroli G, Weeks A, et al: Umbilical vein injection for the routine management of the third stage of labour, *Cochrane Database Syst Rev* (4) CD006176. DOI:10.1002/14651858.CD006176, 2006.

NICE (National Institute for Health and Clinical Excellence): *Intrapartum care. Care of healthy women and their babies during childbirth*, London, 2007, NICE.

Odent M: Don't manage the third stage of labour, *Pract Midwife* 11(9):313, 1998.

Page D: Breastfeeding learning the dance of latching, *J Hum Lact* 23(1):111–112, 2007.

Pena-Marti GE, Comunian-Carrasco G: Fundal pressure versus controlled

cord traction as part of the active management of the third stage of labour, *Cochrane Database Syst Rev* (4) CD005462. DOI:10.1002/14651858.CD005462, pub2, 2007.

Prendiville WJ, Elbourne D, McDonald S: *Cochrane Database Syst Rev* (3) CD000007. DOI:10.1002/14651858.CD000007, 2000.

Rabe H, Reynolds GJ, Diaz-Rosello JL: Early versus delayed umbilical cord clamping in preterm infants, *Cochrane Database Syst Rev* (4) CD003248. DOI:10.1002/14651858.CD003248, 2004.

Rabe H, Alvarez JR, Lawn C, et al: A management guideline to reduce the frequency of blood transfusion in very-low-birth-weight infants, *Am J Perinatol* 26(3):179–183, 2009.

Soltani H, Dickinson F, Symonds IM: Placental cord drainage after spontaneous vaginal delivery as part of the management of the third stage of labour, *Cochrane Database Syst Rev* (4) CD004665. DOI:10.1002/14651858.CD004665, pub2, 2005.

Soltani H, Dickinson F: Timing of prophylactic oxytocics for the third stage of labour after vaginal birth, *Cochrane Database Syst Rev* (4) CD006173. DOI:10.1002/14651858.CD006173, pub2, 2006.

Spencer PM: Controlled cord traction in the management of the third stage of labour, *Br Med J* 1:1728–1732, 1962.

Ultee CA, van der Deure J, Swart J, et al: Delayed cord clamping in preterm infants delivered at 34–36 weeks' gestation: a randomized controlled trial, *Arch Dis Child Fetal Neonatal Ed* 93:F20–F23, 2006.

Weckert R, Hancock H: The importance of delayed cord clamping for Aboriginal babies: a life-enhancing advantage, *Women Birth* 21 (4):165–170, 2008.

Wickham S: Further thoughts on the third stage of labour, *Pract Midwife* 2(10):14–15, 1999.

Principles of intrapartum skills: examination of the placenta

Examination of the placenta following delivery is an important skill undertaken by the midwife to reduce the occurrence of both postpartum haemorrhage and infection. This chapter describes the structure and appearance of the placenta, discussing the significance of deviations, and concluding with the procedure for undertaking examination of the placenta. It concludes with a brief discussion concerning disposal of the placenta.

LEARNING OUTCOMES

Having read this chapter the reader should be able to:

- describe the structure and appearance of the placenta at term
- describe how the placenta is examined
- discuss the significance of the information obtained from the examination
- discuss the role and responsibilities of the midwife in relation to examining the placenta.

Structure and appearance

The placenta is a disc-shaped structure that has both maternal and fetal surfaces. At term, the placenta weighs approximately 500–600 g (about one-sixth of the baby's weight), has a diameter of 15–20 cm and is 2–3 cm thick. Early cord clamping may result in the placenta being proportionally heavier, whereas delayed cord clamping can produce a placenta that is proportionally lighter, due to the amount of blood transfused from the placenta to the baby at delivery. A larger placenta may be associated with maternal diabetes and multiple pregnancy, a smaller placenta with chronic intrauterine growth restriction.

Occasionally the placenta may develop with an abnormal structure and appearance such as a circumvallate placenta. The placenta enlarges beneath the endometrial surface and the embryonic sac enlarges above it; the endometrium between the two is compressed and obliterated resulting in an acellular membrane, which may affect the attachment of the placenta to the decidua, increasing the risk of placental abruption. The placenta has a thick, grey/white raised ring around the central part of the fetal surface, caused by the fetal membranes folding back on themselves.

Fetal surface of the placenta

The fetal side has a white shiny appearance due to the chorionic plate (a thin membrane continuous with the chorion) and the amnion that cover the surface. The fetal side is composed of 50–60 lobes or cotyledons, which are further divided into 1–5 lobules. Occasionally, the placenta may be divided into two (bipartite) or three (tripartite) separate, distinct lobes, each with an umbilical cord inserted into it. The cord presents as one cord until it is near the placental surface when it divides into two or three to supply each lobe (Fig. 33.1).

Blood vessels, branches of the umbilical vein and arteries are clearly visible, spreading outwards from the point of cord insertion, usually centrally or slightly off centre (Fig. 33.2A,B). A cord inserted at the edge of the placenta – a 'battledore' insertion (Fig. 33.2C) – is usually insignificant, although the attachment may be fragile, increasing the risk of detachment during controlled cord traction. Rarely the cord is inserted into the membranes – a 'velamentous' insertion (Fig. 33.2D) – with vessels running through the membranes to the placenta. The attachment can be very fragile, resulting in detachment during controlled cord traction. The vessels may overlie the cervix ('vasa praevia') and if ruptured during spontaneous or artificial rupturing of the membranes will result in massive fetal haemorrhage.

The umbilical cord contains the two umbilical arteries and the umbilical vein, surrounded by Wharton's jelly, and is covered by the amnion. A cord with fewer than three vessels may indicate a congenital abnormality; the baby should be referred to the paediatrician and a sample of the cord may be required for analysis. The cord is 40–50 cm long (range 30–90 cm), 1–2 cm wide and is twisted

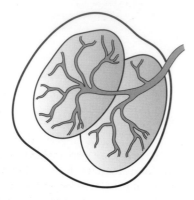

Figure 33.1 • Bipartite placenta

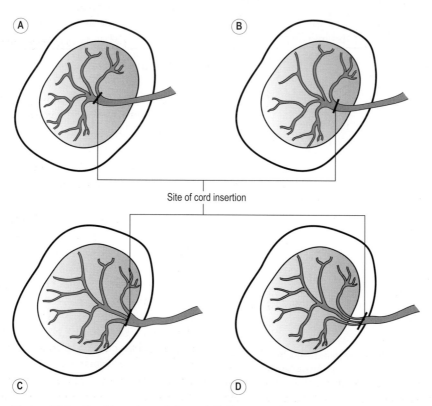

Site of cord insertion

Figure 33.2 • Cord insertions. A Central. B Eccentric. C Battledore. D Velamentous

spirally to provide some protection to the vessels from pressure. A short cord is one measuring less than 40 cm and is usually insignificant unless very short when descent of the fetus through the pelvis will cause the cord to be pulled taut and apply traction on the placenta. A long cord may become wrapped around the fetus or knotted, resulting in occlusion of the vessels. The risk of cord presentation and prolapse increases with a long cord, particularly if the presenting part is poorly applied to the cervix. False knots can occur when the blood vessels are longer than the cord and form a loop in the Wharton's jelly; these are of little significance. A thick or thin cord may be difficult to clamp securely following delivery.

The amnion and chorion comprise the fetal membranes, which appear fused but are not. Stripping one from the other can separate them; the amnion can be pulled back to the cord. The amnion is smooth, translucent and tough, whereas the chorion is thick, opaque and friable. The chorion begins at the edge of the placenta and extends around the decidua. Following delivery, the membranes will have a hole in them through which the baby has been born. If the membranes appear ragged, a piece of membrane may be retained *in utero*. This can affect uterine contractility and predispose to postpartum haemorrhage. It also provides a site for microorganisms to grow, predisposing to infection. The passage of any clots postpartum should be examined for membranes.

Maternal surface of the placenta

The dark red maternal side is composed of 15–20 cotyledons (divided by septa), which have arisen from two or more main stem villi and their branches. During the second and third trimesters, fibrin deposition may occur around the villi resulting in isolated villi infarction. This is usually insignificant unless excessive, affecting the exchange of nutrients and waste products between the maternal and fetal circulation, resulting in intrauterine growth restriction. Calcification due to lime salt deposition on the surface can make it feel gritty; this is insignificant. Occasionally, a cotyledon may be present in the membranes, separated from the placenta but connected by a blood vessel – a 'succenturiate' lobe (Fig. 33.3). If this is retained *in utero*, it predisposes to postpartum haemorrhage and infection as for the retained membrane. The membranes should be

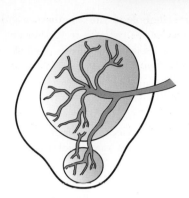

Figure 33.3 • Succenturiate lobe

carefully examined for evidence of missing lobes, suspected if an unexplained hole appears in the chorion, particularly if blood vessels run towards the hole and stop abruptly.

A pale placenta may reflect delayed clamping of the cord, where less blood is retained in the placenta; it could also indicate intrauterine anaemia. Meconium may also be seen on the fetal surface, as may signs of infection and hyperbilirubinaemia. An offensive smelling placenta is often indicative of intrauterine infection.

PROCEDURE: examination of the placenta

- Explain the procedure to the parents and ascertain if they wish to observe the examination.
- Gather equipment:
  - gloves and apron
  - disposable protective cover
  - disposal bag for placenta
  - placenta.
- Wash hands, apply apron and gloves.
- Lay the placenta, fetal surface uppermost, onto the cover (placed on a flat surface) noting the size, shape, smell and colour.
- Examine the cord, noting the length, insertion point and presence of knots.
- Count the number of vessels in the cut end of the cord (if the end has been obliterated, cut off a small portion of the cord and count the vessels in the portion remaining).
- Observe the fetal surface for irregularities.
- Taking hold of the cord with the non-dominant hand, lift the placenta from the surface and

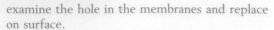
examine the hole in the membranes and replace on surface.

- Spread the membranes outwards, looking for extra vessel or lobes, or unexplained holes.
- Separate the amnion and chorion, pulling the amnion back over the base of the umbilical cord.
- Turn the placenta over, maternal side uppermost.
- Examine the cotyledons, ensuring all are present, noting the size and amount of areas of infarction or blood clots.
- Weigh or swab the placenta if indicated.
- Dispose of the placenta and equipment correctly.
- Wash hands.
- Discuss the findings with the parents.
- Document findings and act accordingly.

Cord blood samples

If cord blood is required (e.g. when the mother is Rhesus negative), McDonald (2009) suggests this should be obtained from the fetal surface of the placenta as soon as possible as the blood vessels are congested and visible. Sampling should be undertaken quickly before the blood clots and is usually undertaken before the placenta is examined.

Cord blood samples required for blood gas analysis should be obtained at delivery as a delay in obtaining the sampling can result in an inaccurate result. This may in part be due to the fact that the placenta continues to perfuse for longer than the clamped cord, gaseous exchange can continue until it separates, thus producing different blood–gas results to those that would be found from the cord or from the baby at birth (Lynn & Beeby 2007). Armstrong & Stenson (2006) found that samples taken 20 minutes after delivery, even with double clamping on the cord, were unreliable.

To obtain samples of arterial and venous blood for blood gas analysis, the umbilical cord should be clamped in two places. Two heparinized syringes are required, one for the venous sample, one for the arterial sample. The larger single, thin-walled umbilical vein is located and the needle is inserted into the vein at a 45° angle, taking care not to puncture through the vein walls. The syringe is filled to the required amount, removed from the vein and any air bubbles removed prior to capping the syringe to avoid the blood leaking out. The syringe is labelled and the procedure repeated for the umbilical artery. There is a choice of two umbilical arteries

recognisable by their round appearance and thicker walls. They are also smaller vessels compared to the vein which can make it harder to obtain a sample, as it is easier to puncture both sides of the vessel. The samples should be stored between 2 and 8°C and be delivered to the laboratory within 15 minutes.

Some parents may request cord blood is obtained for stem cell collection. Fyle (2006) advises this should not occur until after the placenta has delivered and should not be the responsibility of the midwife. The Royal College of Obstetricians and Gynaecologists (RCOG 2006) agrees that collection should be undertaken by a trained individual who is not the midwife or doctor and only after the placenta has been delivered. If blood has been removed from the placenta prior to examination, the midwife should be aware that this can affect the colour and size of the placenta.

In some maternity units the placentae are collected and frozen for research purposes; this may entail either the placenta or cord. Cord blood can be donated to the London Cord Blood Bank and used for a variety of haematological conditions (e.g. leukaemia; Fursland 1998). Histological investigation may be required in certain situations (e.g. multiple deliveries, preterm deliveries, stillbirths, suspected infection).

Disposing of the placenta

The majority of women in the UK will want the midwife to dispose of their placenta, which is usually by incineration (Blackburn 2008); local policy should be followed. However, the woman might want to take her detached placenta home. Many cultures bury the placenta on family ground; some may want to plant a tree over the top. The midwife should ascertain the wishes of the woman regarding disposing of the placenta and, if it is to be taken home, the midwife should ensure it is securely double wrapped and placed in a suitable container.

Some women opt for a lotus birth (full non-severance), whereby the baby remains attached to the umbilical cord and placenta until the cord shrivels and detaches naturally (Blackburn 2008). Following the examination of the placenta, the midwife or family member should wipe off any excess fluids, wash it clean if necessary and pat dry. If the woman is in hospital, the placenta is usually wrapped in cloth, but at home it may be placed in a covered bowl or remain wrapped in cloth and kept close to the baby. It is important that air is able to pass through the cloth/bowl cover as the placenta needs to dry out. If this does not happen it can develop a distinct musky smell (the placenta should then be planted or refrigerated after separating the baby from the cord). It is not unusual to rub the placenta with sea salt to assist with the drying process. The woman may add essential oils (e.g. lavender) with or without powdered herbs (e.g. goldenseal) as these have antibacterial properties (Lotus Birth 2009, Wickham 2009, Wikipedia 2009).

ROLE AND RESPONSIBILITIES OF THE MIDWIFE

These can be summarised as:

- undertaking the examination correctly
- recognising deviations from the norm and instigating referral
- appropriate use of standard precautions
- appropriate record keeping.

Summary

- The placenta has fetal and maternal components; both sides should be examined carefully.

- The placenta should be examined to ensure it is complete; retained products predispose to postpartum haemorrhage and infection.
- Deviations from the norm can indicate underlying problems for the baby, e.g. infection, congenital abnormality.
- Standard precautions should always be followed when handling and disposing of the placenta.
- Women vary in how they want to dispose of their placenta and the woman's wishes should be ascertained and facilitated.

SELF-ASSESSMENT EXERCISES

The answers to the following questions may be found in the text:

1. Describe the general appearance of the placenta at term.
2. What are the differences between the fetal and maternal placental surfaces?
3. Describe the procedure for examining the placenta.
4. List the deviations that can be detected and discuss the significance of each.
5. What are the role and responsibilities of the midwife in relation to the examination of the placenta?

References

Armstrong L, Stenson B: Effect of delayed sampling on umbilical cord arterial and venous lactate and blood gases in clamped and unclamped vessels, *Arch Dis Child Fetal Neonatal Ed* 91(5):F342–F345, 2006.

Blackburn S: Physiological third stage of labour and birth at home. In Edwins J, editor: *Community midwifery practice*, Oxford, 2008, Blackwell, pp 66–86.

Fyle J: Routine commercial umbilical cord blood collection, *RCM Midwives* 9(7):261, 2006.

Fursland E: Blood mothers, *Nurs Times* 94(33):42–43, 1998.

Lynn A, Beeby P: Cord and placenta arterial gas analysis: the accuracy of delayed sampling, *Arch Dis Child Fetal Neonatal Ed* 92(4):F281–F285, 2007.

Lotus Birth: Online. Available: http://www.lotusfertility.com/Lotus_Birth_Q/Lotus_ Birth_QA.html 23 March 2009.

McDonald S: Physiology and management of the third stage of labour. In Fraser DM, Cooper MA, editors: *Myles textbook for midwives*, ed 15, Edinburgh, 2009, Churchill Livingstone, pp 532–554.

RCOG: *RCOG Opinion Paper 2: Umbilical cord blood banking*, Online. Available: http://www.rcog.org.uk/news/rcog-advice-umbilical-cord-blood-banking-and-storage 24 March 2009, 2006.

Wickham S: Online. Available: http://www.withwoman.co.uk/contents/info/lotus.html 23 March 2009, 2009.

Wikipedia: Online. Available: http://en.wikipedia.org/wiki/Lotus_Birth 23 March 2009, 2009.

Principles of intrapartum skills: perineal repair

34

Perineal trauma of some kind is estimated to occur in up to 85% of vaginal deliveries in the UK, with 69% requiring suturing (Kettle et al 2002); perineal repair is associated with short-term discomfort and/ or pain and 20% of women experience long-term problems such as dyspareunia (Kettle et al 2007). This chapter examines the procedure, technique and materials used for perineal repair; the anatomy of the pelvic floor is reviewed and the significance of correct perineal repair is highlighted. The reader is encouraged to read widely in other literary sources to appreciate the associated issues (e.g. prevention of perineal trauma, postnatal perineal care).

LEARNING OUTCOMES

Having read this chapter the reader should be able to:

- state the aims of perineal repair
- discuss the role and responsibilities of the midwife when undertaking perineal repair
- discuss the current evidence for the choice of materials and the technique used
- describe how to infiltrate the perineum
- demonstrate tying a knot, continuous non-locked and subcuticular sutures
- list the factors that should be included with record keeping.

The pelvic floor

As a hammock-shaped arrangement of muscles and fascia, the pelvic floor is the supportive structure in the woman's pelvis. The muscles are arranged in two layers, deep and superficial (Fig. 34.1) extending to and from landmarks in the pelvis, encircling other structures (e.g. the vagina) and forming the

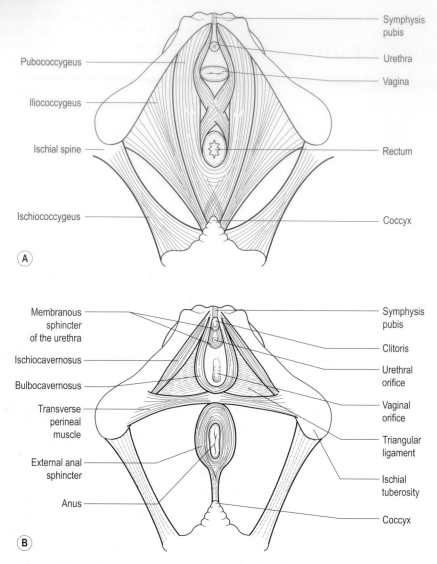

Figure 34.1 • A Deep muscle layer of the pelvic floor. B Superficial muscle layer of the pelvic floor

perineal body. The perineal body is triangular in shape and comprises skin, two superficial muscles (bulbocavernosus and transverse perineal) and one deep muscle (pubococcygeus). It lies between the anus and vagina and is flattened and displaced as the baby is born. The pelvic floor prevents the pelvic organs from prolapsing and is an important component in the correct functioning of the vagina, bladder, uterus and rectum; a damaged or weakened pelvic floor may cause long-term urinary, faecal or sexual morbidity.

Aims of perineal repair

Repairing perineal trauma aims to ensure that the tissues are correctly realigned, haemorrhage is stemmed and dead space (into which bleeding may occur) is reduced. The overall aim is to maintain the integrity of the woman's pelvic floor.

On examining the genital tract immediately post-delivery, the extent of perineal damage is noted and decisions are made as to:

- whether the damage requires repair
- if so, using which materials
- by whom
- in which environment.

Definitions of perineal trauma are based around the structures involved; note that no classification is currently made as to the size of the injury. It may have occurred naturally or be a result of incision (episiotomy). The accepted definitions are:

- first degree: affects skin only
- second degree (tear or episiotomy): affects the skin, posterior vaginal wall and superficial muscle (occasionally deep muscle is affected)
- third degree: affects the same structures as a second degree as well as the anal sphincter and are further classified as:
  - ○ 3a <50% of external anal sphincter torn
  - ○ 3b >50% of external anal sphincter torn
  - ○ 3c injury to both the external and internal anal sphincter
- fourth degree: affects the perineum (as above) and the anal sphincter complex and epithelium (NICE 2007).

However, damage can occur to any part of the pelvic floor, perineal body or vulval tissue, including the vagina and/or labia. Careful examination of the labia is required to determine if the clitoris or urethra have been damaged.

Suturing is the most likely means of repair; there has been some speculative research into the use of tissue adhesive (Adoni & Anteby 1991, Rogerson et al 2000) but there is little evidence this is preferable to suturing, with further research and development required (RCM 2008, Viswanathan et al 2005). The skill of the operator is paramount; midwives can provide good continuity of care for the woman, but care needs to be evidence based, with training and updating and within one's capabilities. Hesitations about the task in hand, for whatever reason, should cause the midwife to refer to an experienced midwife or obstetrician. The health and wellbeing of the woman may be seriously affected in both the short and long term if the repair is poorly completed (Sleep et al 1984). Extensive perineal damage or third- or fourth-degree injury requires repair by a senior obstetrician in theatre with additional analgesia (general or regional anaesthesia). If the urethra is involved, the repair may need to be undertaken by a genitourinary specialist. Bilateral labial grazes that would be in apposition when standing or sitting should also be sutured

so that the labia do not heal together. Arkin & Chern-Hughes (2001) cite a case study in which the labia needed surgically parting some months following abrasions in childbirth. If the woman declines suturing of bilateral labial tears, she should be advised about the risks and encouraged to part her labia daily to reduce the likelihood of fusion. Perineal repair can be undertaken in the home if adaptations are made to accommodate suitable positioning of the woman and midwife (with good light). If the repair is extensive, however, the midwife may consider transfer to a hospital environment.

Current evidence

Draper & Newell (1996) suggest that failure to adhere to evidence-based practice with perineal repair may have wide-ranging consequences in women's lives. The body of research is now extensive (but still increasing) and therefore there is little excuse for diversity in practice. Kenyon & Ford (2004) discuss the process and implementation of an evidence-based accepted protocol in their maternity unit.

To suture or not to suture?

NICE (2007) recommends that first-degree tears where the wound is not in apposition and all second-degree tears should be sutured, although not all women will consent to the procedure. Kenyon & Ford (2004) agree, indicating that the existing studies are small and therefore unreliable and that, at this time, suturing of the vaginal wall and muscle layers is indicated. McCandlish (2001) also suggests that it is time to seek the evidence, but not to change practice until reliable evidence exists.

The midwife should discuss the rationale for suturing, with the advantages and disadvantages, to allow the woman to make a more informed choice. The advantages of suturing include quicker initial healing of the tissues with better wound alignment compared with not suturing (Fleming et al 2003, Langley et al 2006, Leeman et al 2007) and reduced urinary problems (Metcalfe et al 2006) although the RCM (2008) suggests that studies on non-suturing have yielded conflicting results and agree with Metcalfe et al (2006) that further research is required. However, suturing can be a painful procedure in itself, may require the use of lithotomy, which can be difficult for some women (e.g. those with pelvic girdle pain) and may result in increased use of analgesia (Langley et al 2006, Leeman et al 2007). Metcalfe et al (2006) found reported levels of perineal pain were similar between sutured and unsutured women.

The skin, following the Ipswich Trial (Gordon et al 1998), may be left unsutured providing that the skin edges are in apposition with a gap no greater than 0.5 cm. This is considered to reduce dyspareunia at 3 months postpartum, but with no differences in short- or long-term perineal pain. However, Grant et al (2001) found that 1 year later there were no differences in relation to the amount of discomfort or pain experienced, dyspareunia and the time in which sexual intercourse was resumed; the RCM (2008) conclude that there appears to be neither benefit nor disadvantage in relation to suturing or not suturing the skin. Viswanathan et al (2005) advise that it is preferable to leave both the superficial vaginal and perineal skin unsutured.

Choice of material

Fast-absorbing polyglactin sutures are currently considered to be the suture material of choice when compared to chromic catgut and other absorbable sutures as they are associated with less perineal pain, a reduced need for analgesia, less uterine cramping at 24–48 hours and at 6–8 weeks, a significant reduction in the need for suture removal, fewer healing problems in the short term and earlier resumption of sexual activity (Greenberg et al 2004, Kettle et al 2007, Leroux and Bujold 2006, Viswanathan et al 2005). Size 2/0 is indicated for perineal tissue.

Instruments

There is little mention of instruments, except that Bott (1999) recommends that midwives should learn to suture with instruments (needle holder and tissue forceps) rather than fingers, to reduce the risk of injury to the midwife and possible transfer of HIV. The Department of Health (DH 1998) also recommends the use of blunt-ended needles for suturing to reduce these risks further; the American College of Surgeons also support the use of blunt-ended needles when suturing muscle to reduce the risk of needlestick injury (ACS 2007). However, Wilson et al (2008) found no difference in the rate of surgical glove perforation between blunt and sharp needles during perineal repair but the use of blunt needles increased the difficulty of perineal repair.

Technique

Perineal repair is often completed in three stages:

1. posterior vaginal wall
2. perineal muscle layer
3. perineal skin.

The use of a loose continuous suture is currently recommended for all three layers as it results in less short-term pain than interrupted or locked sutures (Kettle et al 2007). Whilst a continuous locked suture has been used to repair the vagina in the past – this was thought to prevent concertinaing of the vaginal wall if the continuous non-locked suture were pulled too tight (Enkin et al 2000) – there have been no randomised controlled trials to confirm this (Kettle et al 2007). Indeed, Kettle et al (2007) agree that tight stitches can restrict the distribution of tissue resulting in increased pain and propose the use of a loose continuous suture as it enables the tension to be transferred throughout the length of the whole stitch thereby reducing pain.

The current evidence may be summarised as:

- if indicated, a perineal wound should be sutured throughout using a rapidly absorbing polyglactin suture, e.g. Vicryl Rapide®, with a loose continuous unlocked suture to the posterior vaginal wall and muscle layer, bringing the skin into good apposition
- if skin closure is indicated, a continuous subcuticular technique should be used
- for good practice (not evidence based) the midwife should consider standard precautions and use instruments to suture with and if possible blunt-ended needles.

Perineal suturing

A successful perineal repair incorporates all of the following principles:

Effective analgesia for the woman

Sanders et al (2002) indicate that pain during suturing is greater than midwives may realise for women who do not have regional analgesia. Where an epidural has been used effectively during labour, a top-up should be given prior to suturing. If this does not achieve effective anaesthesia or regional analgesia has not been used, the perineum should be infiltrated using 20 mL 1% lidocaine (NICE 2007) according to an approved patient group direction; analgesics such as Entonox® are also useful. Following repair, NICE (2007), Kenyon & Ford (2004) and Hedayati et al (2003) recommend rectal diclofenac 100 mg stat., provided this is not contraindicated, as it is associated with less pain during the 24 hours following the repair and less analgesia is required within the first 48 hours.

The woman may find it less painful if she is holding/feeding the baby as this may distract her from the suturing process. It is also important to keep her informed of what is happening, particularly when touching her, as she can still experience pressure sensations despite an effective anaesthetic block.

Asepsis and standard precautions

A sterile suturing pack is used and the midwife wears gloves, apron and any other necessary items for infection control and protection purposes that local protocols suggest. Research into suitable fluids for perineal swabbing remains limited; water is widely used, but not proven (Jessiman 2001). Lubricant may also vary according to local protocols between water-soluble (e.g. KY Jelly®) and chlorhexidine Hibitane® cream.

Alignment of the tissues to encourage granulation and healing

The midwife should be very familiar with the pelvic floor anatomy and therefore be quite certain of the alignment of the tissues. The distinction in colour between the tissues is often very helpful. A good light source and access to the perineum is important for the repair to be completed properly. Occasionally, the midwife may discover on examining the woman that the tear is more extensive than originally thought. This allows decisions to be reviewed; if necessary an obstetrician is called. Whilst the lithotomy position is still widely used in hospitals, its use is not always essential and so is being used less in practice.

It is important that the woman is comfortable and able to open her legs sufficiently. Care must be taken to ensure that the woman does not abduct her legs excessively, and she may find it more comfortable to rest her legs against lithotomy poles.

At home suitable alternatives can be found (e.g. sitting on the edge of the bed with legs supported on chairs). When aligned properly the process of wound healing begins (see Chapter 52); sutures that are too tight or too loose may impede this process.

Cessation of haemorrhage

Suturing must achieve this in each part of the repair, otherwise haemorrhage can continue between the layers resulting in a haematoma or postpartum haemorrhage. Should a bleeding vessel be located, it should be tied off.

Reduction of any dead space

Haemorrhage may occur into areas of dead space resulting in a haematoma; bringing the tissues into apposition reduces the risk of this occurring.

Minimal amount of suture material

Any foreign material in tissue results in a reaction. Fewer knots and less suture material will result in improved healing.

Infiltration of the perineum for repair

Using an aseptic technique, anaesthetic – usually 20 mL 1% lidocaine – is infiltrated into the four aspects of the tear, along the left- and right-hand sides of the vaginal wall and perineum. The tissue is held with tissue forceps while the needle is inserted at point A along to point B (Fig. 34.2). The plunger should be withdrawn to ensure the needle is not within a blood vessel. If blood is seen in the syringe it should be withdrawn and the procedure recommenced using a new needle, syringe and solution (aspiration is repeated each time the position of the needle is changed). If blood is not present, the needle is slowly withdrawn as the anaesthetic is injected along line B to A, the needle is reversed rather than removed so that the distance C to A is also infiltrated. It is then inserted into point D and the process repeated B to D, C to D. It is important to allow time for the anaesthetic to work before commencing suturing.

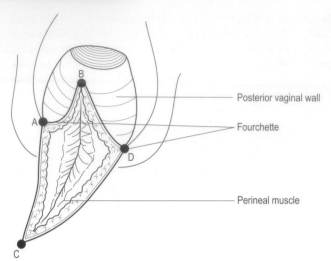

Figure 34.2 • Infiltration prior to suturing

- Posterior vaginal wall
- Fourchette
- Perineal muscle

Using a needle holder

In appearance, the needle holder appears very similar to artery forceps, except that the grooves are designed to retain a better grip of the needle. The suture is placed in the packet in such a way that, as the packet is torn at the right-hand side, the needle is exposed in the correct position to attach the needle to the needle holder without having to remove the suture from the packet. The suture is attached to the needle, the needle being appropriately shaped to reduce tissue trauma and also levelled off approximately one-third of the way along the needle to allow the needle holder to grasp it securely. The needle holder should be placed on the last third of the needle (the part closest to the thread) at right angles to the curve of the needle.

The needle holder is held by the shank with the wrist curved backwards and the needle is inserted into the tissue. The wrist is then turned forwards to guide both the direction and depth of the needle through the tissue. The free end of the needle is secured using tissue forceps whilst the needle holder is removed from the needle and then reclamped on the end of the needle protruding through the tissue. With the palm facing down, the needle is pulled completely through the tissue using a flicking movement of the wrist along the curve of the needle.

Suturing techniques

The basic suturing techniques described are for a right-handed midwife; a left-handed person will need to adapt these principles. Note that where

there is any possible exposure to the needle, tissue forceps should be used to hold the tissue, rather than fingers to reduce the risk of a needlestick injury (Bott 1999).

Tying a knot

The knot is tied three times, to the right with two throws, to the left (one throw) and back to the right (one throw) so that it will not slip and will lie flat (Fig. 34.3). When tying a knot to anchor the suture the short end is cut short and the stitching continues using the long end.

Continuous non-locked suture

This is suitable for use on the posterior vaginal wall and perineal muscles. To ensure that the tear is repaired completely the apex of the tear must be located and clearly visualised – inserting a lubricated tampon may assist by minimising lochial blood loss:

1. The first stitch enters the tissue above the apex, where a knot is tied to anchor it and the short end cut.
2. The next stitch is placed below and parallel to the first one; the left hand applies slight tension to the thread and the needle emerges to the left of the thread that is held (Fig. 34.4).
3. It is continued at approximately 1-cm intervals down the vaginal wall to the fourchette and if required along the perineal muscle layer.

4. If the skin does not require suturing, the suture is tied and a loop is retained to act as the short end.

5. The knot is then tied in the same way and may be buried for comfort.

Burying a knot is achieved by cutting the short end then passing the needle under the suture line to take the knot into the tissue. The long end is then cut (Fig. 34.5).

Subcuticular suture to perineal skin

As the name suggests, the suture is beneath the skin. If the perineal muscles have not been sutured and there is no thread to continue with, a new stitch is begun at the anal end with a knot tied beneath the skin. To do this the needle is inserted deeply on the left-hand side of the tear, emerging (still on the left) superficially just below the skin and a knot tied (Fig. 34.6). The needle is then reversed on the needle holder (the point of the needle emerging to the right of the needle holder), and on the right-hand side of the tear the needle is entered superficially beneath the skin opposite the knot on the left. The needle emerges superficially (still on the right) at approximately the length of the needle. The next bite is taken along the left side of the incision, entering opposite where the last suture emerged on the right (Fig. 34.7). The process is repeated until the fourchette is reached. A loop is retained with the last suture to tie off a knot. Both ends are cut. There should not be any suture material apparent on the outside of the perineum.

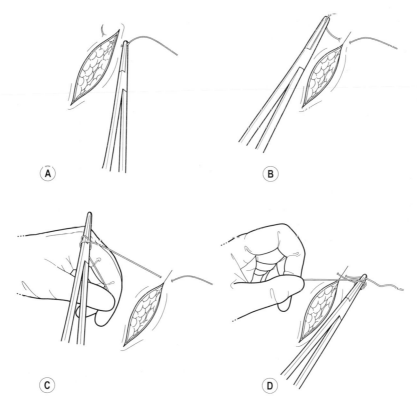

Figure 34.3 • Instrument tied knot: consisting of three throws to 'lock' and prevent slippage. Key: white thread, left side of suture material; black thread, right side of suture material (Adapted with kind permission from Nisbet & Rouse 1992) **A–C** Holding the tissue with tissue forceps, use the needle holder to pass through tissue from right to left, leaving 8–10 cm on the right hand side. **D** Hold needle holder in right hand parallel to tissue, grasp left thread between thumb and index finger of left hand, pass thread in front of and over needle holder.

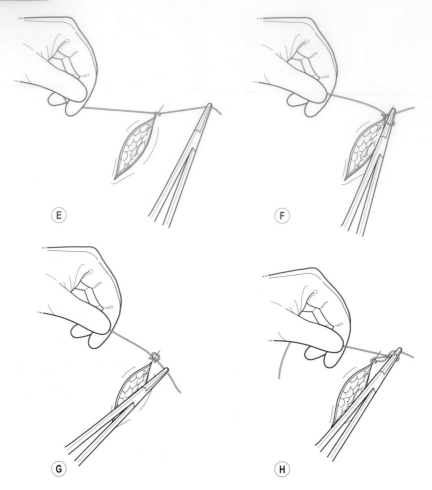

Figure 34.3—cont'd E,F Wind two loops of left suture over needle holder, rotate needle holder from 9 o'clock to 11 o'clock position. G Continue rotating needle holder until 1 o'clock position (right hand should be palm up at this stage), grasp right thread with needle holder as close to the end as possible. H Pull right thread through loops of left thread.

PROCEDURE: perineal repair

- Obtain informed consent.
- Gather equipment and place on a dressings trolley or suitable working surface:
  - ○ sterile repair pack with sterile gown
  - ○ water/lotion
  - ○ plastic apron
  - ○ sterile gloves
  - ○ sterile sutures
  - ○ 20 mL lidocaine with sterile needle (21-g green) and syringe
  - ○ lubricant
  - ○ diclofenac suppository (if not contraindicated)
- Correctly assist the woman into a suitable position and keep her covered. A stool should be available for the midwife to sit on and the light is positioned appropriately.
- With clean hands open the outer covering of the repair pack (an assistant can do this).
- Put on apron and wash and dry hands.
- Open the pack.
- Using an aseptic technique open and place on sterile field other items required, e.g. sutures, swabs,

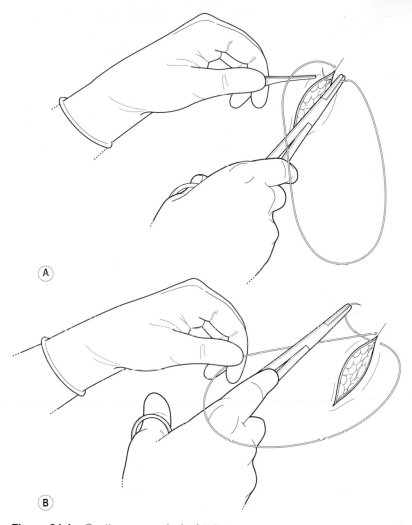

(A)

(B)

Figure 34.4 • Continuous non-locked suture

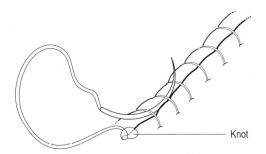

Figure 34.5 • Burying a knot

needle, syringe, gloves, gown, diclofenac suppository and add lotion and lubricant to bowl/gallipots (this can be done by an assistant, if present).

• If using lidocaine, open the ampoule and place within easy reach on a clean surface unless an assistant is present to open and hold the ampoule.

• Uncover the woman as necessary.

• Wash and dry hands.

• Apply gown and gloves.

• Check and count the swabs, needles and instruments.

• Arrange the trolley in a way that suits.

• Draw up the anaesthetic – if no assistant is present the ampoule can be held using a swab to maintain sterility.

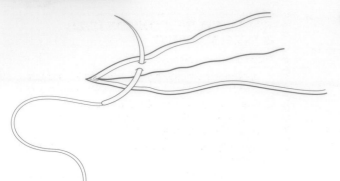

Figure 34.6 • Tying a subcutaneous knot

- Cleanse the vulva using a non-touch technique, working from top to bottom, using each swab only once.
- Establish a sterile field beneath the woman's buttocks, over her legs and abdomen using the sterile towels and fenestrated drape.
- Infiltrate the perineum as described above; time is given for anaesthesia to be achieved.

- Re-examine the genital tract to establish the extent of the trauma and realign the tissues; refer if necessary.
- Insert a lubricated vaginal tampon to absorb the lochial loss so that visibility while suturing is good, attaching the tail to the sterile drapes using artery forceps.

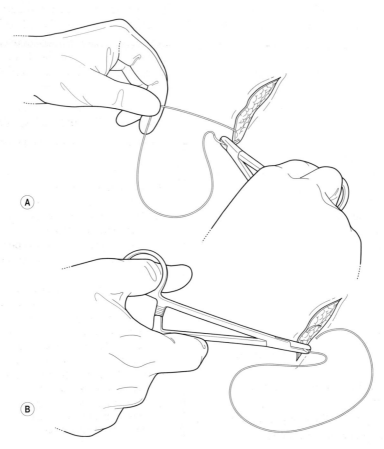

Figure 34.7 • A, B Subcuticular suture to the skin

- Locate the apex, insert the first suture just above it and anchor with a knot.
- Complete a continuous loose non-locked suture down the vaginal wall.
- Locate the perineal muscles and suture with a continuous non-locked suture, securing with a buried knot if the skin is in good apposition (0.5 cm maximum gap). If necessary the deep and superficial muscles can be sutured in two layers.
- If the skin is not in good apposition, complete a subcuticular suture, beginning at the anal end and ending at the fourchette with a subcuticular knot.
- Examine the vagina and perineum to establish that the tissue is in good alignment and that all haemorrhage has stopped.
- Remove the tampon, examine the repair gently and insert one lubricated finger into the anus to establish that the sutures have not gone through the rectal mucosa. Administer rectal analgesia if not contraindicated.
- Remove the drapes and assist the woman into a comfortable position, placing a sanitary towel over the perineum. Advise her with regard to ongoing perineal care.
- Count the swabs, instruments and needles and dispose of sharps correctly.
- Dispose of the equipment and wash hands.
- Document the repair and act accordingly.

Record keeping

The following should be included:

- date and time of the procedure
- nature and extent of the tear
- position of the woman
- anaesthetic drugs used
- tampon inserted and removed
- suture material used
- order of repair
- techniques used to which area
- examinations *per vaginam* and per rectum following the repair
- indication that swab, needle and instrument count are correct
- analgesia administered following procedure
- legible signature of suturing midwife.

ROLE AND RESPONSIBILITIES OF THE MIDWIFE

These can be summarised as:

- appropriate assessment of the wound to establish who should suture, where, with which anaesthetic
- providing the woman with evidence-based information to allow her to make an informed decision regarding suturing
- use of appropriate materials, technique, asepsis and standard precautions
- education and support of the woman before, during and following the procedure
- contemporaneous records.

Summary

- Perineal repair is a very important procedure for which the midwife should be correctly trained and updated and able to acknowledge any limitations, thus referring. Undertaking audit is also good practice.
- Evidence-based practice should be used with regard to the materials and techniques used.
- The repair is a sterile procedure, in which the aims include alignment of the tissue, stemming haemorrhage and reduction of dead space.

SELF-ASSESSMENT EXERCISES

The answers to the following questions may be found in the text:

1. What is the function of the pelvic floor?
2. When might a midwife ask a senior obstetrician to complete a perineal repair?
3. Describe how to successfully infiltrate the perineum prior to perineal repair.
4. List the aims of successful perineal repair.
5. What is the current material of choice for perineal repair?
6. Give a rationale for the technique used when suturing the posterior vaginal wall and the muscle layer.
7. What kind of technique should be used for the perineal skin if suturing is indicated?
8. Summarise the role and responsibilities of the midwife in relation to perineal repair.
9. List all the aspects of the repair that should be included in the records.
10. Find some suitable suturing equipment and demonstrate tying a knot, continuous non-locked and subcuticular suturing.

References

ACS (American College of Surgeons): *Statement on sharps injury*, Available online: http://www.facs.org/fellows_info/statements/st-58 accessed 21 January 2009, 2007.

Adoni A, Anteby E: The use of histoacryl for episiotomy repair, *Br J Obstet Gynaecol* 98:476–478, 1991.

Arkin A, Chern-Hughes B: Case report: labial fusion postpartum and clinical management of labial lacerations, *J Midwifery Womens Health* 47(4):290–292, 2001.

Bott J: HIV risk reduction and the use of universal precautions, *Br J Midwifery* 7(11):671–675, 1999.

DH (Department of Health): *Guidance for clinical health care workers. Protection against infection with blood borne viruses*, London, 1998, The Stationery Office.

Draper J, Newell R: A discussion of some of the literature relating to history, repair and consequences of perineal trauma, *Midwifery* 12:140–145, 1996.

Enkin M, Keirse MJ, Neilson J, et al: *A guide to effective care in pregnancy and childbirth*, Oxford, 2000, Oxford University Press.

Fleming E, Hagen S, Niven C: Does perineal suturing make a difference? The SUNS trial, *Br J Obstet Gynaecol* 110:684–689, 2003.

Gordon B, Mackrodt C, Fern E, et al: The Ipswich Childbirth Study: 1. A randomised evaluation of two stage postpartum perineal repair leaving the skin unsutured, *Br J Obstet Gynaecol* 105:435–440, 1998.

Grant A, Gordon B, Mackrodt C, et al: The Ipswich childbirth study: one year follow up of alternative methods used in perineal repair, *Br J Obstet Gynaecol* 108:34–40, 2001.

Greenberg JA, Lieberman E, Cohen AP, et al: Randomized comparison of chromic versus fast absorbing polyglactin 910 for postpartum perineal repair, *Obstet Gynaecol* 103(6):1308–1313, 2004.

Hedayati H, Parsons J, Crowther CA: Rectal analgesia for pain from perineal trauma following childbirth, *Cochrane Database Syst Rev 2003* (3): CD0003931. DOI:10.1002/14651858.CD003931, 2003.

Jessiman W: Lotions and lubricants, *Pract Midwife* 4(3):23–28, 2001.

Kenyon S, Ford F: How can we improve women's postbirth perineal health? *MIDIRS Midwifery Digest* 14(1):7–12, 2004.

Kettle C, Hills R, Jones P, et al: Continuous versus interrupted perineal repair with standard or rapidly absorbed sutures after spontaneous vaginal birth: a randomised controlled trial, *Lancet* 359(9325):2217–2223, 2002.

Kettle C, Hills RK, Ismail MK: Continuous versus interrupted sutures for repair of episiotomy or second degree tears (Review), *Cochrane Database Syst Rev 2007* (4) CD000947. DOI.:10.1002/14651858.CD000947, pub2, 2007.

Langley V, Thoburn A, Shaw S, et al: Second degree tears: to suture or not? A randomized controlled trial, *Br J Midwifery* 14(9):550–554, 2006.

Leeman LM, Rogers RG, Greulich B, et al: Do un-sutured second degree perineal lacerations affect postpartum functional outcomes? *J Am Board Fam Med* 20(5):451–457, 2007.

Leroux N, Bujold E: Impact of chromic catgut versus polyglactin 910 versus fast-absorbing polyglactin 910 sutures for perineal repair: a randomized controlled trial, *Am J Obstet Gynaecol* 194(6):1585–1590, 2006.

McCandlish R: Routine perineal suturing: is it time to stop? *MIDIRS Midwifery Dig* 11(3):296–300, 2001.

Metcalfe A, Bick D, Tohill S, et al: A prospective cohort study of repair and non-repair of second degree perineal trauma: results and issues for future research, *Evid Based Midwifery* 4(2):60–64, 2006.

National Institute for Health and Clinical Excellence (NICE): *Intrapartum care: care of healthy women and their babies during childbirth*, Clinical guidance 55, London, 2007, NICE.

Royal College of Midwives (RCM): *Suturing the perineum. Midwifery practice guidelines*, London, 2008, Royal College of Midwives.

Rogerson L, Mason GC, Roberts AC: Preliminary experience with twenty perineal repairs using Indermil tissue adhesive, *Eur J Obstet Gynaecol Reprod Biol* 88:139–142, 2000.

Sanders J, Campbell R, Peters T: Effectiveness of pain relief during perineal suturing, *Br J Obstet Gynaecol* 109:1066–1068, 2002.

Sleep JM, Grant A, Garcia J, et al: West Berkshire perineal management trial, *Br J Med* 289:587–590, 1984.

Viswanathan M, Hartmann K, Palmieri R, et al: *The use of episiotomy in obstetrical care: A systematic review*, 2005, Agency for Healthcare Research and Quality. Available online: www.ahrq.gov/downloads/pub/evidence/pdf/episiotomy/episodo.pdf accessed 18 January 2008.

Wilson LK, Sullivan S, Goodnight W, et al: The use of blunt needles does not reduce glove perforations during obstetrical laceration repair, *Am J Obstet Gynecol* 199(6):1097–6868, 2008.

Principles of intrapartum skills: management of birth at home

35

This chapter focuses on the midwife's role and management of labour and delivery in the home setting. It highlights the considerations for care at home that are different from care in hospital; the reader may find it helpful to refer to other relevant chapters (e.g. Chapters 31–33). Safe homebirth is very much a team effort, the woman and her family are at the centre of the care, but it can only be facilitated with midwifery skills, the communication and planning of obstetric services as a whole, effective working with the ambulance service and in some instances active involvement of the general practitioner (GP). Some women will prefer to give birth in a hospital setting; this is as much their choice as home is for other women.

LEARNING OUTCOMES

Having read this chapter the reader should be able to:

- highlight the research-based evidence that relates to safe delivery at home
- discuss the differences in skills and attitudes that the midwife utilises when managing birth at home
- discuss the value and principles of good preparation for all the parties concerned
- list the equipment and information that the midwife needs available
- discuss the overall role and responsibilities of the midwife when caring for labouring women at home
- Discuss the initial assessment necessary if attending a birth that has already happened without medical assistance (born before arrival (BBA)).

Safety

According to the Office of National Statistics (ONS 2008), in 2006 in England and Wales, 2.7% of births took place at home. This is an upward trend; regional variations show that some areas have a much higher figure (BirthChoiceUK 2008). It is also considered that if women were given a truer choice the rate would be nearer 8–10% (DH 2003). It is necessary to make the distinction between planned births at home (often with low risk factors) and unexpected (for whatever reason) delivery at home. For planned home births there is little in the way of randomised controlled trials but meta-analysis of smaller (often observational) studies suggests a greater chance of a normal birth, with lower intervention rates and higher maternal satisfaction when birthing at home compared to hospital (RCOG/RCM 2007).

NICE (2007) are clear that women should be given a choice about where to give birth. This is clarified however by the need for a low risk criterion, with an extensive list for medical or childbirth related disorders that warrant care in an obstetric unit (Box 35.1). Ongoing assessment throughout the pregnancy and labour will be necessary to ensure that the woman remains within the low risk criteria. The emphasis, however, remains on communication and choice. The woman who is fully informed regarding, the likelihood, method, length of time and possible reasons for transfer in labour to an obstetric unit, is more likely to make a 'realistic' plan for her labour.

Midwifery skills

There are many articles of opinion that share highly positive experiences for midwives and their practice as well as the women and families in their care (Cook 2003, Jones 2003, Kitzinger 2001). While midwives may have limited experiences of home birth, those that do often regard it as a professionally enhancing experience. Different skills are needed than when caring for women in hospital including issues such as:

- Needing a full understanding and confidence in labour physiology and a woman's ability to give birth naturally.

- Fundamental midwifery skills using limited equipment, e.g. Pinard stethoscope or Doppler sonicaid use rather than cardiotocography monitor, delivery in alternative positions, management of pain with limited availability of pharmacological preparations.

- 'Active inactivity': women who have planned their birth at home often assume a greater level of control. A midwife may feel a little superfluous but has in fact to remain 'with woman', to keep alert, being active in, for example, observing for signs of the labour progressing, while appearing to be relatively inactive. As a guest in the woman's home, the midwife is obliged to be relaxed, tactful, blending in to the circumstances and events, while still exercising the full range of professional labour care and support. Mood and temperament of the environment affect the finely tuned hormonal interplays that are needed physiologically for labour (Russell 2008). Odent (1996) describes the midwife's role as watching, waiting and trusting the woman's own ability to give birth.

- Flexibility and adaptability are required, e.g. continuing to maintain standard precautions, following aseptic guidelines or maintaining health and safety protocols while working in an unfamiliar environment. Midwives also find that their decision-making skills and professional autonomy are increased.

Box 35.1

Risk factors suggesting a planned birth at an obstetric unit

- Medical disorders: cardiac disease, hypertension, asthma that requires additional treatment, cystic fibrosis, haemoglobinopathy disease, thromboembolic disease or history, platelet disorders, atypical antibodies, known Group B Streptococcus (GBS) needing antibiotics in labour, immune, endocrine and renal disorder, abnormal liver function tests, epilepsy or previous cerebrovascular accident, psychiatric disorder requiring current inpatient care, myomectomy/hysterotomy

- Pregnancy/labour related issues: pre-eclampsia/eclampsia, now or previously, small for gestational age, fetal death, poly-/oligohydramnios, abnormal fetal heart (FH), multiple birth, malpresentation, antepartum haemorrhage, substance misuse, preterm labour or spontaneous rupture of membranes (SROM), haemoglobin <8.5 g/dL, BMI >35 kg/m^2 at booking

- Other factors warranting individual assessment: haemoglobinopathy traits, haemoglobin 8.5–10.5 g/dL, spinal abnormalities, previous fractured pelvis, history of previous baby >4.5 kg, history of extensive perineal trauma, >40 years, parity 6 or more, cone biopsy or fibroids

Adapted and summarised from NICE (2007)

- Management of unexpected situations or emergencies for mothers or babies when assistance may be some miles or minutes away.

It is clear, however, that as well as being professionally well prepared for birth at home, the midwife's personal feelings are significant in the woman's success. Floyd (1995) suggests that a woman has greater success if the midwife has a positive attitude, confidence, competence and willingness. Supervisors of midwives can assist midwives who feel that they are lacking the experience to gain this as part of their annual professional development review.

Preparation

Good preparation is necessary for several agencies involved.

Maternity services

Each service needs to have considered home birth provision within its service as a whole, including the training and updating of midwives, budgetary provision for items such as mobile phones and birthing equipment, and issues such as midwife availability, referral and transport systems. It is likely that risk management assessments are made frequently in relation to the service. Provision should be made for women who fall outside of the low risk criteria but continue to choose the home birth option. The supervisor of midwives will provide advice and support in this situation (Jones 2003). Protocols should include whether midwives are expected, for example, to site intravenous cannulae in an emergency.

The midwife

It can be helpful if the midwife knows the geography and socioeconomic demography of the area. This can highlight potential risk factors to personal safety. Equally, good working relationships with others in the healthcare team can make the management of problems smoother and enhance the communication that facilitates the woman's care. Knowing which second midwife to call and how to access the supervisor of midwives is essential information which should be easily to hand. The Royal College of Midwives (RCM 2002) rightly points

out that midwives are fully equipped to manage normal birth; the essence is to manage it confidently at home with good judgements and actions in the event of abnormality. All professional competencies, e.g. 'drills and skills' for emergencies and the like (including community management), must be undertaken as per the mandatory requirement, the need for such skills may be greater at home and the midwife is responsible for her practice whatever the environment (NMC 2004). Cannulation and suturing skills are also advisable.

Equipment (sphygmomanometer, Entonox®, suction apparatus, etc.) should all be stored, used and serviced correctly (see Chapters 5, 24, 55 and 56, respectively), with the midwife ensuring that she is very familiar with the equipment carried and its location. Keeping items together (e.g. equipment for primary postpartum haemorrhage management or resuscitation) means that they are easily accessible and easily moved around the home with the woman. Pethidine is rarely used, but may be supplied from the NHS Trust, via a GP, or via a midwife's private prescription following authorisation by a supervisor of midwives (see Chapter 18). Other medicines that the midwife carries, such as oxytocic agents, naloxone, lidocaine, may be administered according to the agreed patient group direction as for any other woman. Other equipment for the birth should include the items suggested in Box 35.2. Further details can be obtained from the RCM (2003). Items such as the delivery pack may be kept at the woman's home in advance, but this may depend on local protocols and the midwife's discretion. The midwife will need to supply her own food and drinks.

The woman and her family

Clearly, for a planned home birth the woman is likely to be well prepared. RCM (2003) recommends obtaining items such as plastic sheeting, towels, rubbish bags, light foods and drinks, alternative sources of heating and lighting, massaging equipment, appropriate clothing for mother and baby, pillows and pethidine, amongst other things. Gwillim (2009) recommends a birthing covering of 1×1.25 m, this being polythene covered with layers of newspaper and an old sheet, all of which are glued into place and can be disposed of afterwards. Family poverty should not be a hindrance to home birth and, as such, the midwife may need

---

Box 35.2

Equipment suggested for managing labour and birth at home

- Antenatal equipment including Pinard stethoscope and/or sonicaid and gel, sphygmomanometer, thermometer, venepuncture equipment, sharps box, swabs and medium, reagent sticks, blood and midstream urine (MSU) bottles, pen torch, scissors, tape measure, gloves (sterile and non-sterile), documentation such as continuation sheets, blood forms
- Labour equipment including sterile delivery and vaginal examination packs, aprons and other personal protective equipment, urinary catheters, amnihook, speculum and lubricating gel cannulation equipment, fluids and giving sets, razor, suturing equipment, torch, incontinence pads, drugs (including spare Entonox®), suppositories, container for placenta, rubbish bags, water thermometer, documentation for

labour care including birth notification and emergency management cards
- Resuscitation equipment for woman and baby including oxygen (with tubings, airways, bags and masks), suction with neonatal and maternal suckers, stethoscope, stop-watch, heat source and possibly endotracheal tubes and laryngoscope depending on local protocol, blood glucose sticks and lancets
- Postnatal equipment including weighing scales, equipment for neonatal examination and documentation such as neonatal examination forms, child health record, postnatal exercises and advice, transfer of care documentation, cord clamp cutter, baby labels, vitamin K

---

to assist in providing some of the items needed. The woman should be fully aware of how and when to contact the midwife. A prebirth home visit that looks at all the practicalities – proposed room for birth, unobtrusive space for equipment, resuscitation area, location of telephone or presence of a mobile phone with sufficient battery charge and signal, etc. – is helpful in reassuring all parties.

Principles of managing birth at home

Safe care begins with knowing how the midwife will be notified and whether there is a requirement to notify anyone else of the call-out, e.g. labour ward or second midwife.

Assessment on arrival

Is labour progressing? Can the midwife leave and return later at a given time or rest in another room for a while? Is a second midwife needed for an imminent birth? This assessment should also include a history of the labour so far, with all assessments being recorded on a partogram or in the woman's records. Fetal and maternal well-being need to be established, abdominal examination is necessary; vaginal assessment may be according to the clinical indicators and the woman's wishes.

Establish a working area

It is helpful to establish space for equipment and resuscitation (portable, if possible) and a table for writing records. Take the opportunity to inform the second midwife of likely schedule (if not already contacted).

Ongoing labour care

This is as for any labouring woman, including all assessments for labour progress, fetal and maternal well-being. It is likely that the woman will naturally be mobile and utilise the furniture and supporters around her for pain relief. She may also take regular baths or showers, eat and drink as she feels appropriate, pass urine as needed and use other techniques (e.g. doing the ironing), to help and distract. As labour progresses the midwife is more likely to observe the 'in on self' effect as the woman has less conversation and more of an intensity about her. The midwife will utilise the 'active inactivity' described above and is likely to begin intuitively to understand how the woman is progressing. If water labour or birth is planned the reader is encouraged to read Chapter 36.

Second stage of labour

The woman is likely to push physiologically using the furniture, etc. available to her; the midwife remains vigilant as to signs of second stage onset, fetal and maternal wellbeing and indicators of progress (see Chapter 31 for greater detail). The second midwife should ideally be called if not already present. The midwife should be mindful of her own care (e.g. back strain) when needing to adapt to the woman's position.

Third stage of labour

Many women may opt for expectant management at home; this requires that the midwife understands the physiology and is competent to undertake its management (see Chapter 32). The placenta remains the woman's property; however, often the midwife removes it from the home in a suitable container and disposes of it as for hospital births. If the woman wishes to keep it she should be encouraged to bury it deeply in the garden or seek advice from the Environmental Health Department. The midwife will need to improvise to examine the genital tract with sufficient light and visibility; if suturing is required chairs may be needed to support her legs and something firm may be needed beneath the woman's buttocks. All equipment is dealt with as for hospital births and returned to the hospital.

Care of the newborn

There is little difference in the care of the newborn at home. If resuscitation is required the decision to call help is made swiftly and the midwife follows the usual guidelines (see Chapter 56). Provision is made in the next 24–48 hours for a qualified person to undertake the neonatal examination.

Transfer to hospital

The midwife must have referral systems and numbers in place; often, referral is to the nearest consultant delivery suite or to a consultant obstetrician directly. Advice may also be sought from the supervisor of midwives and calls may be made directly to ambulance control on agreed numbers. Transfer to hospital is made using an ambulance (often paramedic) in the event of an emergency, a non-urgent transfer may be made using the woman's own transport, but this may depend on local protocols. GPs are often, by agreement, bypassed in such circumstances. The woman may find referral very hard and it is appropriate to discuss the likely criteria with her in advance as well as at the time. Building a relationship, and therefore

trust, with the woman antenatally is likely to make transfer a little easier for her. If an emergency transfer, it can be helpful to have a card written out (filling in the details at the last minute) that a member of the family can read from when speaking to ambulance control. Leaving the front door open and a light on can save valuable time. In some areas ambulance controls are notified in advance of the planned home births. If a paramedic attends, the midwife should be aware that the woman is still the midwife's 'case' and that full responsibility remains with the midwife, not the paramedic.

Documentation

This is as thorough as for any hospital birth, including all discussions, referrals and actions. Partograms, birth notifications, etc. may all be left in the woman's home in advance. The parts of the records that require computerisation will be undertaken by the midwife on return to the unit.

Other practitioners

Occasionally, women may bring in their own assistants such as aromatherapists. The midwife should ensure that, as the professional responsible, the woman and practitioner have sensible working limits and that if for any reason the midwife needs the therapy to stop, this is understood.

Communicating when there are difficulties

Occasionally, women choose options that the midwife feels less comfortable about, for example, poor lighting from candles only. Good preparation, continuity of care and opportunities to build a good trusting relationship with the woman in advance will smooth the management of such issues.

Self-appraisal and audit

Clinical governance ensures that the service is effective via audit, but this also aids midwives to appreciate the quality of their care and to review any areas that can be improved. Self-appraisal will help less experienced midwives to develop confidence in home birth management, along with the support of a supervisor of midwives.

Born before arrival (BBA)

When unplanned births occur at home the midwife may be called after the ambulance service. It is necessary to make some swift assessments:

- Baby: does it need resuscitating? Is it cold? What is it's gestation? Where was it born? (sometimes into the toilet). Has it been fed?
- Mother: Was it a precipitate labour? Placenta in or out? Bleeding? State of perineum?

Care of (often) shocked people is necessary, decisions are made as to whether transfer into hospital is necessary once the initial assessment and management have been undertaken. Records are completed as for any other birth and communication with colleagues must be of a high standard.

- A range of new and existing skills are utilised; maintenance of skills such as resuscitation and emergency drills is essential.
- Preparation, by all parties involved, contributes to the safety and delivery of care. This includes issues such as drugs, equipment, accessibility to other healthcare professionals and referral systems.
- Many aspects of home care mirror hospital care but the midwife often needs to utilise her professional autonomy to the full. This is particularly the case when the unexpected occurs or the woman is outside of the low risk criteria.
- Care should be taken to protect the midwife's personal safety.

ROLE AND RESPONSIBILITIES OF THE MIDWIFE

These can be summarised as:

- professional, thorough labour care planned and undertaken in an unfamiliar environment but according to all rules and protocols that govern safe and effective practice
- recognising deviations from the norm and instigating referral.

Summary

- Providing labour care at home for healthy women with a planned home birth can be a highly satisfying experience for the midwife and the family.

SELF-ASSESSMENT EXERCISES

The answers to the following questions may be found in the text:

1. Summarise the current guidelines relating to the safety of birth at home.
2. Compile a low risk criterion to identify women suitable for home birth.
3. Discuss the skills needed by the midwife to undertake safe home births.
4. List the items needed for a home birth.
5. Summarise the differences between caring for a labouring woman at home and caring for one in hospital.
6. To whom will a midwife refer if a deviation from the norm occurs?
7. Discuss what assessments would be made initially on arrival at a BBA.

References

BirthChoiceUK: *Regional statistics*, Available online, www. Birthchoiceuk.com January 2009, 2008.

Cook M: A 'beautiful' birth, *MIDIRS Midwifery Dig* 13(4):447–448, 2003.

DH (Department of Health): *Changing Childbirth*, London, 2003, HMSO.

Floyd L: Community midwives' views and experience of home birth, *Midwifery* 11:3–10, 1995.

Gwillim J: Home birth. In Chapman V, Charles C, editors: *The Midwife's labour and birth handbook*, ed 2, Oxford, 2009, Wiley-Blackwell, pp 83–92.

Jones D: Midwifery supervision and home births, *Midwives* 6(9):386–388, 2003.

Kitzinger S: Becoming a mother, *MIDIRS Midwifery Digest* 11(4):445–447, 2001.

NICE (National Institute for Health and Clinical Excellence): *Intrapartum care: care of healthy women and their babies during childbirth*, Clinical Guideline 55, London, 2007, NICE.

NMC (Nursing and Midwifery Council): *Midwives rules and standards*, London, 2004, NMC.

Odent M: Why labouring women don't need support, *Mothering* 80:47–51, 1996.

ONS (Office for National Statistics): News release: home births continue gradual increase, 25 September 2008. Available online, www. statistics.gov.uk January 2009, 2008.

RCM (Royal College of Midwives): *47 Home birth handbook, Vol. 1:*

Promoting home birth, London, 2002, RCM Trust.

RCM (Royal College of Midwives): *Home birth handbook, Vol. 2: Practising home birth*, London, 2003, RCM Trust.

RCOG/RCM (Royal College of Obstetricians and Gynaecologists/ Royal College of Midwives): *Home Births Joint Statement No.2*. Available online, www.rcog.org.uk April 2009, 2007.

Russell K: Watching and waiting:the facilitation of birth at home. In Edwins J, editor: *Community midwifery practice*, Oxford, 2008, Blackwell publishing, pp 25–46.

Principles of intrapartum skills: management of birth in water

36

CHAPTER CONTENTS

For some time there have been serious advocates for the use of water for labouring women. There is now clearer guidance and a distinction made between its use at varying stages of labour (NICE 2007, RCOG/RCM 2006). However, subjecting the use of water in labour to rigorous research methods is not an easy process and there are still unanswered questions, particularly with regard to neonatal outcome (Rafferty 2008). This chapter reviews this evidence and summarises the necessary aspects of care. A fuller understanding will be gained if it is read in conjunction with Chapters 30–32.

LEARNING OUTCOMES

Having read this chapter the reader should be able to:

- highlight the current evidence
- discuss the benefits of water use in labour
- outline a low risk criteria and indicate the situations in which water use is prohibited or dubious
- list the items of equipment necessary
- discuss the aspects of care pertinent to labouring in water
- discuss the midwife's role and responsibilities.

Introduction

Women may choose informally to bath or shower often prior to seeking professional help in labour. This is clearly different from deep water immersion in a birthing pool. Service providers are obliged to draw up protocols that aim to provide safe and effective care when deep water is used. Such protocols cover both pools in hospitals and birthing centres, and care by midwives in the woman's home where a pool may be hired in. The distinction is also made between the use of water for analgesic purposes during the first stage of labour and actual birth in the water. Midwives should be familiar with their local protocols for these two separate issues, and should be updated both in undertaking and assisting at pool births (RCOG/RCM 2006).

Considered benefits of water use

In the first stage of labour water is known to:

- shorten the length of first stage
- aid relaxation and coping strategies
- reduce the need for pharmacological analgesia and medical intervention.

During the second stage of labour:

- aid perineal stretching and therefore reduce perineal trauma
- reduce birth intervention
- provide a gentle transition to extra uterine life for the baby
- more likely to facilitate expectant management of the third stage of labour.

(Summarised from MIDIRS 2008)

Both the NICE guidelines (2007) and RCOG/RCM joint statement (2006), in the light of currently available evidence, endorse labouring in water for pain relief purposes in the first stage of labour where an inclusion/exclusion criteria exists. The RCOG/RCM (2006) are prepared to state too, that 'healthy women with uncomplicated pregnancies at term ... should be able to proceed to water birth if they wish'. NICE (2007) is less sure, stating that 'there is insufficient high quality evidence to either support or discourage giving birth in water'. Other commentators would agree that there are some outstanding issues; Cluett et al (2002) recommended that research was still needed into clinical outcomes, the economic impact and the physiological effects of water use in labour. The debates about water temperature, cervical dilatation and infection risks continue. However, the benefits of water use (as listed above) are being recognised and therefore pool use is on the increase (Garland 2006).

Who is suitable to use a birthing pool?

Firstly, any woman who has been given all the available information and wishes to use the pool is considered. Secondly, the inclusion/exclusion criteria should be applied when assessing her risk factors. Historically, low risk criteria have been proposed; however Burns & Kitzinger (2001) suspect that in

particular instances other conditions may be permitted, e.g. hypertension or vaginal birth after caesarean. At this time the following are proposed as safe criteria:

- established labour with singleton fetus and cephalic presentation (Chapman & Charles 2009)
- uncomplicated pregnancy of >37 weeks gestation (Burns & Kitzinger 2001)
- spontaneous rupture of membranes less than 24 hours.

Situations in which the use of water is contraindicated include:

- maternal dislike
- maternal pyrexia
- opiate use in labour of less than 2 hours ago (NICE 2007)
- any known cause for concern for mother or fetus (Burns & Kitzinger 2001).

Situations for which there is debate (no real evidence available):

- known infection (e.g. group B streptococcus). The use of universally applied standard precautions and adherence to cleansing protocols make this questionable
- the need for electronic fetal monitoring. Equipment is available to monitor continually in water but this raises a number of issues – primarily whether suspected fetal distress is (as suggested above) a known cause for concern for the fetus
- previous caesarean birth
- high body mass index; the woman may be harder to remove from the pool in the event of an emergency
- prolonged rupture of membranes, when the risk of ascending infection is considered higher
- thin meconium where continuous fetal monitoring is not indicated.

Despite having low risk criteria, the midwife should always be alert to any obstetric or neonatal emergency, removing the woman from the pool swiftly and undertaking the correct management measures.

When is a good time to enter the pool?

In 1998, Odent recognised that the relaxation offered by water and the lack of gravity could cause a non-established labour to cease. Most women were therefore prohibited from entering the water until 5 cm dilated. However, Garland (2006) notes that an uncomfortable woman, whatever her dilatation, is likely to relax in the water; Cluett et al (2004) noted that such labours often then progress. Garland (2006) considers that the next hour is the most critical time to observe for signs of progress, if the labour is slowing the woman can be asked to mobilise again for a while.

Equipment

There should be space around the pool on each side and the means to fill, reheat and empty it. A thermometer is necessary, as is a sieve (to remove debris from the water) and an aqua Doppler. A mirror and torch may both be useful where lighting is dim. The midwife can also benefit from a kneeler or stool and the woman may appreciate a float to rest on. Midwives should protect themselves; for example, the woman can float to the surface for fetal auscultation, reducing the risk of damage to the midwife's back. Gauntlet gloves may also be useful. The midwife must ensure, whether in hospital or at home, that the means to call for assistance and resuscitation equipment are all to hand. A hoist or other equipment should be available to aid the woman in leaving the pool quickly, a mattress or other means of lying down comfortably should be available, absorbent non slip floor coverings (e.g. old towels) and a good supply of drying towels are all essential. A birthing stool may be helpful for land management of the third stage. Access to Entonox® may be necessary. Pool use at home should include a trial run, ensuring that birthing partners are also comfortable with their role.

Principles of care

Assessments of maternal and fetal wellbeing

As with homebirth (see Chapter 35) midwives have the opportunity to exercise their autonomy in a generally low intervention environment. The need to have confidence in the physiology of labour and the woman's ability to give birth naturally are significant features. All labour observations, care and documentation are undertaken as for any other labour, just as referrals are made if there is any deviation from the norm. The woman's temperature should be recorded hourly. The woman will need to leave the pool to pass urine and the midwife may decide in accordance with the other clinical signs as to the frequency and need for vaginal examinations. These may be on land or in the water. The aqua Doppler is used throughout to assess fetal wellbeing. The woman is encouraged to adopt positions that are comfortable. She may use Entonox®, and other complementary therapies; it is important that she remains well hydrated.

Water depth and temperature

The birthing pool needs to be able to accommodate water to the level of the woman's breasts when sitting. There is significant debate as to the water temperature; at this time NICE (2007) recommends assessing and recording the water temperature hourly, it should not exceed 37.5°C. Anderson (2004), in her review of literature and physiology, concludes that the woman's preference is the best guide to correct water temperature. The RCOG/RCM (2006) concur with this. It is often necessary to remove water when adding water for temperature adjustment purposes in order to retain a similar water level. Chapman & Charles (2009) also indicate that the cooler water is on the surface and that therefore good mixing is necessary prior to taking the water temperature.

The birth

It is advisable to have a second midwife in attendance, but this may vary according to local protocol. The woman is likely to push physiologically and is more likely to have a 'hands poised' (McCandlish et al 1998) delivery (avoiding any stimulation to the baby) with the midwife giving gentle verbal instruction (if necessary), while utilising the mirror and possibly torch, to see advancement of the presenting part. It is not necessary to assess for the presence of the umbilical cord around the neck; interference can again cause premature stimulation. The baby should be born fully underwater, hence the need to retain the water level and to encourage the woman to keep her buttocks beneath the water. Once born the baby is brought to the surface without any unnecessary delay, where respiration can begin in air. Garland (2006) notes that often after delivery in water a baby's respiratory response is naturally slower; if, however, there are obvious respiration difficulties it is necessary to clamp and cut the cord, removing the baby for resuscitation (see Chapter 56).

When bringing the baby to the surface, care should be taken in case of a short umbilical cord. Anderson (2000) cites a number of instances in which the cord has snapped on bringing the baby above the water level. Cord clamps should be readily available and the midwife should be alert to the need to act quickly. The baby should rest with its head above water, retaining its body heat, at approximately the level of the mother's uterus until management of the third stage begins.

Third stage of labour

If clinically appropriate and desired by the woman, a physiological third stage can be completed in the pool. Blood loss may be harder to estimate and therefore the woman's clinical condition should be considered as part of the assessment. Active management is possible in water, but many midwives may not feel confident about this. When convenient, the mother and baby are brought out of the pool and care continues as for any other birth (e.g. neonatal assessment, examination of the mother's genital tract). It should be noted that on leaving the pool care is needed to keep the mother and baby warm, attention must be paid to containing her *per vaginam* blood loss with sanitary towels, and floor coverings are needed to reduce the risk of slipping on the wet floor.

Infection control

As for any birth, measures are taken to maintain asepsis; however, there is often less intervention and so water cleanliness becomes one of the priorities. The sieve is used to remove any debris, but if the amount is significant, particularly following a vomit, it is advisable to ask the woman to leave the pool temporarily while decontamination takes place. Hired pools often have a disposable liner, but cleaning of the pool is also necessary. Plumbed pools should also be thoroughly cleansed after each use. Burns & Kitzinger (2001) recommend a chlorine-releasing agent of 10 000 parts per million; local protocols may approve other solutions, but they should all be effective against HIV and hepatitis B and C. Jacuzzi-style pools should be avoided.

Emergencies

In the event of an emergency, assistance is called and the woman is helped/removed from the pool quickly and the appropriate management commenced. It is vital that midwives undergo frequent 'drills and skills' practices to have competence in managing emergency situations with a pool birth. In the event of a shoulder dystocia lifting one leg onto the side of the pool or stool often facilitates the delivery. If, however, the woman needs to leave the pool with the shoulders undelivered, care should be taken not to knock the baby's head on the side of the pool. This action is often sufficient to rotate the fetus and facilitate delivery.

ROLE AND RESPONSIBILITIES OF THE MIDWIFE

These can be summarised as:

- thorough, safe labour care as for any birth, but with added considerations for the comfort and safety of the woman, baby and midwife when using the medium of water for analgesia or birth
- contemporaneous record keeping.

Summary

- Clearer guidance now exists to support women and midwives in their use of water for all the stages of labour. There are some outstanding issues and further research is still needed.
- Low risk protocols recommend which women can utilise water. Care is taken to ensure that the pool is appropriately filled; water and maternal temperature should be recorded hourly, the water should not exceed 37.5°C.
- A water birth is a low intervention birth, the baby is brought to the surface without delay; care is taken to avoid the cord snapping.

SELF-ASSESSMENT EXERCISES

The answers to the following questions may be found in the text:

1. What is the current evidence with regard to the use of water for labour and birth?
2. List the items of equipment necessary for birth in water.
3. Describe how the midwife would manage the second stage of labour in water.
4. List the considerations that a midwife should be mindful of when caring for a woman labouring in water.

References

Anderson T: Umbilical cords and underwater birth, *Pract Midwife* 3(2):12, 2000.

Anderson T: Time to throw the water birth thermometer away? *MIDIRS Midwifery Dig* 14(3):370–374, 2004.

Burns E, Kitzinger S: *Midwifery guidelines for use of water in labour*, Oxford, 2001, OCHRAD, Oxford Brookes University (eburns@brookes.ac.uk).

Chapman V, Chales C: Water for labour and birth. In Chapman V, Chales C, editors: *The Midwife's labour and birth handbook*, ed 2, Oxford, 2009, Wiley-Blackwell, pp 93–105.

Cluett ER, Nikodem VC, McCandlish EE, Burns EE: Immersion in water in pregnancy, labour and birth, *Cochrane Database Syst Rev* (2): CD000111. DOI:10.1002/14651858. CD000111, pub2, 2002.

Cluett ER, Oickering RM, Getliffe K, et al: Randomized control trial of labouring in water compared with standard of augmentation for management of dystocia in first stage of labour, *Br Med J* 328 (7435):314–318, 2004.

Garland D: 'On the crest of a wave': Completion of a collaborative audit, *MIDIRS Midwifery Dig* 16(1):81–85, 2006.

McCandlish R, Bowler U, van Asten H, et al: A randomised control trial of care of the perineum during second stage of normal labour, *Br J Obstet Gynaecol* 105(12):1262–1272, 1998.

MIDIRS: *The use of water during childbirth. Informed Choice leaflet (11) for professionals*, Bristol, 2008, MIDIRS.

NICE (National Institute for Health and Clinical Excellence): *Intrapartum care: care of healthy women and their babies during childbirth. Clinical Guideline 55*, London, 2007, NICE.

Odent M: Use of water during labour – updated recommendations, *MIDIRS Midwifery Dig* 8(1):68–69, 1998.

Rafferty L: Time to make a splash – a literature review on the use of water for labour and birth to inform service provision, *MIDIRS Midwifery Dig* 18(4):523–528, 2008.

RCOG (Royal College of Obstetricians and Gynaecologists)/RCM (Royal College of Midwives): *Immersion in water during labour and birth*, Joint Statement No. 1, London, 2006, RCOG/RCM.

Assessment of the baby: assessment at birth

37

The assessment of the baby at birth is two-fold: the first is an immediate assessment undertaken to assess the adjustment from intrauterine to extrauterine life, using the Apgar scoring system; the second is a complete physical examination to confirm normality and detect deviations from the norm. This chapter focuses on the principles of assessment of the baby, considering the different ways the condition of the baby is assessed at birth. The midwife is involved in assessing the baby as part of the care of the baby at birth (NICE 2007). This provides an indication of how well the baby is making the adjustment to extrauterine life and whether any assistance is required.

LEARNING OUTCOMES

Having read this chapter the reader should be able to:

- discuss the Apgar score and how it is used in practice
- describe the examination of the baby at birth, identifying how normality is confirmed
- discuss the role and responsibilities of the midwife in relation to assessment of the baby at birth.

The Apgar score

Devised by Dr Virginia Apgar in the 1950s, this provides a means of assessing the condition of the baby at birth in relation to five variables: respiratory effort, heart rate, colour, muscle tone and reflex irritability. The score is initially assigned at 1 minute, to allow time for the changes to begin. Further scores are undertaken at 5 and 10 minutes. The score can be assessed more frequently if any of the scores are low and resuscitation is required, to provide an indication of the effectiveness of resuscitation measures undertaken (e.g. at 3 and 5 minutes). Low 1-minute scores have no correlation with future outcome. The 5-minute score provides an indication of

Table 37.1 The Apgar scoring system: the five classifications used and the criteria for scoring 0–2

Sign	0	1	2
Appearance (colour)	Blue, pale	Body pink, limbs blue	All pink
Pulse (heart rate)	Absent	<100	>100
Grimace (response to stimuli)	None	Grimace	Cry
Activity (muscle tone)	Limp	Some flexion of limbs	Active movements, limbs well flexed
Respiratory effort	None	Slow, irregular	Good, strong cry

neonatal mortality but poor long-term prediction of future outcome (AAP & ACOG 2006, O'Donnell et al 2006, Pinheiro 2009).

Each variable is assigned a score of 0, 1 or 2, thus the baby is given a total score out of 10. A mnemonic, APGAR, can be used to remember the five variables (Table 37.1). A score of 7–10 at 1 minute suggests the baby is in a good condition. A score of 4–6 indicates moderate depression, requiring some degree of resuscitation but may also be due to other factors such as prematurity, effects of maternal drugs, congenital malformation, etc. (AAP & ACOG 2006). A baby who scores 0–3 is severely depressed (Mead 1996) and is usually already undergoing resuscitation, possibly ventilation. An Apgar score assigned during resuscitation is not equivalent to that obtained from a baby who is breathing spontaneously and there is no accepted standard for reporting Apgar scores for babies who are being resuscitated (AAP & ACOG 2006, Pinheiro 2009).

It is difficult to anticipate which babies will have a low Apgar score at birth. Dijxhoorn et al (1986) suggest changes in the fetal heart rate do not compare well with Apgar scores at delivery. This may explain why some emergency caesarean sections undertaken because of serious concerns regarding the fetal heart rate deliver a baby with a total Apgar score of 9 or 10. A persistently low Apgar score on its own should not be considered a specific indicator of intrapartum asphyxia.

The Apgar score is a subjective scoring system and is therefore vulnerable to bias. Ideally, it should not be assigned by the person undertaking the delivery, however this is not always feasible when only one midwife is in attendance at the birth. At the time of birth, the midwife delivering has to consider the condition of both the mother and the baby. This can result in retrospective scoring, influenced by subsequent events. Additionally, Letko (1996) suggests midwives could be less objective due to their involvement with the outcome. Although the Apgar score could be jointly assigned by all present at delivery, O'Donnell et al (2006) suggest there is poor interobserver reliability.

Other factors can influence the score; for example, assessment of colour can be affected by lighting, skin pigmentation, haemoglobin levels, degree of peripheral perfusion, maternal drugs, trauma, congenital abnormality, infection, hypoxia and hypovolaemia (AAP & ACOG 2006, Letko 1996). Skin pigmentation generally develops from the fifth day of life in non-Caucasian babies (Silverton 1993); however, if the skin is darkly pigmented, the appearance can be assessed by observing the mucous membranes, the palms and the soles – these should be pink. The preterm baby is likely to have lower Apgar scores than the term baby due to neurological immaturity resulting in poor muscle tone, slower reflexes and a bluish-red colouring of the skin. Low scores are inversely related to body weight and are limited in predicting morbidity and mortality (AAP & ACOG 2006).

Assessing the Apgar score

- Observe the appearance, e.g. is the baby pink all over (2), is the body pink but the extremities blue (1), or is the baby pale or blue all over (0)?
- Estimate the heart rate by palpating the umbilicus or placing two fingers across the chest over the apex, count the rate for 6 seconds then multiply by 10. Determine whether the heart rate is above 100 (10 beats or more over

the 6-second period) (2), under 100 (less than 10 beats in 6 seconds) (1) or absent (0). A baby who is pink, active and breathing is likely to have a heart rate above 100.

- The response of the baby to stimuli should be noted. This could be in response to being dried or handled or, for a baby who is being resuscitated, it may be the response to facemasks or airways used. Determine whether the baby cries in response to stimuli (2), whether it is trying to cry but is only able to grimace (1) or whether there is no response (0).
- Observe the muscle tone of the baby by observing the amount of activity and degree of flexion of the limbs: are there active movements using well-flexed limbs (2), is there some flexion of the limbs (1) or is the baby limp (0)?
- Finally, observe the respiratory effort made by the baby: is it good and strong (often seen in conjunction with a crying baby) (2), is respiration slow and irregular (1) or is there no respiratory effort (0)?

PROCEDURE: Apgar scoring

- Ensure the lighting is sufficient to allow good visualization of colour; have good access to the baby.
- Note time of delivery, wait 1 minute then undertake first assessment, assess the five variables quickly and simultaneously, totalling the score.
- Act promptly and appropriately according to the score, e.g. a baby scoring 0–3 requires immediate resuscitation (it may already have commenced if the baby is obviously compromised at birth).
- Repeat at 5 minutes; the score should increase if previously 8 or below.
- Repeat again at 10 minutes.
- Document findings and act accordingly.

Birth examination

The midwife is required to undertake a complete physical examination at birth to confirm normality and detect deviations from the norm (NMC 2004). This is usually undertaken after the first hour of life to enable the baby to have a long period of skin-to-skin contact between mother and baby and after his first feed (NICE 2007). However, it is important not to allow the baby to become cold, and the examination may be delayed if the baby has a low temperature, or is unwell. While this examination should detect obvious abnormality, it can miss other abnormalities, particularly those that only become apparent in the first days of life. For this reason, a further physical examination is also undertaken in the UK by the paediatrician or suitably trained midwife during the first 48 hours of life. The heart, lungs and hips are examined during this subsequent physical examination.

While it is not necessary to undertake the examination in exactly the same order as detailed below, it is important that the examination is thorough and complete; the midwife should develop a systematic approach to the examination.

Principles of newborn examination

- Explain the procedure to the parents and gain their informed consent.
- Wash and dry hands to minimise the risk of infection to the baby; gloves are worn if there is risk of coming into contact with blood or body fluids.
- Ensure adequate lighting to allow clear visualisation; have good access to the baby, preferably in the presence of one or both parents.
- Check the baby is warm; to maintain the temperature only uncover the part of the baby being examined and re-cover quickly.
- Examine the baby systematically and thoroughly.

The head

Look for signs of moulding and caput succedaneum, as these may result in the head appearing asymmetrical and will influence the measurement of the head circumference. The head should be examined for visible signs of trauma (e.g. lacerations from a fetal scalp electrode, forceps marks) and for signs of bruising – this may increase the risk of physiological jaundice occurring.

Feel along the suture lines and fontanelles – are they of normal size and appearance? Widely spaced sutures may be indicative of a preterm baby, lack of moulding or hydrocephalus. Narrowly spaced

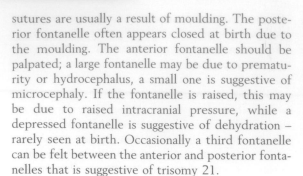

sutures are usually a result of moulding. The posterior fontanelle often appears closed at birth due to the moulding. The anterior fontanelle should be palpated; a large fontanelle may be due to prematurity or hydrocephalus, a small one is suggestive of microcephaly. If the fontanelle is raised, this may be due to raised intracranial pressure, while a depressed fontanelle is suggestive of dehydration – rarely seen at birth. Occasionally a third fontanelle can be felt between the anterior and posterior fontanelles that is suggestive of trisomy 21.

Head circumference

The head circumference may be measured at birth, using the occipitofrontal circumference; the measurement around the occiput and forehead. However, due to the changes that occur at birth, this measurement is likely to change over the next 48 hours; for this reason, it is better to record the head circumference 2–4 days after birth (Johnston et al 2003).

Shape of the face

The shape of the face should appear symmetrical; the size and position of the eyes, nose, mouth, chin and ears should be noted in relation to each other. Moderate facial asymmetry is associated with prolonged second stage, forceps delivery, macrosomia and birth trauma (Stellwagen et al 2008).

Eyes

Examine the eyes to ensure two are present and assess their size, shape and any slanting. Cataracts may be noticeable by a cloudy appearance of the cornea. Any discharge should be noted; this is not normal and could be indicative of infection. The presence of conjunctival haemorrhage, usually acquired during the second stage of labour, should also be noted. The pupils should be examined and should appear round. Occasionally, a keyhole shape is present (coloboma), which could be indicative of an underlying retinal defect.

Nose

The shape of the nose and width of the bridge should be observed; this should be greater than 2.5 cm in the term baby. It is not unusual for the nose to be squashed at birth; if so, this should be noted, particularly if it is affecting the baby's ability to breathe. The nostrils should not flare; if they do, this is usually indicative of respiratory illness.

Mouth

Observe the mouth; the lips should be formed and symmetrical. Asymmetry could be indicative of facial palsy. A small mouth may be due to micrognathia, often associated with underlying abnormality. The area between the lips and the nose should be examined for the presence of a cleft lip. The inside of the mouth should be visualised using a good light source; this is more easily achieved when the baby is crying or by pressing gently on the chin or the angle of the jaw to encourage the baby to open his mouth. The palate should be observed for intactness, particularly at the junction of the hard and soft palate where a cleft palate may occur and the palate should be high and arched. Digital examination should only be undertaken if a submucous cleft palate is suspected (Habel et al 2006). While looking in the mouth, the presence of white spots on the gums or palate (usually due to Epstein's pearls or teeth) should be noted, as should the length of the frenulum.

Ears

Examine the ears to ensure two are present and they are fully formed, in the correct position. The ears of the term baby should contain enough cartilage to allow the ears to spring back into position when moved forward gently. The pinna should be well formed with defined curves in the upper part. Correct positioning of the ears is determined by tracing an imaginary line from the outer canthus of the eyes horizontally back to the ears; the top of the pinna should be above this line. Low set ears may be associated with an underlying chromosomal abnormality (e.g. trisomy 21). The external auditory meatus should be examined to ensure patency. The presence of accessory skin tags or auricles should be noted and may be associated with renal abnormalities (Rose 1994).

Neck

Babies have short necks, which should be examined for symmetry. Move the fingers around the neck to detect the presence of any swelling (e.g. cystic hygroma, sternomastoid tumour). The baby should be able to move the head to both sides well past the shoulder 100–110° from the midline and flex the head 50–60° laterally towards his ear. Limited lateral movement is associated with torticollis (Stellwagen et al 2008). Webbing is unusual and could be indicative of a chromosomal abnormality (e.g. Turner's syndrome); redundant skin folds at the back of the neck are suggestive of trisomy 21.

Clavicles

Using the index finger, feel along the clavicles to ensure they are intact, particularly if there was a breech presentation or shoulder dystocia – both increase the risk of a fractured clavicle, resulting in little or no movement in the associated arm.

Arms

Both arms should be the same length; this can be confirmed by straightening the arms down the side of the baby and comparing the two together. Both arms should be moving freely; spontaneous arm movements can be elicited by stroking the forearm or hand. Lack of movement may be associated with underlying trauma (e.g. fractures, nerve damage) or to poor motor control associated with neurological impairment. The number of digits should be counted and examined for the webbing between them. Polydactyly or syndactyly should be noted. The palm should be straightened and the number of palmar creases noted; a single crease might be associated with chromosomal abnormality (e.g. trisomy 21). Look at the nails for the presence of paronychia as these may become infected or get caught on bedding, causing them to tear and bleed.

Chest

Examine the chest for symmetry of movement with respiration. The respiratory rate can be counted if needed and any signs of respiratory distress (e.g. sternal recession, intercostal recession) reported to the paediatrician immediately. The nipples and areolae should be well formed in the term baby and appear symmetrical on the chest wall but should not be widely spaced (this may be indicative of any underlying chromosomal abnormality). Any accessory nipples should be noted. The breasts may appear enlarged; this is normal and of little significance unless there are signs of infection.

Abdomen

Observe the abdomen, which should appear rounded and move in synchrony with the chest during respiration, inspecting the area to ensure it is intact and gently palpating to ensure there are no abnormal swellings. The umbilical cord should be securely clamped; this should be inspected to ensure there are no signs of haemorrhage.

Genitalia

With boys, the length of the penis should be assessed – this is usually about 3 cm – and the position of the urethral meatus confirmed. The foreskin should not be retracted as it is adherent to the glans penis and physically retracting it at this age can lead to phimosis. The scrotum should be gently palpated for the presence of two testes.

For girls, the vulva should be examined by parting the labia gently to ensure the presence of the clitoris, and the urethral and vaginal orifices. A mucoid discharge may be present which is normal.

Legs

Examine the legs and feet to assess symmetry, size, shape and posture. Confirm that the legs are the same length by straightening them together and comparing the two and then by bending the legs at the hips and knees and comparing length (McCarthy et al 2005). Both legs should be moving freely; lack of movement may be associated with underlying trauma (e.g. fractures, nerve damage) or to poor motor control associated with neurological impairment. The position of the feet in relation to the legs should be noted as both positional and anatomical deformities may cause the feet to be turned inwards or outwards, upwards or downwards. Some of these deformities will require corrective treatment. The shape of the feet should be noted, including oedema or a 'rocker bottom' appearance. The number of toes should be counted and examined for webbing between them by separating them; polydactyly or syndactyly should be noted.

Spine

Examine the spine by turning the baby over, looking for any obvious abnormality such as spina bifida and also for any swelling, dimpling or hairy patches; these could indicate an abnormality of the spinal cord or vertebral column. Assess the curvature of the vertebral column by running the fingers lightly over the spine. This may be easier to do by straddling the baby over one hand, while using the other hand to feel the spine (ensure the head is supported). Gently part the cleft of the buttocks, look for any dimples or sinuses and confirm the presence of the anal sphincter.

Skin

During the examination, the condition of the skin should be observed. The colour should be noted, as should the presence of any rashes or marks (e.g. birthmarks, bruising). Any obvious swelling or spots should be examined and recorded. A Mongolian blue spot may be evident in some babies, particularly those with an Asian or African ancestry. This appears like bruising, usually over the sacral area. This should be observed over the next few days to enable the midwife to differentiate between the possibility of the discoloration being a bruise or a Mongolian blue spot.

Elimination

The passage of urine or meconium should be recorded as it indicates patency of the renal and lower gastrointestinal tract respectively.

Weight

The weight of the baby should be recorded in kilograms; this can be undertaken at the beginning or end of the examination provided the baby is warm.

Length

The crown–heel length of the baby may be recorded; this is not routinely undertaken and is difficult to measure accurately. The length is measured in two stages using a non-stretchable tape measure: from the crown (top part of the head) to the base of the spine, and from the base of the spine to the heel. A second person may be required to straighten the legs. Length can also be measured by placing the baby on a disposable paper sheet and marking the paper where the top of the baby's head is. The baby's legs are then straightened without moving the paper from under the baby and a mark placed where his feet are positioned. The baby can then be lifted from the sheet and the distance between the two marks measured. Alternatively, specialised calibrated equipment may be used, providing a more accurate measurement. The head and feet must be in contact with the equipment, with the legs fully extended (Fig. 37.1).

Once the examination is completed, the baby should be returned to his mother for further skin-to-skin contact or dressed and left comfortable either with the parents or securely in the cot. The findings should be recorded in the appropriate documentation, reporting any deviations to the midwife in charge or paediatrician. The parents should be informed of the findings.

PROCEDURE: birth examination

- The procedure is explained to the parents and informed consent gained.
- Wash and dry hands, put on gloves if required.

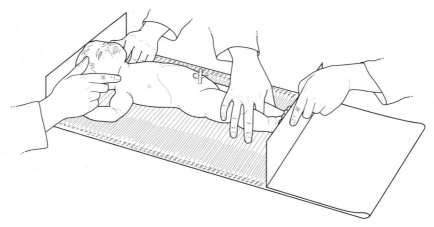

Figure 37.1 • Measuring the length of the baby using specialised calibrated equipment (Adapted from Farrell & Sittlington 2009)

- Ensure the lighting is good and the baby is warm.
- Examine the baby methodically, beginning with the head, face and neck, then the clavicles, arms, hands, chest and abdomen; finally the genitalia, legs, feet and spine are examined.
- The colour, tone and activity of the baby are noted throughout the examination.
- The passage of urine and meconium is recorded.
- Other observations undertaken include the head circumference, length and weight.
- The baby is placed skin-to-skin with his mother or dressed following the procedure.
- Discuss the findings with the parents.
- Document findings and act accordingly.

ROLE AND RESPONSIBILITIES OF THE MIDWIFE

These can be summarised as:

- being able to competently assess the baby at birth, using the Apgar score, and understanding the significance of the score
- undertaking the birth examination thoroughly and competently, referring as necessary
- contemporaneous record keeping.

Summary

- Assessment of the baby at birth is an important skill undertaken by the midwife.
- Apgar scoring is quick and easy to undertake, but is subjective and influenced by factors such as lighting and skin pigmentation.
- Birth examination is a thorough physical examination that detects obvious abnormalities; some abnormalities may not be apparent until the baby is older; subsequent examinations should be undertaken as required.

SELF-ASSESSMENT EXERCISES

The answers to the following questions may be found in the text:

1. How would a baby who scores 1 for each category of the Apgar score be recognised?
2. What factors influence the score awarded at birth?
3. Describe the top to toe examination of the baby undertaken by the midwife at birth.
4. What are the role and responsibilities of the midwife in relation to the assessment of the baby at birth?

References

AAP (American Academy of Pediatrics), ACOG (American College of Obstetricians and Gynecologists): The Apgar score. Policy statement, *Pediatrics* 117 (4):1444–1447, 2006.

Dijxhoorn MJ, Visse GHA, Fidler VJ, et al: Apgar score, meconium and acidaemia at birth in relation to neonatal neurological morbidity in term infants, *Br J Obstet Gynaecol* 893:217–222, 1986.

Farrell P, Sittlington N: The normal baby. In Fraser DM, Cooper MA, editors: *Myles textbook for midwives*, ed 15, Edinburgh, 2009, Churchill Livingstone, p 772.

Habel A, Elhadi N, Sommerlad B, et al: Delayed detection of cleft palate: an audit of newborn examination, *Arch Dis Child* 91:238–240, 2006.

Johnston PGB, Flood K, Spinks K: *The newborn child*, ed 9, Edinburgh, 2003, Churchill Livingstone.

Letko MD: Understanding the Apgar score, *J Obstet, Gynaecol Neonatal Nurs* 25:299–303, 1996.

McCarthy J, Scoles P, MacEwen G: Developmental dysplasia of the hip (DDH), *Curr Orthop* 19:223–230, 2005.

Mead M: The diagnosis of foetal distress: a challenge to midwives, *J Adv Nurs* 23:975–983, 1996.

NICE (National Institute for Health and Clinical Excellence): *Intrapartum guidelines. Care of healthy women and their babies during childbirth*, London, 2007, NICE.

NMC (Nursing and Midwifery Council): *Midwives rules and standards*, London, 2004, NMC.

O'Donnell CPF, Kamlin OF, Davis PG, et al: Interobserver variability of the 5-minute Apgar score, *J Pediatr* 149(4):486–489, 2006.

Pinheiro JMB: The Apgar cycle: a new view of a familiar scoring system, *Arch Dis Child Fetal Neonatal Ed* 94:F70–F72, 2009.

Rose SJ: Physical examination of the full-term baby, *Br J Midwifery* 2(5):209–213, 1994.

Silverton L: *The art and science of midwifery*, New York, 1993, Prentice Hall.

Stellwagen L, Hubbard E, Chamber C, et al: Torticollis, facial symmetry and plagiocephaly in normal newborns, *Arch Dis Child* 93(10):827–831, 2008.

Assessment of the baby: daily examination

38

The daily examination of a baby in the postnatal period monitors the early changes and ensures optimum progress. Any deviations from the norm can be identified and appropriate action taken. It is known as the daily examination to identify it as a different examination from the birth examination.

It isn't however undertaken every single day, but according to identified clinical need. This chapter considers how the daily examination of a baby is undertaken and the role and responsibilities of the midwife in relation to this.

LEARNING OUTCOMES

Having read this chapter the reader should be able to:

- describe the observations that may be made as part of the daily examination of the baby, identifying how normal progress is recognised
- discuss the role and responsibilities of the midwife in relation to daily examination of the baby.

Principles of the daily examination

Parental care

Facilitating optimal infant health and development relies significantly on the skills, education and care given by the parents. The midwife works with families through the ante- and intrapartum periods to culminate in the beginnings of infant health and wellbeing. The midwife teaches by example (e.g. hand washing) as well as with verbal (wherever possible, evidence based) suggestions. In undertaking a daily examination for the baby the midwife relies on communication with the parents to appreciate the complete picture. Equally, it is a time for guiding and advising parents, when necessary, but ultimately in supporting and encouraging them in their new role.

Consent

As the baby cannot give consent for the examination, the midwife should explain the procedure to the parents and gain their consent. This may not be granted if, for example, the baby is now asleep, having been awake all night. The midwife undertakes a risk assessment, based on detailed conversation, to appreciate whether a physical examination must be undertaken or whether it can be postponed until later. The examination should ideally be undertaken when one or both parents are present.

Reducing infection risks

The baby is a 'compromised host' at birth, at risk from infection that can affect morbidity and mortality. Standard precautions should be utilised (see Chapter 8), it is important to avoid cross-infection from other sources; hand hygiene should be scrupulous (see Chapter 9). If contact with body fluids is anticipated then personal protective equipment is used (e.g. gloves and apron).

Examination of the newborn

As mentioned above, the daily examination is not a copy of the examination undertaken at birth, but is a daily assessment of progress thereafter. It therefore relies on the fact that all body systems have been screened, any deviations from the norm are known about and so daily progress is assessed accordingly. It should be undertaken methodically, in a good light and a warm environment.

Initial observations

Observations on entering a woman's personal environment (hospital or home) can give immediate indicators as to the situation and provide the midwife with prompts when giving care advice:

- parents may immediately begin to express problems or anxieties
- how they are feeling may be apparent by looking: peaceful, tired, tearful, happy, wearing nightclothes, etc.
- how the parent(s) handle and react to the baby
- environmental factors such as heat/cold, the presence of smoke, pets, other relatives/siblings/ visitors – their reactions or concerns, general level of hygiene.

The following observations are likely to lead into detailed discussion:

- The baby's behaviour: is the baby active, sleepy, contented, unsettled, does the baby cry a lot, what is the cry like, can the baby be pacified easily?
- Feeding patterns: does the baby wake for feeds? What is the approximate feeding pattern? (This will vary according to feeding method.) If breastfeeding, is the mother happy that the baby latches correctly and achieves an effective feed? If formula feeding, are amounts taken appropriate for age? Is the mother fully conversant with sterilising and preparing feeds (see Chapters 43 and 44)? Is the baby settled after a feed? Is there any vomiting or posseting? In the event of vomiting green bile, or any projectile vomiting, a direct referral is made to a paediatrician.
- Elimination: do the number and nature of wet and soiled nappies suggest that feeding is progressing and body systems are functioning normally?
- Are the parents feeling confident about other aspects of baby care, e.g. skin care, managing unsettled periods?
- Do the parents have any other concerns or questions at this time?

General observation of the baby

Observing the baby before undressing it can reveal several potential problems:

- Under-/overclothed: advice may be needed as to correct temperature management when indoors.
- Respirations: the respiratory pattern is noted (often irregular in newborn babies, see Chapter 6), with a normal respiratory rate of 40–60 per minute expected when the baby is at rest with no signs of respiratory distress. It may be higher if the baby has been crying. Chest movement should be symmetrical (this is often better assessed when the baby is undressed), nasal flaring should not be seen.
- Obvious signs of vomiting or posseting (see above).

- Skin colour: the baby should appear pink all over, indicating good peripheral perfusion. When the baby has darkly pigmented skin, signs of peripheral perfusion can be assessed by observing the mucous membranes, the palms and the soles. Cyanosis with or without signs of respiratory distress should be reported to the paediatrician immediately. If the baby appears pale, this should be reported, as it could be indicative of underlying illness. It is not unusual for babies to develop physiological jaundice, seen as a yellow discoloration of the skin (and sometimes the sclera and mucous membranes). Physiological jaundice usually appears from the third day and may deepen over the next couple of days before beginning to subside by the seventh day. If the jaundice appears severe and widespread, especially if the baby is very sleepy or not feeding, the serum bilirubin level should be estimated. Clinical estimation of the degree of jaundice can be inaccurate and is influenced by the type of lighting, the reflective ability of objects around the baby and the peripheral blood flow (Johnston et al 2003).
- Limb movement: when the baby is active all four limbs should be moving without any signs of discomfort. If the baby was a breech presentation antenatally it is likely that his legs continue to maintain an extended position.
- Head shape: signs of birth trauma may be noted. The head is examined in greater detail as the examination progresses (see below).

Following the initial observations, discussions with the parents and general observations, the midwife then undertakes a 'top to toe' examination of the baby. Care is taken to only expose the parts that are being assessed so that the baby does not cool. On picking up the baby the midwife will appreciate the baby's body temperature and whether he is irritable on handling.

Physical examination

Head

Using the fingertips, feel along the suture lines and fontanelles. Moulding should have resolved within the first 24 hours of birth. The anterior fontanelle should be palpated, and should be level. If raised, this may be due to raised intracranial pressure; a depressed fontanelle is suggestive of dehydration. While feeling around the head, note any new swellings. A cephalhaematoma first appears between 12 and 36 hours and is likely to increase in size, taking up to 6 weeks to disappear. Any bruised or traumatized areas noted at or since birth should be examined to ascertain that healing is occurring and there are no signs of infection.

Eyes

Inspect the eyes to ensure they are clear, with no signs of discharge. If a discharge is present, the eyes should be cleaned (see Chapter 13) and a swab taken if indicated (see Chapter 11). The parents should be shown how to clean the eye. Refer to the paediatrician if necessary. Jaundice may be noted in the sclera, as discussed above.

Mouth

The mouth should be looked at using a good light source and should be clean and moist; the presence of white plaques should be investigated as these could be indicative of a monilial infection (if breastfeeding, the mother's nipples should also be assessed). If the baby has fed recently, sucking blisters may appear on the lips. Although this gives the appearance that the skin is peeling from the lips, no treatment is needed

Skin

Skin colour should be assessed as discussed above. The skin should also be examined for any rashes, spots, bruising or signs of infection or trauma. Erythema toxicum appears as a blotchy red rash and is of little significance, as are milia. However, septic spots should be identified early and treatment instigated if required. Look also for areas of excoriation that may occur due to friction with bedding or clothes, or in cases of excoriation of the buttocks, may be due to an ammoniacal burn or fungal infection. The nails should be examined for paronychia. If the baby was postmature the skin may be dry, parents should be reassured that no treatment is necessary (see Chapter 13). On exposure of the baby's trunk (non-infective) engorged breasts may be noted. Parents need reassuring that no treatment is necessary and that as hormone levels fall the problem will resolve. In the event of redness or signs of infection, the baby should be referred to the paediatrician.

Umbilicus

The umbilical cord and umbilicus should be examined daily for signs of separation and to exclude infection (see Chapter 13). The cord usually separates within 5–16 days; a small stump of cord may be left in the umbilicus, which should be examined daily. Early signs of infection may be detected by redness around the umbilicus; the cord may also smell offensive and become sticky.

Nappies

Effective elimination acts as a guide for neonatal health, particularly for effective feeding. In the first few days of life term babies micturate 15–60 mL/kg per day. This increases in the subsequent days to one or more episodes of voiding per feed (Blackburn 2007). In reality, two or more voids should be seen on days 1–2, three or more on days 3–4 and five or more by days 5–6. After 1 week of age, six or more voids should be seen, the volume having increased during the week so that nappies are increasingly heavy (McNally et al 2008). Disposable nappies can be torn open at the back to reveal urine within the crystals if in doubt about the presence of a void.

Meconium is seen for the first 2 days, a changing stool is present on days 3–4 followed by a yellow stool thereafter. A baby that is being fed effectively should defecate at least twice a day. The elimination pattern should be consistent with age and effective feeding, deviations from the norm encourage the midwife to initially consider whether additional feeding support is required. A yellow stool may be seen earlier than day 5 if feeding is particularly good.

The presence of urates is sometimes seen in the nappy, often as orange or red crystals. Parents need reassurance that this is not a major complication, but care should be taken to ensure that feeding is giving the baby sufficient fluid and nutrition.

Female infants may have a small pseud menstruation: a tiny mucousy red bleed may seen. It is caused by the effects of mater hormones within the baby's system and is harml

Weight

A healthy term baby undergoes a diuresis from intra to extra uterine adaptation. This results in a physiological weight loss of 5–10% of its birth weight within the first 3–4 days. Birth weight is generally regained by 2 weeks of age. It is important that correctly calibrated electronic scales are used each time. A weight loss of greater than 10% of birth weight would give cause for concern. If this was accompanied by suboptimal urine and stooling then feeding would need careful investigation.

However, Crossland et al (2008) indicate that actually there is little accurate knowledge known about the weight changes in healthy term babies up to 2 weeks of age. In their small study, babies were weighed each day for 2 weeks. They concluded that feeding problems should be considered if weight is not increasing by 6 days, but some healthy babies took 17 days to regain their birth weight. Iyer et al (2008) implemented an early weighing protocol in which babies were weighed 72–96 hours after birth. They found a higher detection rate for hypernatraemic dehydration and so increased breastfeeding rates. Equally, Kudumula et al (2009) implemented weighing on days 3, 5 and 10 and report the same findings as Iyer et al (2008). In each instance the mothers that needed additional support for feeding were identified and assisted.

Identity

If the daily assessment is being undertaken in hospital then it is important to establish that the baby is wearing identity bands according to local protocol.

Screening

Undertaking the examination as a whole is a form of screening for normality. Specific haematological screening, e.g. newborn blood spot screening or serum bilirubin may be undertaken with parental consent. Newborn blood spot screening should be undertaken on day 5. Chapter 39 discusses this in greater detail.

er the examination

n the examination is complete, the baby should dressed and the findings recorded in the appro- e documentation. The results should form the basis of advice given to the parents regarding the progress and subsequent care of the baby. Any deviations from the norm should be acted on accordingly and appropriate care instigated.

PROCEDURE: daily examination of the baby

- Make a mental note of anything significant on entering the woman's personal environment (see above).
- Discuss the progress of the baby with the parents, allaying their anxieties if necessary.
- Explain procedure, gain informed consent.
- Wash hands (apply gloves only if contact with body fluids is anticipated), undertake a general observation of the baby.
- Ensure there is good light and a warm environment, undress the baby and undertake the 'top to toe' examination described above.
- Weigh the baby if indicated.
- Redress the baby and give back to the parents.
- If day 5, newborn blood spot screening may be taken with consent. The baby would be redressed but with a foot exposed, the baby will be with a parent or with the midwife, depending on preference (see Chapter 39).
- Discuss the findings with the parents.
- Document the findings and act accordingly.

ROLE AND RESPONSIBILITIES OF THE MIDWIFE

These can be summarised as:

- undertaking all aspects of the daily examination thoroughly and competently, referring as necessary
- education and support of parents
- contemporaneous record keeping.

Summary

- The midwife examines the baby daily as part of the care provided to the mother and baby during the postnatal period.
- The midwife uses skills of communication and observation to ensure that optimal infant health is achieved. It also provides an opportunity to discuss detailed care and advice.

SELF-ASSESSMENT EXERCISES

The answers to the following questions may be found in the text:

1. Describe the different aspects of the daily examination of the baby.
2. What would the midwife do if the baby's mouth had visible white plaques?
3. How should the midwife advise a mother that has seen urates in the baby's nappy?
4. What are the role and responsibilities of the midwife in relation to the daily examination of the baby?

References

Blackburn ST: *Maternal, fetal and neonatal physiology: a clinical perspective*, ed 3, St. Louis, 2007, Saunders.

Crossland DS, Richmond S, Hudson M, Smith M, Abu-Harb M: Weight change in the term baby in the first 2 weeks of life, *Acta Paediatr* 97:425–429, 2008.

Iyer NP, Srinivasan R, Evans K, Ward L, Cheung JWA, Mattes JWA: Impact of early weighing on neonatal hypernatraemic dehydration and breast feeding, *Arch Dis Child* 93(4):297–299, 2008.

Johnston PGB, Flood K, Spinks K: *The newborn child*, ed 9, Edinburgh, 2003, Churchill Livingstone.

Kudumula V, Asokkumar A, Akinsoji O, Babu S: Breastfeeding malnutrition in neonates: a step towards controlling the problem, *Arch Dis Child* 94(3):246, 2009.

McNally S, Napier K, Welford H: *What's in a nappy? NCT Information sheet*, London, 2008, NCT.

Assessment of the baby: capillary sampling

39

This chapter considers capillary blood sampling from the baby. The most common method of obtaining blood samples from the neonate is via a heel prick (Barker et al 1994). The midwife undertakes this as part of routine screening, and also to detect or confirm deviations from the norm (e.g. serum bilirubin or serum glucose estimations).

LEARNING OUTCOMES

Having read this chapter the reader should be able to:

- describe the procedure for obtaining a capillary blood sample from the heel
- discuss the factors that need to be considered, highlighting those which enhance the procedure
- describe in detail the specific considerations for taking a reliable newborn blood spot screening
- discuss the role and responsibilities of the midwife in relation to capillary sampling.

Underpinning anatomy

The blood is obtained from the capillaries contained within the skin. The arterial venous network of the skin is located at the junction of the lower dermis and upper subcutaneous tissue. The skin should be punctured only to the depth of this junction to facilitate blood flow; a deeper puncture can have serious complications. If the calcaneus (heel bone) is punctured, there is a risk of osteochondritis or osteomyelitis resulting. The distance between the skin and bone can vary depending on where on the foot measurement is taken (with the narrowest distance being at the posterior curve of the heel) and the weight and gestation of the baby.

Another consideration is the position of plantar arteries and nerves, which should be avoided. Puncturing the arteries can result in haemorrhage and increases the risk of introducing infection, which could result in septicaemia. Puncturing the nerves can result in permanent damage to the nerve.

Blumenfeld et al (1979) estimated the distance from the surface of the skin to the arterial–venous network to be 0.35–1.6 mm (at postmortem). Jain & Rutter (1999) attempted to replicate this work with live babies and argue that none of the babies in their study had a distance of less than 3 mm between capillaries and skin, and thus argue that any part of the plantar surface would be suitable for pricking. However, more research is necessary and this is not yet incorporated into current practice. Automated lancets (generally) puncture to a depth of 2.4 mm or less (often 1 mm).

How to avoid puncturing the calcaneus, plantar arteries and nerves

* Use the lateral and medial portions of the heel as puncture sites [UK National Screening Committee (UKNSC) 2008].
* Draw an imaginary line from midway between the fourth and fifth toes laterally and medially from the middle of the big toe as the calcaneus rarely extends beyond these (Fig. 39.1) (these points are also furthest away from the arteries and nerves).
* The correct depth of puncture can be achieved using a 'measured' lancet.

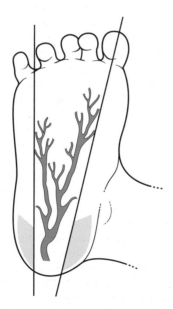

Figure 39.1 • Heel sites for capillary sampling in the baby

* Select a new puncture site for each collection.
* Use a good technique to avoid having to repeat the procedure.

Newborn blood spot screening tests (previously known as the Guthrie test)

Blood spot screening is offered to all babies and should be taken between 5 and 8 days after birth (the day of birth being day 0), ideally on day 5. Testing at this stage is necessary to instigate treatment as early as possible. Many disorders could be found from these blood spots; however, screening programmes have to consider issues such as sensitivity and reliability, cost effectiveness and likely benefit. Hence, at this time, the UKNSC (2008) recommends screening from blood spot tests for:

* phenylketonuria (PKU)
* congenital hypothyroidism
* sickle-cell and thalassaemia
* cystic fibrosis
* medium chain acyl CoA dehydrogenase deficiency (MCADD).

The blood spot form is accompanied by its own glassine envelope. A type of blotting paper is used for the drops of blood; this allows the blood to soak through to the required depth for accurate testing. There are four circles, each one needs to have one drop of blood in it that fills the circle fully. Inaccurate results may be obtained if the blood:

* is multilayered
* is multispotted (several smaller drops fill the circle)
* has been forced out of the heel by squeezing
* is contaminated (water, alcohol, heparin or any other substance in close proximity)
* has not soaked through.

Repeat tests are requested if:

* a specific condition (e.g. cystic fibrosis) requires it
* the test was taken before 4 days of age
* the specimen card has errors or omissions
* the test was taken less than 72 hours after a transfusion
* it is an insufficient or contaminated sample
* there has been a delay in it reaching the laboratory (UKNSC 2008).

Historically, there has been guidance with regard to ingestion of milk feeds for certain days before testing, presence of antibiotics and gestational age. The UKNSC is clear that testing should be undertaken on day 5 irrespective of these things.

One of the UKNSC's standards (2008) is that the form should be completed fully, contemporaneously and with the baby's NHS number (ideally a bar-coded label given to parents on discharge from hospital). Parents also need to be able to give informed consent for the test; the UKNSC recommends the leaflet 'Newborn blood spot screening for your baby' (downloadable), suggesting that it is given antenatally and then discussed again at least 24 hours prior to the test. In the event of declining the test 'DECLINE' should be written on the form, and it should be forwarded to the laboratory as for any others. Parents should receive the result before their 6- to 8-week neonatal assessment.

Bilirubin estimation

A capillary sample may be taken to estimate the level of unconjugated bilirubin in the blood of a jaundiced baby. In some maternity units, the sample is then sent to the pathology laboratory, whereas other maternity units have the equipment (centrifugal machine) to undertake the test themselves. Usually two thin, preheparinized capillary tubes are filled with blood. Care should be taken to avoid getting air in the capillary tubes as this may result in the blood dispersing totally from the tubes during spinning, necessitating a further blood test.

Blood glucose estimation

This is usually undertaken as a diagnostic test when hypoglycaemia is suspected or as a screening test in babies considered to be 'at risk' of developing hypoglycaemia. The midwife should be familiar with the equipment used to estimate the level of glucose in the blood. Increasingly blood glucose is being estimated via a venepuncture sample rather than a capillary sample as the results are more accurate. Cleansing of the skin with alcohol-impregnated wipes affects the accuracy of the results.

Factors to consider when undertaking capillary sampling

Preparation

Informed consent should be gained (see above for newborn blood spot screening) whatever the nature of the test, along with an indication of how and when to expect the results.

The need to warm the foot in advance (with extra socks or warm water (Permalloo & Chapple 2008)) is contentious. The UKNSC (2008) supports not warming the foot, as do Barker et al (1996). In their trial warming had no effect on the time taken, baby's response or need for second specimen. Hassan & Shah (2005) illustrate a case of scalding that occurred when a warm water nappy had been wrapped around the foot. The use of extra clothing, however, would appear to have anecdotal support (Stewart et al 2005).

Position and comfort of the baby

Despite giving informed consent many parents will still find these kinds of procedures difficult to cope with. Most parents will appreciate explanations of what's going to happen, the baby's expected response and what they can do to assist. Others may choose to absent themselves and allow the midwife to continue alone. In both instances reassurances are necessary, part of the baby's comfort will come from its parents' response.

The baby may be held either across the lap or against the shoulder by the mother, another person or the midwife undertaking the test. Alternatively, the baby can be laid on a flat surface (e.g. cot, changing mat on the floor). Upright positions are better as gravity can assist with the direction of blood flow and make it easier to collect the blood from the foot. Breastfeeding during the procedure places the baby in an ideal position. Whatever position is chosen, the baby should be held securely to prevent excessive movement of the foot, which may interfere with the collection of the sample, and to ensure that the person undertaking the test has hands free to hold the equipment, the foot and subsequently the card/testing equipment. It may be easier to wrap the baby in a blanket to prevent the baby's limbs moving too much, although some babies will object to this.

There are a number of behavioural responses to pain seen within the baby, which include facial expressions, body movements and crying characteristics. Facial expressions consisting of brow bulge, eye squeeze, nasolabial furrow and open lips can be seen in the majority of babies within 6 seconds of the heel prick. Facial expressions are considered more specific than body movements (which also occur in response to wiping the heel with a medicated swab) and crying (premature infants are less likely to cry) (Harrison & Johnston 2002). For many babies, however, this elicits a crying response with some becoming very distressed. This may inhibit blood flow as the leg muscles contract and impede circulation. Physiological responses including an increase in the heart and respiratory rate may also be seen, although it is not known if this is due to the pain of the procedure or the effects of being handled. The midwife should consider how the pain and discomfort can be reduced.

For the baby who is breastfeeding when the procedure is performed, very little pain symptomatology may be noticed, particularly when this is combined with skin-to-skin contact (Gray et al 2000). Not all studies confirm this although it is difficult to compare studies; in Carbajal et al's (2003) study, breastfeeding was stopped 2 minutes before the procedure was undertaken.

Oral sucrose reduces the pain behaviour exhibited (Bilgen et al 2001, Overgaard & Knudsen 1999). While Stevens et al (2003) agree that sucrose is safe and effective, they suggest an optimal dose has not yet been identified and repeated use of sucrose in babies requiring several capillary samples should be investigated. Use of sucrose in the very low birthweight baby, where the condition is unstable or the baby is ventilated, also needs to be investigated further (Stevens et al 2003). Some parents may be opposed to the idea of administering sucrose to their baby. The midwife should be aware of alternative, more physiological methods of reducing the pain experience (skin-to-skin contact, talking, massaging, cuddling, non-nutritive sucking (Simpson 2004). Overgaard & Knudsen (1999) found that making sure the baby was quiet and relaxed prior to the capillary sampling had a similar effect to sucrose administration.

The use of a local anaesthetic gel has been proposed for neonatal venepuncture (Moore 2001) and heel pricks (Bellini et al 2002), although Jain et al (2001) found it to be ineffective. If this is to be used it is important to ensure it is suitable for use in neonates and will not cause vasoconstriction as this will increase the difficulty in obtaining a sample and increase the pain felt by the baby.

Cleansing and puncturing the foot

For newborn blood spot screening, the UKNSC (2008) suggests that the heel should be cleansed with either alcohol or water, and should be dried carefully to prevent contamination of the specimen. Alcohol should not be used if the specimen is for glucose monitoring. Automated lancet devices may be reusable (with disposable lancets or blades attached) or disposable. They puncture or incise the skin to a predetermined depth and are recommended for use. Some of the devices allow the midwife to choose the penetration depth; this is preferable when undertaking the procedure on a preterm or low birthweight baby.

Safety

The use of standard precautions is indicated, apron and gloves should be worn. The use of lancets that withdraw, or can be removed with a 'firing' or non-touch action, all help to reduce the risks of percutaneous injury for the midwife. A sharps box must be on hand to use immediately when undertaking neonatal capillary sampling.

Facilitating blood flow

Newborn babies have a sluggish circulation or vasoconstriction (acrocyanosis) that may affect not only the amount of blood obtained but also the measurement of some blood tests. The baby should be kept warm, with only the foot exposed during the procedure. The need or otherwise to warm the foot is discussed above. Holding the foot downwards encourages blood flow. If the blood is not flowing well, the heel may be gently squeezed and released; however, blood spot results are affected if the blood is diluted by interstitial fluid in this way. The risks of haemolysis and bruising are also increased.

Blood collection

After puncturing the foot patience should be employed to allow a large drop of blood to collect. Permalloo & Chapple (2008) suggest that 15 seconds allows for this, longer may see the blood clotting. Some practitioners wipe away the first drop of blood to avoid contamination from the skin or apply petroleum jelly just below the puncture site to help the blood collect in a large globule. There is no discussion or researched evidence for either of these actions.

- Newborn blood spot screening: ensure that one large drop of blood drops onto the top side of the card into each circle.
- Blood glucose: one large drop of blood is placed onto/into the reagent strip (depending on the type of monitor used).
- Bilirubin estimation: the end of the capillary tube is placed in the drop of blood and one finger is placed on the other end of the tube. The blood is drawn into the capillary tube and the finger removed to facilitate the passage of the blood down the tube, taking care not to allow the blood to spill out the other end. When full, the tubes are sealed, often with plasticine.

Stopping the bleeding

When sufficient blood has been obtained, pressure should be applied to the site using gauze or cotton wool, to stem blood flow and decrease the risk of haematoma formation and bruising. When the bleeding has stopped, a plaster may be applied, although this is not essential.

Record keeping and specimen despatch

As well as the specimen card (discussed above) records are completed that indicate when the test was taken and for the newborn blood spot screening, when it was sent to the laboratory. Completed newborn blood spot screening cards should be sent via 1st class mail within 24 hours of being taken (ideally in a prepaid envelope). All other specimens should be processed or despatched promptly.

PROCEDURE: obtaining a capillary sample

- Gain informed consent from the parents; determine if they will be present and who will hold the baby.

- Gather equipment:
  - automated lancet
  - apron and non-sterile gloves
  - alcohol-impregnated swab, if indicated
  - collecting equipment
  - cotton-wool ball or gauze swab
  - plaster to cover puncture site
  - portable sharps box.
- Wash hands, apply apron and gloves.
- Position the baby appropriately, considering the comfort of the baby.
- Inspect the foot to select the best site, avoiding underlying nerves and bone.
- Encourage the baby to be calm and relaxed.
- Wipe with alcohol-impregnated swab if indicated; leave to dry for at least 30 seconds.
- Hold the ankle with the non-dominant hand with the foot flexed.
- With the dominant hand pierce the skin with the lancet; put used lancet in sharps box.
- Hold the foot downwards, wait patiently for a large drop of blood to accumulate (approximately 15 seconds), collect the specimen as required (see above).
- If completing a newborn blood spot screening allow the next drop of blood to form and then drop onto the card, continue in this way until all four circles are filled. Allow the spots to air dry (away from direct sunlight or heat) before placing in the envelope.
- Using a cotton-wool ball or gauze swab, apply pressure to the site; apply plaster if required.
- Return the baby to the parents if they were not holding him during the procedure.
- Dispose of equipment correctly and wash hands.
- Document the results and act accordingly.

ROLE AND RESPONSIBILITIES OF THE MIDWIFE

These can be summarised as:

- recognising the need for capillary blood sampling
- undertaking the procedure correctly and safely at the correct time
- education and support of the parents
- contemporaneous record keeping.

Summary

- Obtaining a capillary blood sample from the baby should be undertaken only when required, as there are risk factors associated with this procedure.
- The reliability of the results depends upon the accuracy of the procedure. When undertaking a newborn blood spot screening (day 5) care should be taken not to contaminate the specimen, to fill each circle with one large drop of blood, to fully complete the request card and to ensure its prompt despatch.
- The midwife should be aware of the measures that can facilitate a non-traumatic experience for mother and baby.

SELF-ASSESSMENT EXERCISES

The answers to the following questions may be found in the text:

1. List the indications for undertaking capillary blood sampling.
2. When obtaining a capillary blood sample from the heel of the baby, how can the risk of damage to the underlying nerves and bone be minimised?
3. When obtaining a capillary blood sample from the heel of the baby, how can blood flow be encouraged?
4. When undertaking newborn blood spot screening list the factors that could warrant requiring a repeat specimen.
5. How can the amount of pain felt by the baby be reduced?
6. What are the role and responsibilities of the midwife in relation to capillary sampling?

References

Barker DP, Latty BW, Rutter N: Heel blood sampling in preterm infants: which technique? *Arch Dis Child (Fetal Neonatal Ed)* 71(3):206–208, 1994.

Barker DP, Willetts B, Cappendijk VC, et al: Capillary blood sampling: should the heel be warmed? *Arch Dis Child* 74:F139–140, 1996.

Bellini CV, Bagnoli F, Perrone S, et al: Effect of multisensory stimulation on analgesia in term neonates: a randomised controlled trial, *Pediatr Res* 41(4):460–463, 2002.

Bilgen H, Ozek E, Cebeci D, et al: Comparison of sucrose, expressed breast milk and breast-feeding on the neonatal response to heel prick, *J Pain* 2(5):301–305, 2001.

Blumenfeld TA, Turi GK, Blanc WA: Recommended site and depth of newborn heel skin punctures based on anatomical measurements and histopathology, *Lancet* 1:230–233, 1979.

Carbajal R, Veerapen S, Couderc S, et al: Analgesic effect of breast feeding in term neonates: randomised controlled trial, *Br Med J* 326:13–15, 2003.

Gray L, Watt L, Blass EM: Skin-to-skin contact is analgesic in healthy newborns, *Pediatrics* 105(1): 460–463, 2000.

Harrison D, Johnston L: Bedside assessment of heel lance pain in the hospitalized infant, *J Obstet Gynaecol Neonatal Nurs* 31(5): 551–557, 2002.

Hassan Z, Shah M: Scald injury from the Guthrie test: should the heel be warmed? *Arch Dis Child Fetal Neonatal Ed* 90(6):F533–F534, 2005.

Jain A, Rutter N: Ultrasound study of heel to calcaneum depth in neonates, *Arch Dis Child* 80:F243–245, 1999.

Jain A, Rutter N, Ratnayaka M: Topical amethocaine gel for pain relief of heel prick blood sampling: a randomised double blind controlled trial, *Arch Dis Child (Fetal Neonatal Ed)* 84:F56–F59, 2001.

Moore J: No more tears: a randomized controlled double-blind trial of amethocaine gel vs. placebo in the management of procedural pain in neonates, *J Adv Nurs* 34(4): 475–482, 2001.

Overgaard C, Knudsen A: Pain-relieving effect of sucrose in newborns during heel prick, *Biol Neonate* 75:279–284, 1999.

Permalloo N, Chapple J: Newborn screening revisited: what midwives need to know. In Edwins J, editor: *Community Midwifery Practice*, Oxford, 2008, Blackwell, pp 107–131.

Simpson C: Congenital anomalies, fetal and neonatal surgery, and pain. In Henderson C, Macdonald S, editors: *Mayes' Midwifery*, ed 13, Edinburgh, 2004, Baillière Tindall, pp 670–683.

Stevens B, Yamada J, Ohlsson A: Sucrose for analgesia in newborn infants undergoing painful procedures. In *Cochrane Library*, Issue 3. Update Software, Oxford, 2003.

Stewart RJ, Franck L, Hardelid P: National guidelines on blood sampling for newborn screening, *Electron lett* 2005. Available online. http://fn.bmj.com/cgi/eletters/90/6/F533 January 2009.

UKNSC (UK National Screening Committee): *Antenatal and newborn screening programmes*, 2008. Available online. www.newbornbloodspot.screening.nhs.uk January 2009.

Assessment of the baby: developmental dysplasia of the hips

40

CHAPTER CONTENTS

Developmental dysplasia of the hips (congenital dislocation of the hips) encompasses a continuum of abnormalities in the immature hip of the baby that ranges from mild dysplasia to full dislocation (Storer & Skaggs 2006). Mild dysplasia may not become clinically apparent until adulthood (Dezateux & Rosenthal 2007) but when it is untreated can lead to long-term complications such as pain in the hips, knees and lower back, gait disturbances and degenerative hip changes and is a leading cause of arthritis in the hip (Dezateux & Rosenthal 2007, Mahan & Kassler 2008). This chapter considers the assessment for developmental dysplasia, including discussion of who should undertake the assessment, when and how.

LEARNING OUTCOMES

Having read this chapter the reader should be able to:

- describe how the hips are examined to detect developmental dysplasia
- discuss the role and responsibilities of the midwife in relation to this screening test.

Developmental dysplasia

Developmental dysplasia of the hips (DDH) occurs in approximately 1 per 1000 births (McCarthy et al 2005) although there are cultural differences which increase the incidence. Risk factors for developing DDH include:

- Breech presentation: the risk increases further with a vaginal breech birth compared to elective prelabour caesarean section (Dezateux & Rosenthal 2007, Lowry et al 2005, Mahan & Kassler 2008, McCarthy et al 2005, Storer & Skaggs 2006).
- Family history (Dezateaux & Rosenthal 2007, Mahan & Kassler 2008, McCarthy et al 2005, Storer & Skaggs 2006).
- Female infants: possibly related to increased joint laxity in response to maternal hormones such as relaxin (Dezateux & Rosenthal 2007, Lowry et al 2005).
- Swaddling where the hips are adducted: this is more common in countries/cultures where swaddling for long periods is undertaken, e.g. Saudi Arabia, Japan, Turkey, Navajo Indians, Lapp populations (Dezateux & Rosenthal 2007,

Mahan & Kassler 2008). The incidence decreases when babies are able to flex and abduct their hips when swaddled (Mahan & Kassler 2008).

- Ethnicity: increased in Caucasian babies (McCarthy et al 2005).
- High birthweight babies (Dezateux & Rosenthal 2007).
- Oligohydramnios (Dezateux & Rosenthal 2007).

Situations where the hips of the fetus/baby are maintained in prolonged periods of extension and adduction increase the incidence of DDH. McCarthy et al (2005) suggest that other musculoskeletal disorders of malpositioning or uterine crowding may also be present (e.g. talipes, torticollis).

When to assess for developmental dysplasia of the hips

The stability of the hips can be assessed at birth; some babies' hips will appear to be dislocatable whereas others are actually dislocated. However, there is an ongoing debate about whether DDH should be assessed at birth or when the baby is older as the majority of cases of DDH detected at birth resolve spontaneously in the first week of life (Mahan & Kassler 2008). There is also concern that repeated Barlow hip tests may cause dislocation in an otherwise normal hip; despite these concerns there appear to be no reported increases in hip laxity (Mahan & Kassler 2008). Isolated hip clicks are considered not to be pathological although they are a frequent cause of referral – this may be decreased by leaving the assessment until the baby is older (Mahan & Kassler 2008). It is important though to detect this condition early to prevent long-term damage to the acetabulum that will result in shortening of the leg. While it may be difficult to detect dislocatable hips at birth due to the lax ligaments, currently it is recommended that all babies should be examined by a competent practitioner before they are discharged from the hospital. For babies born at home, this should be undertaken within the first 48 hours. While the paediatrician often performs this role, midwives in the UK are increasingly undertaking the examination, having undergone further training and assessment to be deemed competent (NMC 2004). If the hip is dislocatable, undertaking the test itself may be a cause of further damage. It is therefore very important that

the test is done gently without excess force, but accurately, to avoid unnecessary repeat tests. Any baby who has a hip that is dislocatable should be referred to a paediatric orthopaedic surgeon.

Testing for developmental dysplasia of the hips involves looking at the appearance of the legs and the skin folds of the thighs, and then physically abducting the legs using either the Barlow or the Ortolani test, feeling for a palpable 'clunk' during the procedure. The range of abduction can also be assessed, as a limited range may be indicative of DDH.

Appearance of the legs and thigh skin folds

This is part of the initial birth examination, but should be repeated prior to examination of the hips. The length of both legs should be the same; if one is shorter, this could be indicative of the head of the femur being located outside of the acetabulum. However, it can be difficult to measure the legs accurately. With the baby lying supine, the legs should be flexed at the hips and knees and the length of the legs compared. If one is shorter than the other, this is highly suggestive of DDH (this is also referred to as the Galeazzi or Allis sign; McCarthy et al 2005). The legs should then be held together and straightened as much as possible and the thigh creases examined, which should be symmetrical. Asymmetry is suggestive of developmental dysplasia, particularly if it is ascertained that this leg is shorter than the other. However, it should be remembered that bilateral developmental dysplasia can occur, in which case the thigh creases will appear to be symmetrical, as both femur heads will be displaced from the acetabulum. This assessment is not as reliable as the physical abduction tests, and therefore should not be used in isolation, but to provide further information to assist the diagnosis.

Barlow's test

The rationale underpinning this test is to try to push the head of the femur out of the acetabulum in a backward direction. If achieved, this will be accompanied by a 'clunk' (Fig. 40.1). The normal hip is not dislocatable; no clunk will be felt. It should only be undertaken when the baby is relaxed to avoid undue force being used (McCarthy et al 2005).

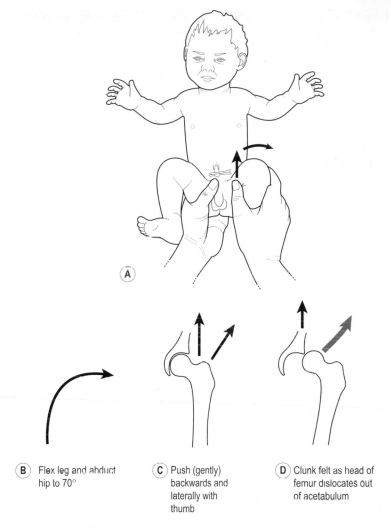

A

B Flex leg and abduct hip to 70°

C Push (gently) backwards and laterally with thumb

D Clunk felt as head of femur dislocates out of acetabulum

Figure 40.1 • Barlow's test (Adapted from Farrell & Sittlington 2009)

PROCEDURE: undertaking the Barlow's test

- Gain informed consent from the parents, undertaking the examination in the presence of one or both parents.
- Wash and dry hands; apply gloves if necessary.
- Place the baby on a flat, firm surface, with good access to the baby.
- Ensure the baby is warm, then undress the baby from the waist down, removing the nappy.
- Position the legs in adduction.
- Examining the hips one at a time, hold the knee and hip in a flexed position and place a thumb on the inner aspect of the thigh (over the inner trochanter) and the index and middle fingers over the outer part of the thigh (over the greater trochanter of the femur at the hip).
- Abduct the leg gently downwards to try to dislocate the hip by pushing down towards the supporting surface then gently pulling the leg upwards (if dislocatable, a 'clunk' is felt at this point as the head of the femur dislocates from the acetabulum and moves back towards it; this procedure is not possible if the hip is not dislocatable). Repeat with other leg.
- Redress the baby.
- Wash and dry hands.
- Discuss the findings with the parents.
- Document the findings and act accordingly.

Ortolani's test

The rationale for this test is that if the hip is unstable, the head of the femur will try to relocate in the acetabulum during the procedure as pressure is applied on the trochanter from behind, accompanied by a 'clunk' (Farrell & Sittlington 2009) (Fig. 40.2). The normal hip is not dislocatable; no clunk will be felt. As for the Barlow's test, it is important the baby is relaxed when undertaking this procedure.

PROCEDURE: undertaking the Ortolani's test

- Gain informed consent from the parents, undertaking the examination in the presence of one or both parents.
- Wash and dry hands; apply gloves if necessary.
- Place the baby on a flat, firm surface, with good access to the baby.

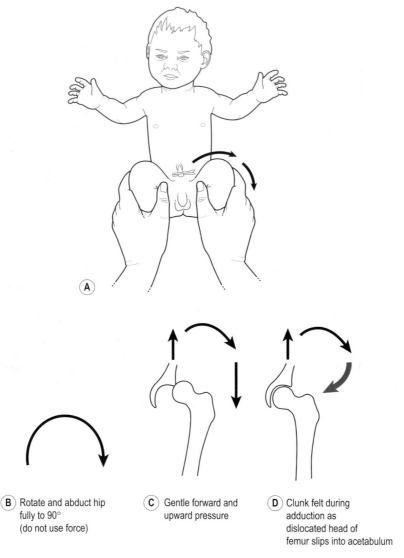

B Rotate and abduct hip fully to 90° (do not use force)

C Gentle forward and upward pressure

D Clunk felt during adduction as dislocated head of femur slips into acetabulum

Figure 40.2 • Ortolani's test (Adapted from Farrell & Sittlington 2009)

- Ensure the baby is warm, then undress the baby from the waist down, removing the nappy.
- Examine the hips one at a time, taking hold of each leg, placing the thumb on the inner aspect of the thigh (over the inner trochanter) and the index and middle fingers over the outer aspect of the thigh (greater trochanter of the femur at the hip).
- Flex the knees and the hips 90° and abduct the leg gently (a 'clunk' is felt as the head of the femur dislocates from the acetabulum; if no clunk is felt, but the leg cannot be abducted fully, developmental dysplasia is also indicated).
- Redress the baby.
- Wash and dry hands.
- Discuss the findings with the parents.
- Document the findings and act accordingly.

ROLE AND RESPONSIBILITIES OF THE MIDWIFE

These can be summarised as:

- being able to undertake the procedure correctly and safely, if appropriately trained
- education and support of the parents
- referral as necessary
- contemporaneous record keeping.

Summary

- The appropriately trained midwife or paediatrician should undertake assessment for developmental dysplasia prior to discharge from hospital, or within 48 hours of a home confinement.
- There are two tests that can be used to assess the ability of the femur head to dislocate: Barlow and Ortolani.

SELF-ASSESSMENT EXERCISES

The answers to the following questions may be found in the text:

1. When would the midwife undertake the test for developmental dysplasia?
2. Describe the two methods of assessment.
3. What is the significance of the clunk?
4. What are the role and responsibilities of the midwife in relation to the assessment of developmental dysplasia?

References

Dezateux C, Rosenthal K: Developmental dysplasia of the hip, *The Lancet* 369:1541–1552, 2007.

Farrell P, Sittlington N: The normal baby. In Fraser DM, Cooper MA, editors: *Myles textbook for midwives*, ed 15, Edinburgh, 2009, Churchill Livingstone, pp 778–779.

Lowry CA, Donoghue VB, O'Herlihy C: Elective caesarean section is associated with a reduction in developmental dysplasia of the hip in term breech infants, *J Bone Joint Surg* 87B(7):984–985, 2005.

Mahan ST, Kassler JR: Does swaddling influence developmental dysplasia of the hip? *Pediatrics* 121(1):177–178, 2008.

McCarthy J, Scoles P, MacEwen G: Developmental dysplasia of the hip (DDH), *Curr Orthop* 19:223–230, 2005.

NMC (Nursing and Midwifery Council): *Midwives rules and standards*, London, 2004, NMC.

Storer SK, Skaggs DL: Developmental dysplasia of the hip, *Am Fam Physician* 74(8):1310–1316, 2006.

Principles of infant nutrition: breastfeeding

41

There can be no doubt as to the suitability of human milk for human infants. However, the 2005 Infant Feeding Survey (Bolling et al 2007) suggested that only 21% of babies were being exclusively breastfed at 6 weeks of age in the UK. Colson (2005a) questions the advice and care given to breastfeeding women over the last few decades and suggests that the relationship of particular maternal/child positions stimulate innate breastfeeding behaviours and so significantly aid the initiation of breastfeeding (Colson 2007b). Colson (2007b) terms this new approach to breastfeeding initiation as biological nurturing. This will be reviewed in this chapter as well as the traditional approach to breastfeeding practice. Also discussed are basic breast anatomy,

feeding cues and patterns, assessing for effective feeding and problem solving. The chapter ends by discussing the safe expressing and storage of breast milk.

LEARNING OUTCOMES

Having read this chapter the reader should be able to:

- briefly describe the anatomy of the breast and the physiology of lactation
- describe how to facilitate correct attachment at the breast using: (1) the traditional approach; and (2) the concept of biological nurturing
- compare and contrast the traditional and biological nurturing practices
- discuss the recognition and significance of feeding cues, feeding patterns and effective attachment
- discuss correct expressing and storage of breast milk.

Understanding lactation

Each breast functions independently. Each has a rich blood, nerve and lymphatic supply and is comprised of glandular tissue and fat. Support is provided from ligaments. The proportions of fat and glandular tissue vary for each woman, glandular tissue increases in pregnancy under hormonal influences in preparation for lactation. In some women the proportion of glandular tissue to fat is 2:1.

The glandular tissue is an extensive convoluted ductal network separated into lobes. These are subdivided into lobules; within each lobule are alveoli, each of which is a cavity lined with acini cells surrounded by myoepithelial cells. Under the influence of prolactin milk is produced in the acini cells. When the infant suckles (under the influence of oxytocin) the milk is propelled into the network of ducts by the muscular contraction of the myoepithelial cells. The lactiferous ducts branch to join other larger ducts, eventually opening out onto the surface of the nipple. Recent research (Geddes 2009) suggests that there are 4–18 ducts opening onto the nipple, the average being 9. The network of ducts has been identified much nearer to the surface of the breast than originally thought and the milk collecting areas (lactiferous sinuses) were not visualised, suggesting that milk is transported freshly through the ducts on demand.

Colostrum is present from about the sixteenth week of pregnancy but it is the loss of placental hormones that initiates the rise in oxytocin and prolactin and therefore the availability of increasing volumes of milk for the newborn infant. Colson (2007a, 2008) suggests that practice should protect and encourage the mechanisms that stimulate breastfeeding hormones in order to ensure effective transfer of nutrition from mother to child. These include prolonged cuddling and baby holding, skin-to-skin contact, privacy, feeding in biological nurturing positions (below) and maintaining the physical environment in a calm, warm, safe manner (minimal neocortical stimulation).

Milk is supplied according to demand, consequently it is the effective removal of milk from the breast according to the baby's appetite that stimulates the milk supply. The milk is thought to change during the feed (and change over time as the infant grows) so that both the hunger and thirst are satisfied.

Successful attachment at the breast

There is no doubt in any part of the literature that an incorrect attachment at the breast potentially both damages the nipples and prevents effective transfer of milk. Mohrbacher & Stock (2003) suggest that correct attachment means that the nipple extends beyond the hard palate in the mouth (and therefore does not traumatise the tissue) whilst the ducts beneath the areola are compressed to eject the milk. The baby sucks initially with quick short sucks that soon change to slow deep ones.

The mother may experience a 'toe curling' sensation initially as the nipple is drawn out, thereafter the feed should be painless (Mohrbacher & Stock 2003).

The traditional approach

Traditional practice encourages the mother to adopt an upright position, using pillows on her lap so that the baby is close to her ('tummy to mummy'), the baby's nose being level with the nipple. As the baby's mouth opens with a wide gape (and natural extension of the head), the mother brings the baby swiftly onto the breast (Fig. 41.1). The baby is then supported across the shoulders and/or back.

The biological approach

Biological nurturing first encourages the mother to adopt a comfortable, well-supported semi-recumbent position. Mother and baby are in skin-to-skin contact (or lightly dressed), the baby lies on the mother's abdomen, 'tummy *on* mummy' and is fully supported by her body contours or (depending on position) the baby's feet might be supported by the bed or pillows. The atmosphere should be relaxed and unhurried, with plenty of time for caressing and cuddling. These positional interactions release innate reflexes in the baby (Colson et al

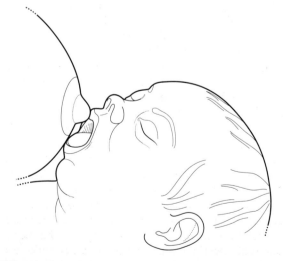

Figure 41.1 • The wide gape. Note, too, the slightly extended head, proximity of top lip/nose to nipple, position of bottom lip and direction that nipple enters the mouth

2008) (including moderately preterm and small-for-gestational-age infants; Colson et al 2003), which encourage the baby, in his or her own time, to find the breast, self-attach and effectively feed. Babies often manoeuvre themselves into the optimal position. Colson (2005b) notes that if a baby has not self-attached successfully at the breast a modification in body lie (the direction of the baby's position) can facilitate this. In her studies, babies adopted a similar lie for feeding to their in-utero position – longitudinal, transverse or oblique. Between feeds the baby may sleep in this position or in arms but Colson et al (2003) proposed that unrestricted access to the breast, including feeding whilst asleep, for at least the first 3 days of life may increase breastfeeding duration.

Summary

Although there are significant differences, it can be considered that some aspects of the two approaches – traditional and biological – complement each other. Skin-to-skin contact is practised after birth in many maternity services, whatever the method of feeding. It is recognised to aid both physiological stability (Mohrbacher & Stock 2003) and thermoregulation (Christensson et al 1992). Biological nurturing continues (and expands on) these principles into the days following, to aid the initiation of breastfeeding. Rooming in, unrestricted feeding on demand, exclusive breastfeeding and the like (WHO/UNICEF 1989, Baby Friendly Initiative (BFI) undated) are all consistent with biological nurturing (Colson 2005b). Colson (2005b) also recognises that some mothers will still need more traditional guidance but 'hands off' assistance (Inch et al 2003) to achieve correct positioning and attachment at the breast.

In both instances, as the mother gains confidence, experimentation with different positions becomes easier. Many biologically nurtured babies are able to self-attach quickly, and often without having to crawl to the breast. As a concept, Colson (2005b) notes that confidence often occurs more quickly when biologically nurturing, the mother can have the confidence that her baby and her body can work together to effectively feed her child. As well as the mutual health benefits for mother and child, there is pleasure – a commodity that Colson (2005a) suggests should be the marketing pitch for breastfeeding.

Feeding cues

A baby who has unrestricted access to the breast is able to latch as and when the reflexes are released, but for all babies feeding is better facilitated when feeding cues are recognised. As the baby's sleep begins to lighten, rapid eye movements can be seen beneath the eyelids and, with some movement of the arms and legs, this is often one of the first feeding cues. The baby might make sucking sounds, begin to 'fidget' and begin to root or suck fingers before beginning to cry. Crying is a late feeding cue; a crying baby is harder to attach to the breast and so may eventually lose interest and go back to sleep. A feed might be missed and this could be detrimental to the baby, the mother and the breastfeeding success.

Expected feeding patterns in the newborn

The bioavailability of colostrum and breast milk, combined with the size of the baby's stomach, means that breastfed babies feed frequently. The midwife does need to establish that frequent feeding is not because of a poor latch or other breastfeeding difficulty. Frequent feeding (nutritive or non-nutritive) encourages hormonal surges, an increase in milk supply, uterine contraction and the reduction of physiological jaundice. Mothers can be reassured that such patterns, particularly in the first few days, are physiologically normal; effective feeding is achieved by 8–12 feeds in 24 hours (Mohrbacher & Stock 2003). Cluster feeding is also common: the baby feeds frequently over a short time period then may not feed for 4–5 hours (Mohrbacher & Stock 2003).

Assessing effective feeding

The midwife remains responsible to ensure neonatal and maternal wellbeing whichever method of breastfeeding practice is utilised. The skills of observation and communication are necessary, with the ability to recognise deviations from the norm and to employ sensitive problem solving. If there is any doubt as to whether a baby is feeding effectively the following aspects should be considered:

- Does the latch appear and feel to be appropriate? As the baby feeds, the midwife observes the jaw rhythmically moving; sometimes the ears are seen to move at the same time. The mouth is wide, sometimes the areola can be seen above the nipple, but little (depending on size) will be seen beneath the nipple. The lower lip is curled down. Chin and breast are in close contact and feeding is quiet (gulping or clicking indicates a poor fix). The baby will suck and then pause, during which time he will remain on the breast. Sucking begins spontaneously within a few seconds, prompting is not required. Swallowing may be seen and heard. The baby will come off spontaneously when finished and should then be offered the other breast.
- Does the baby appear satisfied on completion of the feed?
- Is there adequate urine and stooling for the baby's age? (see Chapter 38 for specific detail). There should also be a less than 10% birthweight loss and appropriate weight gain (approximately 450 g per month).
- Does the mother experience the sensation of the breast being lighter and softer after feeding? Neither the breasts nor nipples should be sore or uncomfortable, the nipple should not have changed shape or appearance as the baby comes off the breast.
- Does the mother look any different when feeding? Colson (2007a) recognises the role of oxytocin in creating a particular complexion for the mother. As oxytocin surges the mother can be seen to be flushed, peaceful, relaxed and slightly disconnected from the environment. This can be discreetly observed as an indicator of effective feeding.

Problem solving

A large proportion of breastfeeding problems can be traced back to a poor attachment at the breast. Insufficient milk supply, sore or cracked nipples, mastitis and engorgement are all linked to feeding technique. If the baby is latched on correctly and permitted to demand feed, the nipples will not be traumatised, the milk will be drained properly so that engorgement and mastitis do not occur, and the supply of the milk will match the demand. Hence, these problems can be overcome with

further support and education to ensure that the technique is appropriate. For the mother who has not tried biological nurturing, the midwife can advocate this practice. Where there are ongoing breastfeeding difficulties, sitting and observing the feeding from the onset of the feed can provide valuable indicators as to how the problem can be overcome. The international Baby Café initiative (Rogers & Hickman 2008) provides both professional and peer support. Cup feeding (see Chapter 42) can sometimes be utilised to support periods of breastfeeding difficulty or after the separating of a tongue tie. All women should understand how to express and store breast milk.

Expressing breast milk

There may be occasions when it is necessary to express breast milk. These include separation from the baby, problems attaching the baby at the breast, sleepy reluctant feeders and a clinical need to increase the milk supply.

Expressing may be undertaken manually by hand or by using a hand or electric pump. Hand expression is effective and cheap.

Hand expression

Milk flow is aided by:

- The application of warmth (flannels, shower, bath) to the breasts.
- Relaxed peaceful environment in which the baby (or photograph) is near.
- Gentle massage of the breasts using the fingers of clenched fist to 'roll' down the breast towards the nipple. The nipple should then be gently rolled between the finger and thumb to stimulate the oxytocin.
- Leaning forwards and gently shaking the breasts.

To express the milk the breast is cupped in the hand with the thumb above the nipple and fingers below, approximately at the edge of the areola. Where the ducts branch significantly (often felt as pea-like structures under the skin; Brown 2005) the fingers and thumb should press backwards initially, then inward and forward, easing the milk from the ducts. The position of the hand should be moved around the breast to ensure all lactiferous ducts are emptied. A sterilised, wide-necked receptacle is needed to collect the milk in. As the flow slows (after a few minutes) expressing should be switched to the other breast. As that one slows, the first breast is then commenced again. This pattern encourages a repeated 'let down' of the milk and should be continued until both breasts are empty. Expressed breast milk can be kept at room temperature for 6 hours, between 5 and 10°C for 3 days, refrigerated at 0–4°C for 8 days or frozen at −18°C for 6 months (BFN 2009).

ROLE AND RESPONSIBILITIES OF THE MIDWIFE

These can be summarised as:

- evidence-based practice with good communication to provide information, support and encouragement to facilitate the woman's ability to successfully breastfeed
- monitoring of the health and wellbeing of the mother and child, employing problem solving strategies should the need arise
- contemporaneous record keeping.

Summary

- Traditional practice utilising an upright maternal sitting position and the teaching of positioning and attachment skills has been challenged by the concept of biological nurturing.
- Biological nurturing (Colson 2005b) encourages the mother to adopt a comfortable, semi-recumbent

position. In amongst lots of baby holding and, if appropriate, skin-to-skin contact, babies use their innate reflexes to move towards the breast and self-attach. This can happen whether the baby is awake or asleep.

- Correct attachment at the breast is vital, both to facilitate nutrition and to prevent breastfeeding problems. Midwives need to be able to facilitate this (by whichever approach the woman uses) and to utilise problem solving strategies accordingly.
- Demand feeding should be supported and encouraged. Midwives should be familiar with the ways to assess that effective feeding is taking place.

SELF-ASSESSMENT EXERCISES

The answers to the following questions may be found in the text:

1. Describe the basic anatomy and physiology of the lactating breast.
2. Discuss how this knowledge is used to promote successful breastfeeding.
3. How can the mother recognise when the baby is ready to feed?
4. Describe to a woman how to successfully attach her baby at the breast using the traditional approach.
5. Describe the features of biological nurturing.
6. Describe the markers used to assess effective breastfeeding.
7. What advice would you give to a woman who needs to hand express?

References

BFI (UNICEF Baby Friendly Initiative): undated, *The UNICEF UK Baby Friendly Initiative Information leaflet*. Online. Available: http://www.babyfriendly.org.uk.

BFN (The Breastfeeding Network): *Expressing and Storing Breast Milk*, Paisley, 2009, BFN. Online. Available: http://www.breastfeedingnetwork.org.uk, 23 June 2009.

Bolling K, Grant C, Hamlyn R, Thornton A: *Infant Feeding survey 2005*, London, 2007, The Information Centre. Online.

Available: http://www.ic.nhs.uk, 24 March 2009.

Brown SJ: Changes in breast anatomy, *Midwifery Matters* 104:13–15, 2005.

Christensson K, Siles C, Moreno L: Temperature, metabolic adaptation and crying in healthy full term newborns cared for skin-to-skin or in a cot, *Acta Paediatr* 91:488–493, 1992.

Colson S: Maternal breastfeeding positions: have we got it right? (1), *Pract Midwife* 8(11):24–27, 2005a.

Colson S: Maternal breastfeeding positions: Have we got it right? (2), *Pract Midwife* 8(11):29–32, 2005b.

Colson S: Biological Nurturing (2) The physiology of lactation revisited, *Pract Midwife* 10(10):14–19, 2007a.

Colson S: Biological Nurturing (1) A non-prescriptive recipe for breastfeeding, *Pract Midwife* 10(9):42–48, 2007b.

Colson S: Bringing nature to the fore, *Pract Midwife* 11(10):14–19, 2008.

Colson S, de Rooy L, Hawdon J: Biological nurturing increases duration of breastfeeding for a vulnerable cohort, *MIDIRS Midwifery Digest* 13(1):92–97, 2003.

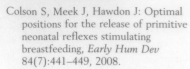
Colson S, Meek J, Hawdon J: Optimal positions for the release of primitive neonatal reflexes stimulating breastfeeding, *Early Hum Dev* 84(7):441–449, 2008.

Geddes D: Ultrasound imaging of the lactating breast: methodology and application, *Int Breastfeed J* 4(4): 2009.

Inch S, Law S, Wallace L: Hands off! The breastfeeding best start project (1), *Pract Midwife* 6(10):17–19, 2003.

Mohrbacher N, Stock J: *The breastfeeding answer book*, rev ed 3. Illinois, 2003, La Leche League International.

Rogers M, Hickman I: Organisation of a Baby Café: an innovative approach, *Pract Midwife* 11(5):40–43, 2008.

WHO/UNICEF (World Health Organization/United Nations Children's Fund): *Protecting, promoting and supporting breastfeeding: the special role of maternity services*, A joint WHO/UNICEF statement, Geneva, 1989, WHO.

Principles of infant nutrition: cup feeding

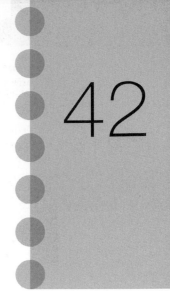

CHAPTER CONTENTS

Cup feeding is considered to be a viable alternative to using a teat for a breastfed baby, but it is important that the technique is correct. This chapter considers the indications for cup feeding, the potential dangers and the correct technique. It should be read in conjunction with Chapters 41 and 43.

LEARNING OUTCOMES

Having read this chapter the reader should be able to:

- discuss the advantages, disadvantages and indications for cup feeding
- describe the correct technique
- summarise the midwife's role and responsibilities in relation to cup feeding.

Advantages of cup feeding

The ideal way for a baby to feed is to be effectively breastfed. However, when this is not possible, for whatever reason, cup feeding provides a method of feeding that:

- promotes tongue action consistent with breast-feeding
- removes the possibility of nipple/teat confusion
- encourages initial digestion of the milk in the mouth that would not occur if fed via a nasogastric tube.

Disadvantages

Point 9 of the UNICEF 'Ten steps to successful breastfeeding' charter (WHO/UNICEF 1989) says that a breastfed baby should not have a teat or pacifier (on the understanding that developing the different muscles used with a teat makes attaching to the breast more difficult). Conversely, Flint et al (2007) concluded that at 3–6 months of age it made no difference to breastfeeding status whether a baby was fed with a cup or a teat. The Baby Friendly Initiative (2008) points out the flaws that might have skewed these conclusions and recommends that, until further evidence is available, the evidence behind the need to avoid teats and pacifiers is stronger.

It is also recognised (Thorley 2008) that term babies can become addicted to cup feeding if not put regularly to the breast; they can also lose the skills needed to breastfeed if the cup feeding technique is incorrect.

Indications

Cup feeding is recognised to have two valuable uses:

1. As an interim measure for full-term babies when breastfeeding is not yet established (e.g. birth trauma, sore nipples, use of opiates in labour, maternal infant separation, mild palate deformities). Samuel (1998) describes the way in which babies mature their sucking action and cites examples of the ways in which cup feeding aided term babies that initially lacked the skill.

2. For the preterm infant without sufficient suck/swallow coordination, who can easily tire if breast- or bottle-fed. Lang et al (1994) suggest it to be appropriate from 30 weeks' gestation. However, Freer (1999) demonstrated that preterm infants underwent greater physiological instability when cup feeding than breastfeeding and so encourages caution.

Cup feeding can be helpful in situations such as the special care baby unit, where expressed breast milk can be given in the mother's absence. Samuel (1998) notes that less is taken from a cup than a bottle; the baby's stomach is therefore not overdistended and the feeding pattern is likely to be similar to a baby-led breastfeeding pattern. The cups should be sterilised as for any other feeding equipment used for a baby (see Chapter 43).

The baby should be supported in an upright position and should lap or sip, rather than having the milk poured into his mouth. The danger of aspiration into the lungs is greater if the baby is not upright and not permitted to control the flow (Thorley 1997). The procedure should not be hurried.

Parents can be taught to cup feed easily and may gain greater confidence in relation to their subsequent feeding method, having had the opportunity to learn (Samuel 1998). Term babies often dribble, calculations of the amount taken should consider this, and parents need to be aware that this is normal.

PROCEDURE: cup feeding

- Ensure that the baby is alert and interested.
- Gather equipment:
  - ○ expressed breast milk
  - ○ sterilised cup
  - ○ bib/napkin
  - ○ baby's records.
- Wash hands.
- Sit comfortably with the baby in an upright sitting position, well swaddled (to prevent hands knocking the cup) with the bib in place.
- Place the cup (about half full, if possible) lightly on the baby's bottom lip, reaching the corners of his mouth, with the level of milk touching his lips. Begin slowly.
- Retain the cup in this position (throughout any pauses) allowing the baby to lap by bringing his tongue forwards. Avoid the temptation to pour the milk in.
- The baby will determine the pace and cease feeding when no longer hungry.
- Ensure that the feed time has been pleasurable with lots of comfort and social interaction for the baby. Return the baby to a safe environment once finished.
- Wash and sterilise the cup, wash hands.
- Complete documentation.

ROLE AND RESPONSIBILITIES OF THE MIDWIFE

These can be summarised as:

- recognising the need to use cup feeding as a valuable interim measure to support breastfeeding
- teaching a safe and correct technique
- support and encouragement of parents
- record keeping.

Summary

- Cup feeding is a valuable interim measure; it is important that the baby and the cup are both positioned correctly and that the baby laps at his own pace.

SELF-ASSESSMENT EXERCISES

The answers to the following questions may be found in the text:

1. Discuss the advantages and disadvantages of cup feeding.
2. List the circumstances when it is indicated.
3. Describe how to correctly cup feed a baby.
4. Summarise the role and responsibilities of the midwife when cup feeding.

References

Flint A, New K, Davies M: Cup feeding versus other forms of supplemental enteral feeding for newborn infants unable to fully breastfeed, *Cochrane Database Syst Rev* (2): CD005092. DOI 10.1002/14651858. CD005092.pub2, 2007.

Freer Y: A comparison of breast and cup feeding preterm infants, *J Neonatal Nurs* 5(1):16–20, 1999.

Lang S, Lawrence C, Orme R: Cup feeding: an alternative method of infant feeding, *Arch Dis Child* 71:365–369, 1994.

Samuel P: Cup feeding, *Pract Midwife* 1(12):33–35, 1998.

The Baby Friendly Initiative: *Cup feeding versus other forms of supplemental enteral feeding for newborn infants unable to fully breastfeed*, 2008. Online. Available: http://www.babyfriendly.org.uk/ newsletter/email_updates/research/ research_update_030707htm, June 2008.

Thorley V: Cup feeding: problems created by incorrect use, *J Hum Lact* 13(1):54–55, 1997.

Thorley V: *Cup feeding*, 2008. Online. Available: http://www.breastfeeding. asn.au/bfinfo/cupfeeding.html, June 2008.

WHO/UNICEF (World Health Organization/United Nations Children's Fund): *Protecting, promoting and supporting breastfeeding: the special role of maternity services*, A joint WHO/ UNICEF statement, Geneva, 1989, WHO.

Principles of infant nutrition: sterilisation of feeding equipment

43

Utmost care should be taken to protect babies against any potential sources of infection because of the immaturity of their immune system. All feeding equipment should be carefully sterilised; traces of milk can harbour and multiply bacteria quickly. The effects of gastroenteritis can be life threatening to a newborn baby and fungal infection can be difficult to treat. This chapter considers the correct use of the different sterilising techniques and the role of the midwife in relation to this.

LEARNING OUTCOMES

Having read this chapter the reader should be able to:

- describe all of the ways in which effective sterilisation can be undertaken

- discuss the role and responsibilities of the midwife.

Sterilisation advice

Ackerley (2001) indicates that the advice given regarding sterilisation of feeding equipment needs to be given to all new mothers, regardless of feeding method at that time. Formula-feeding mothers need it immediately; breastfeeding mothers may or may not need it, but might have difficulty comprehending it fully if they are emotionally distressed because breastfeeding has failed or if they are very tired. The preparation of formula feeds is one area of practice that has changed significantly in recent years; mothers with older children need sterilisation and feed preparation advice just as much as first-time mothers. Compliance with the advice is likely to be greater if the reasoning is also discussed. Mainstone (2004) argues that this advice should be a part of general home infection-control measures and so should be taught in the woman's usual domestic residence. Particular care should be taken if the woman's first language is not English.

Cleaning feeding equipment

All equipment needs to be thoroughly cleansed before being sterilised, regardless of sterilisation method. Retained milk will harbour bacteria and may survive the sterilisation process. Gilks et al (2008) reviewed the literature with regard to decontamination of feeding equipment for neonatal intensive care use. They concluded that no method of sterilisation was guaranteed to sterilise (to disinfect instead) but that this was heavily dependent on whether or not the equipment had been thoroughly cleaned first. The recommended cleaning technique (adapt according to equipment used, e.g. cup or breast pump) is as follows:

- dispose of any leftover feed immediately
- dismantle the bottle completely
- wash all parts using hot soapy water and a bottle brush, or use a dishwasher
- turn teats inside out and use the teat end of the bottle brush or a teat brush to clean all surfaces
- squeeze water through teat holes
- rinse items thoroughly under running cold water tap to remove soap (DH 2007).

Methods of sterilisation

Choices may be made according to convenience and costs, both of the initial outlay and of ongoing use. There are four different methods of sterilisation:

1. boiling
2. chemical
3. steam: microwave
4. steam: electrical.

Boiling

Boiling in the home can be a hazardous activity and therefore is often considered a short-term interim measure. Prolonged use of boiling may destroy the teats; boiling them alone for 5 minutes is acceptable. A large saucepan with a lid is required and a trivet in the base of the pan prevents the bottles from burning. It is clearly an inexact science, there is no consensus as to how long items should be boiled for, the information supplied by NHS Direct (2008) currently says 'for at least 10 minutes', whereas Ackerley (2001) suggests 20 minutes.

PROCEDURE: sterilisation by boiling

- Immerse the clean equipment fully in cold water in the saucepan, ensuring that there are no air pockets.

- Put the lid on the pan and place on the heat; bring to the boil.
- When clearly boiling, time for at least 10 minutes (NHS Direct 2008); do not add anything else to the pan.
- After 10 minutes, turn off the heat; leave undisturbed in the saucepan until required.
- Wash hands and remove items carefully when cool enough to handle, but within 12 hours.

Chemical

Various preparations – tablets, liquids and crystals – are commercially available for chemical sterilisation, usually using cold tap water. However, it should be noted that sodium hypochlorite (often the chemical used) achieves a high level of disinfection rather than sterilisation (Atkinson 2001). The dangers of not washing and rinsing the equipment thoroughly are again reiterated. Metal parts of any description must not be placed in the fluid, but should be boiled. The manufacturer's instructions should be followed carefully, particularly to ensure that the concentration achieved is correct. They generally use similar principles.

PROCEDURE: chemical sterilisation

- A large enough container should be available with a well fitting lid and floating cover.
- Have thoroughly washed hands and a clean working surface.
- Prepare the sterilising solution using the correct amounts of water and chemical to produce fluid of the correct concentration.
- Fully immerse the clean utensils, ensuring there are no trapped air bubbles; put on the cover and lid.
- Leave the container undisturbed for 30 minutes (times may vary); if anything needs to be added to or removed from the solution during this time the 30 minutes begins again from the time of addition/removal.
- Leave the container undisturbed until required.
- When the equipment is required, wash hands, remove the items carefully, handling them by the aspects that will not come into contact with the baby or milk.

- Either shake the excess off the equipment or rinse them with recently boiled, cooled water (DH 2007).
- Use them immediately.
- Change the sterilising solution every 24 hours.

Microwave

Non-metallic equipment can also be sterilised in a microwave using a specific microwave steriliser, prescribed amount of tap water and suitable feeding equipment. Models vary, and so the manufacturer's instructions should be followed carefully. It should be remembered that the timings often include standing time. The length of time that the undisturbed items are sterile for varies according to steriliser model, these would appear to be between 3 and 24 hours. Sterilising in a microwave without recommended equipment is inappropriate.

Electric steam sterilisers

Feeding equipment can be sterilised by steam using an electric steriliser. The manufacturer's instructions should be followed carefully, particularly ensuring that the correct amount of water is placed in the steriliser. The equipment does need to have complete contact with the steam and so should be loaded with open ends facing downwards. The cycle varies (3–15 minutes); the items should be used immediately. Items not required immediately should be resterilised before use (DH 2007).

Recontamination

There are many ways in which feeding equipment can be recontaminated after sterilisation. Clean hands are essential, especially after changing nappies

and toileting, food preparation and nose blowing (Ackerley 2001). The work surface should be clean and uncluttered and as the feeds are prepared it is essential that no part of the bottle or teat that has contact with the milk or baby should be touched. Sterilised tongs are useful, particularly for placing teats through the bottle top.

ROLE AND RESPONSIBILITIES OF THE MIDWIFE

These may be summarised as:

- careful education and support of the woman, with good documentation and ongoing review
- knowledge and application of best practice principles.

Summary

- The four recognised methods of sterilisation are: boiling, chemical, microwave and electrical steam. Items must be thoroughly cleaned and rinsed before sterilisation.
- It is important that the technique is undertaken correctly whichever method is chosen; babies need to be protected from potential infection.

SELF-ASSESSMENT EXERCISES

The answers to the following questions may be found in the text:

1. Discuss why sterilisation of feeding equipment is necessary.
2. Describe how to sterilise feeding equipment when boiling.
3. Demonstrate how to sterilise feeding equipment using chemical sterilisation.
4. Discuss the different methods of steam sterilisation.
5. Summarise the role and responsibilities of the midwife in relation to effective equipment sterilisation.

References

Ackerley L: Bottle feeding: how to give advice on hygiene, *Prof Care Mother Child* 11(6):152–155, 2001.

Atkinson A: Decontamination of breast milk collection kits: a change in practice, *MIDIRS Midwifery Dig* 11(3):383–385, 2001.

DH (Department of Health): *Bottle feeding*, Revised November 2007, London, 2007, Department of Health.

Gilks J, Gould D, Price E: Decontaminating breast pump collection kits for use on a neonatal unit, *MIDIRS Midwifery Dig* 18(2): 256–259, 2008.

Mainstone A: Domestic hazard analysis of infant feeding utensils, *Br J Midwifery* 12(6):368–372, 2004.

NHS Direct: *Bottle feeding*, 2008 (update 21/1/08). Online. Available; http://www.nhsdirect.nhs.uk/ articles/article.aspx?articleId=641, April 2009.

Principles of infant nutrition: formula feeding

44

When a mother chooses or is advised not to breast-feed, the midwife has an important role in facilitating infant nutrition using formula milk. This chapter considers the significance of correct feed reconstitution, potential dangers, feeding technique and the midwife's role and responsibilities. This chapter needs to be read in conjunction with Chapter 41 (breastfeeding) and Chapter 43 (sterilisation of feeding equipment).

LEARNING OUTCOMES

Having read this chapter the reader should be able to:

- discuss the principles of correct formula milk preparation and the dangers of incorrect reconstitution
- describe how to feed a baby using formula milk
- summarise the role and responsibilities of the midwife.

Formula feeding

Numerous skills are needed to achieve safe infant nutrition when using formula milk. In recent years the practice around reconstitution of the milk has changed notably, with the preparation of 24 hours worth of feeds no longer being an acceptable practice. Equally, Bean (2001) points out that in the campaign to increase breastfeeding rates, information and support for bottle feeding mothers is lost and therefore is increasing the risks for a formula-fed infant. Given that only 21% of UK babies are being exclusively breastfed at 6 weeks of age (SACN 2008) this is clearly an issue.

What are the risks?

This text does not have the scope to examine the risks in detail, but they are multifaceted. Minchin (2000) suggests that the production and manufacture of artificial milk has many unanswered questions – its composition, the role of genetically modified ingredients, the potential hazards in manufacture, to name but a few. Marchant & Rundall (2008) would agree, adding the concerns over misleading advertising claims too. The Department of Health is clear in its guidelines (DH 2007) that formula milk may contain bacteria, and even a simple literature search reveals the health dangers known of formula feeding, and the health benefits to mother and child of breastfeeding. The long-term consequences of a formula-fed nation are not yet fully realised. Added to these risks are the actual reconstitution of the milk both in the home and outside it. Parents may also not appreciate the dangers of choking, how much milk to give, frequency of feeds, etc. The Baby Friendly initiative is clear that women should make infant feeding choices based on accurate and full information of all possible options; it is incorrect to think that Baby Friendly status means that midwives cannot even talk about formula feeding.

Formula milks

Infant formula milks are generally either whey or casein dominant. Whey dominant is considered to be closer to human milk, while casein dominant may be more satisfying for the baby. Neither milk, however, is sterile or can be compared with the suitability of breast milk for the newborn baby, despite advances to add prebiotics and the like to enhance immunity. Formula milk may be ready prepared, but is generally cheaper in powdered form for reconstitution. Other types of formula are available for particular circumstances (e.g. preterm babies, milk allergy, vegetarianism, organic preference); in some instances such a milk is prescribed.

Each packet of formula milk powder is supplied with a plastic scoop that is suitable for use with that packet only. Reconstitution instructions should be followed correctly, the general rule in the UK being one level scoop of powder for each fluid ounce (28 mL) of water. The expiry date should be checked before the powder is used.

Equipment required

The following equipment is suggested:

- Infant feeding bottles with tops, covers and teats: wide-necked bottles are often easier to clean. The scale on the side should be clearly visible. Standard flow teats are acceptable (drip rate of 1 drop per second). The woman may make different choices later, according to her baby's needs.
- Sterilising equipment (see Chapter 43).
- Bottle and teat brushes (non-metallic), hot water and soap.

- Sterilisable tongs or tweezers.
- Plastic spatula or leveller if not integral in milk packet.
- A safe water supply with kettle or means of boiling water.
- Equipment for use out of the home, e.g. flask and container for milk powder (possibly a cool bag, depending on situation).

Feeding preparation

Potential hazards

Gastroenteritis in babies is reported to cost the NHS £35 million per year (MIDIRS 2003), hence one of the reasons to focus on the correct preparation of formula feeds. Dangers include:

- Unclean equipment that has been not been properly sterilised and is then recontaminated (see Chapter 43 for additional guidance).
- A reconstituted feed. This is a breeding ground for bacteria and so needs to be:
  - prepared freshly at the time of need, *not* made in advance and stored
  - prepared with fresh tap water that has been boiled only once, then left to cool for a maximum of 30 minutes: the water temperature will still be about 70 °C and so care should be taken to avoid scalding. In the event of an unsafe water supply bottled water may be used, but it should be boiled as for tap water (DH 2008)
  - cooled under cold running water to the required temperature: if feeding outside of the home pre-prepared formula is recommended, or a freshly sterilised bottle with the powder in a sterilised container and freshly boiled water in a clean flask. The milk would still need to be cooled under cold running water. If needing to take a prepared feed to somewhere specific, e.g. to a child minder, the guidance suggests taking a freshly prepared feed (that's been rapidly cooled and stored in the back of the fridge) in a cool bag with ice packs. On arrival it should be stored in a fridge and used within 4 hours (DH 2007).
- Incorrectly reconstituted feeds: this can lead to obesity, electrolyte imbalance and constipation

(excess powder) or malnutrition (insufficient powder).

- Feeding the baby with a left-over feed: unfinished feeds need to be disposed of within 2 hours of starting. The equipment needs to be washed immediately.

PROCEDURE: preparation of a formula milk feed

- Fill the kettle with the amount required of fresh cold water, put on to boil. Once boiled leave to cool for a few minutes undisturbed (maximum 30 minutes).
- Wash hands, work on a clean, uncluttered surface without distractions. Stand the sterilised feeding bottle on the work surface, leaving the top and teat in the steriliser. If using chemical sterilisation, the items may be shaken or rinsed with cooled boiled water.
- Fill the bottle to the appropriate level, this is best judged at eye level.
- Take a scoop of powder without compressing it, level it using the leveller and add to the water. Continue to add scoops of powder until the correct number has been added. Do not add anything else.
- Place the teat over the bottle handling it only at the bottom edge. Place the screw ring over and tighten, put on a sterilised bottle cover. Shake the milk gently to ensure appropriate mixing of the contents, the powder should be fully dissolved.
- Hold the bottle under cold running water until the feed is cooled to an appropriate temperature. Check it by testing a few drops on the inside of the woman's wrist. The milk should be warm, but not hot.
- Use immediately. Discard unfinished feeds straight away and thoroughly wash all equipment used in hot soapy water prior to sterilising.

Feeding technique

The principles of demand feeding should be upheld: the baby will feed when hungry, taking as much or as little as desired. Babies fed with formula milk often have a regular feeding pattern, approximately 4 hourly, but this may vary. Feed times should be enjoyable and relaxed, when either parent can feed.

The baby should be held securely, close to his parent, in a similar position to breastfeeding, so that eye contact can be maintained.

The teat needs to be over the baby's tongue and the bottle tipped up far enough for air to be excluded from the teat. The teat should administer regular drops, rather than a stream of milk (Ellis & Kanneh 2000). The baby will suck and pause, retaining the teat in his mouth. A bib may catch any of the dribbles. The baby may be winded once or twice during the feed, often by just sitting the baby upright. Rubbing or patting of the back may assist winding. Occasionally, a small amount of milk is regurgitated with wind; this is a normal process. A baby should never be left to 'prop' feed alone; the danger of choking is enormous.

The baby will cease feeding when he has had sufficient milk. The midwife should record the amount of feed taken, the total amount over a 24-hour period acting as an indicator of sufficient nutrition. The baby should be settled between feeds, gain weight and pass urine and stools normally (see Chapter 38). The stool may be firmer and slightly more offensive than that of a breastfed baby. Increasing the amount of feed is necessary when the baby is draining the full amount in the bottle. An additional ounce is reconstituted.

ROLE AND RESPONSIBILITIES OF THE MIDWIFE

These can be summarised as:

- knowledge and application of best practice advice with regard to formula milks, their reconstitution and storage
- education and support of parents to ensure safe infant nutrition and feeding technique
- recognition of a healthy formula-fed infant
- contemporaneous record keeping.

Summary

- It is important that formula milk is reconstituted and cooled correctly before feeding the baby.
- The dangers of contamination are high; sterilised feeding equipment, a safe water supply and a careful reconstitution technique must all be used.
- The midwife has an important role in facilitating parents to develop a safe feeding technique, and in recognising a healthy formula-fed baby.

SELF-ASSESSMENT EXERCISES

The answers to the following questions may be found in the text:

1. Describe how to assist parents to safely feed a baby using formula milk.
2. Describe how a feed is correctly reconstituted.
3. Discuss the possible dangers of incorrect reconstitution?
4. How would you advise a mother to prepare a formula feed when away from home?
5. Summarise the midwife's role and responsibilities when caring for a woman and baby when the baby is being fed with formula milk.

References

Bean N: Is breast always best? *Pract Midwife* 4(11):34–36, 2001.

Department of Health: *Bottle feeding*, Revised November 2007, London, 2007, Department of Health.

Ellis M, Kanneh A: Infant nutrition: part two, *Paediatr Nurs* 12(1):38–43, 2000.

Marchant S, Rundall P: Safe and appropriate infant nutrition: why does it matter? *MIDIRS Midwifery Dig* 18(4):566–570, 2008.

MIDIRS: *Breast or bottle feeding. Informed choice leaflet (7) for professionals*, ed 3, Bristol, 2003, MIDIRS.

Minchin M: Artificial feeding and risk, *Pract Midwife* 3(3):18–20, 2000.

SACN (Scientific Advisory Committee on Nutrition): *Infant Feeding Survey 2005: A commentary on infant feeding practices in the UK*, London, 2008, TSO.

Principles of infant nutrition: nasogastric feeding

45

CHAPTER CONTENTS

Nasogastric tubes (NGTs) may be used in both adults and babies. An NGT is, as the name suggests, a tube that passes through the nose (or mouth (oro-gastric)), into the oesophagus and through into the stomach. They have two main uses:

1. placing food or medication into the stomach
2. removing substances from the stomach.

This chapter considers, for a baby, nasogastric tube insertion, correct tube positioning, feeding technique and tube removal.

LEARNING OUTCOMES

Having read this chapter the reader should be able to:

- highlight the potential risks of naso- and orogastric feeding tubes

- detail the steps that are taken to ensure that the tube is correctly placed
- describe how one is inserted and removed safely
- describe how a baby is fed using a nasogastric tube
- summarise the role and responsibilities of the midwife.

Considerations

Feeding via a nasogastric tube is the most unnatural method of feeding. An important part of digestion begins in the mouth, this is missed when using a tube. Jones & Spencer (1999) also note that signifi-cant fat globules can adhere to the inside of the tube and so render lesser nutrition than is expected. In 2005, the National Patient Safety Agency (NPSA) also issued an alert to the fact that deaths had occurred because of the misplacement of nasogas-tric tubes. Inadvertently placing a tube into the lungs can cause death, either in the short term or from aspiration pneumonia in the longer term. Babies with nasogastric tubes also have an increased risk of vomiting and gastric reflux, issues that also make feeding less pleasurable. Consequently, naso-gastric tubes are used for feeding only when neces-sary. The midwife is most likely to see their use in special care baby units or babies under transitional care; the midwife also has a role in educating and supporting parents who need to undertake nasogas-tric feeds in the home.

The use of nasogastric tubes in adults in mater-nity settings tends to relate to the need to empty the stomach. Occasionally if a general anaesthetic is needed in an emergency a nasogastric tube may be used to empty the stomach to reduce the risk of silent inhalation on intubation. Women who are 'nil by mouth' with a complication (e.g. paralytic ileus) may need continuous drainage of the stomach using a nasogastric tube. Inserting a tube into an adult is very similar except that the woman (if permitted) assists by taking sips of water so that as she swallows the tube is advanced into her stomach.

Safety

The NPSA (2005) revised the guidelines for all age groups with regard to ensuring the tube is in the correct place. Tubes may migrate to the oesophagus, duodenum or lungs, or become coiled or kinked within the oral cavity. Several previously advocated methods are no longer valid. The following methods *should not be used* to assess an NG tube position:

- Auscultation (listening over the stomach with a stethoscope as air is inserted down the tube): sounds may be heard even if the tube is in the lungs.
- Placing the end of the tube in water and watching for bubbles: air may come from both the stomach and lungs.
- Blue litmus paper: its sensitivity to detect between pH variations of gastric and bronchial secretions is insufficient.
- The baby's condition: respiratory distress is not necessarily seen if the tube is in the lungs.
- The presence of aspirate in the tube: this may be still there from the last feed; it is also difficult to assess visually the differences between gastric and bronchial aspirate.
- Presence of securing tape in the same place: a tube can migrate without causing changes to the tape; the tube may also not have been placed correctly on insertion.

The NPSA (2005) has issued specific guidance for the use of naso- and orogastric tubes in neonates:

- The position of the tube should be checked on insertion, before administering any feed or medication, following any episodes of vomiting, retching or coughing or if there is any visible indication that the tube may have moved, e.g. loose tape, change in length of visible tube. All tubes should have markings and be marked on insertion. If continuous feeds are happening, tube checking should be undertaken 15–30 minutes after the end of the feed, before the next one is commenced.

- It should be assessed using aspirate withdrawn from the stomach using pH indicator strips or paper. Only one sort of paper should be available, not different types or from different manufacturers. It should be stored correctly and used by placing the aspirate onto the paper, not drawing the paper through the aspirate. The result should be clearly distinguishable and appear within 10–15 seconds.
- The gastric aspirate should be pH 5.5 or below. A raised gastric aspirate (above pH 6) may be found in the presence of amniotic fluid in a baby less than 48 hours old, in the presence of gastric acid reducing medications and if milk is in the baby's stomach (taking 1- or 2-hourly feeds). In the event of a raised pH senior assistance should be sought, a risk assessment undertaken and documented prior to any further action. Waiting 15–30 minutes before aspirating again, or replacing (advancing or retracting by 1–2 cm) or reinserting the tube may resolve the problem. Referral is needed if the aspirate is still greater than pH 5.5.
- It is noted that some babies may consistently have a raised pH. A multidisciplinary approach is needed in assessing their risks of not feeding with the chances of tube displacement. All decisions should be clearly documented. The NPSA (2005) flow chart illustrates the steps that are taken.
- In the event of not being able to aspirate from the tube the baby should be turned onto their left side, 1–2 mL of air may be injected using a 30 or 50 mL syringe (Wilkes-Holmes 2006) and the tube may be retracted or advanced slightly, as discussed above. These measures aim to dislodge a tube that is caught in the gastric mucosa. If aspiration is still not possible repassing the tube may be considered; care is undertaken as for a raised gastric pH (above).
- X-ray may be used to ascertain that an NG tube is correctly placed. However, this could only be if the baby was being X-rayed for other reasons and if the X-ray was being read by someone suitably qualified. It should also be noted that if deemed to be correct, it is only correct at the time of the X-ray.
- Despite careful checking Wilkes-Holmes (2006) is clear that there is no completely reliable bedside method to confirm tube position; midwives should always be alert to this.

PROCEDURE: inserting a paediatric nasogastric tube

- Gain informed consent from the parents and gather equipment:
  - sterile nasogastric or Ryles tube, size FG 6 (for a baby weighing >1.7 kg) with line markings
  - sterile 30 or 50 mL syringe
  - sterile water
  - tape
  - pH indicator paper with comparison chart
  - non-sterile gloves.
- Position the baby in a good light and a safe place, e.g. in the cot or held by an assistant; swaddle tightly so that hands are kept from the face.
- Wash hands and apply gloves.

- Without touching the skin, hold the tip near to the nose, measure the distance from the nose to the ear and then from the ear to the xiphisternum (Fig. 45.1), noting the distance markers on the tube.
- Lubricate the tip in the water, pass the tube through the smaller nostril, gently but smoothly; if resistance is felt, stop and try the other nostril, observing the condition of the baby throughout. Stop and remove the tube if there is any gasping or cyanosis.
- Once the tube has been passed through the appropriate length, hold the tube in place, attach the syringe and withdraw approximately 0.5 mL of gastric aspirate.
- Test the aspirate with the pH indicator paper; the result should be pH 5.5 or below. If the aspirate is

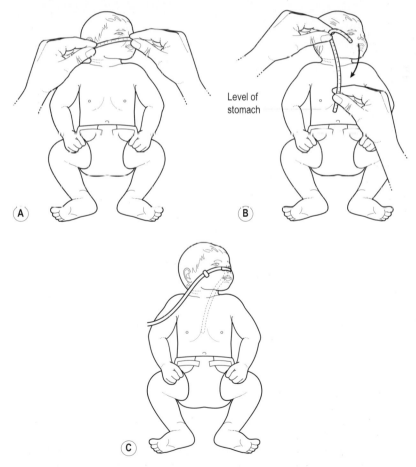

Level of stomach

Figure 45.1 • Measuring the length of the nasogastric tube prior to insertion. A Measure from nose to ear. B Then from ear to xiphisternum, noting the distance markers on the tubing (C)

hard to withdraw, the tube may have been occluded by mucus on insertion; 1–2 mL air may be injected first and then the aspirate withdrawn.

- Once the position is confirmed, remove gloves, tape the tube in place across the baby's cheek.
- Dispose of equipment correctly.
- Wash hands.
- Document and act accordingly.

Administering a tube feed

Breast or formula milk may be used. The amount may be specifically prescribed or calculated based on the baby's daily requirements according to weight, gestation and age. The feed is usually intermittent (bolus); the tube is flushed after each administration and the milk stored and prepared in a sterile way.

PROCEDURE: administering a tube feed

- Gain informed consent from the parents, wash hands and gather equipment:
  - 2 × 30 mL sterile syringes and 1 × 5 mL
  - pH indicator paper (with comparison chart)
  - milk, at room temperature
  - non-sterile gloves
  - sterile water for oral use.
- Position the baby in a good light and a safe place; the baby may be cuddled by one of his parents and interaction should take place as for any other kind of feed.
- Wash hands and apply gloves.
- Establish that there aren't any obvious signs of the tube having moved.
- Attach a syringe and withdraw 0.5–1 mL of gastric aspirate, place it onto the paper and await the result. If pH 5.5 or less, continue. If pH >5.5, follow the guidelines discussed above.
- Remove the plunger from the other syringe, attach the syringe to the tube, but occlude the tube by compressing it gently.
- Pour the required amount of milk into the syringe, holding it in an upright position.

- Release the occlusion on the tube so that the milk begins to flow into the stomach.
- Regulate the flow by occluding and pausing if it is too fast, or by raising or lowering the syringe height. The feed should be leisurely and enjoyable, as for any other feed.
- Observe the baby's condition throughout and stop the procedure if necessary, e.g. coughing, vomiting, hypoxic or bradycardic episodes.
- Follow the feed with 3 mL of sterile water drawn up using the 5 mL syringe to cleanse the tube once the feed is completed (Naysmith & Nicholson 1998).
- Close off the tube, remove gloves, dispose of the equipment and wash hands.
- Complete the records.

Removal of a nasogastric tube

Local protocols will indicate the length of time a nasogastric tube may be retained. Mears (2001) highlights the physiological distress to preterm babies when having a tube changed. She notes that a tube may be left *in situ* for 5–7 days rather than 2 days. Equally, to avoid the trauma of unnecessary reinsertion, ensure that removal is definitely indicated before removing it. Unfortunately, babies frequently remove their own nasogastric tubes unless the tube is well secured.

PROCEDURE: removal of a nasogastric tube

- Obtain informed consent; position the baby in a good light and a safe place.
- Wash hands and apply gloves.
- Remove the tape from the face.
- Pull out the tube smoothly and quickly, place into a bag for disposal (the baby may sneeze).
- Check the tube is complete, dispose of equipment correctly and wash hands.
- Complete documentation and act accordingly. Ensure that the baby feeds normally following the procedure.

ROLE AND RESPONSIBILITIES OF THE MIDWIFE

These can be summarised as:

- undertaking all the techniques safely and competently in line with current best practice
- appropriate support and education of parents
- observation of the baby during and following all procedures; referral if indicated
- contemporaneous record keeping.

Summary

- Nasogastric tubes have a role in feeding babies when oral feeding is not possible.
- The tube must be confirmed to be in the stomach on every occasion. The currently advocated method is the use of pH indicator paper, confirming a pH of 5.5 or less.
- The condition of the baby must be observed throughout. Efforts should be made to make feed times pleasurable.

SELF-ASSESSMENT EXERCISES

The answers to the following questions may be found in the text:

1. Discuss the possible risks of feeding via an NG tube.
2. Describe how to safely insert a nasogastric tube and confirm its position.
3. Describe how to undertake a milk feed using an NG tube.
4. Describe how to remove an NG tube.
5. Summarise the role and responsibilities of the midwife in relation to each of these aspects of care.

References

Jones E, Spencer A: Successful preterm breastfeeding, *Pract Midwife* 2(1):54–57, 1999.

Mears M: Changing nasogastric tubes in the sick and preterm infant: a help or hindrance? *J Neonatal Nurs* 7(6):202–206, 2001.

NPSA (National Patient Safety Agency): *How to confirm the correct position of naso and orogastric feeding tubes in babies under the care of neonatal units*, 2005, August 2005. Online. Available: http://www.npsa.nhs.uk/nrls/alerts-and-directives/alerts/feedingtubes/, 2 April 2009.

Naysmith MR, Nicholson J: Nasogastric drug administration, *Prof Nurse* 13(7):424–427, 1998.

Wilkes-Holmes C: Safe placement of nasogastric tubes in children, *Paediatr Nurs* 18(9):14–17, 2006.

Principles of phlebotomy and intravenous therapy: maternal venepuncture

46

CHAPTER CONTENTS

Venepuncture is the puncturing of a vein with a needle, usually to obtain specimens of blood for laboratory analysis, but may also include the administration of drugs intravenously in an emergency. The ability of a midwife to undertake venepuncture facilitates individualised and holistic care for the woman from the same practitioner. This chapter considers the indications for venepuncture, the rationale for correct preparation and the procedure. The role and responsibilities of the midwife are summarised.

LEARNING OUTCOMES

Having read this chapter the reader should be able to:

- discuss the indications for venepuncture
- describe how venepuncture is undertaken safely and positively

- discuss the rationale for the choice of vein and equipment used
- highlight the possible complications and how they can be avoided
- summarise the role and responsibilities of the midwife.

Indications

- Antenatal 'booking' bloods.
- Assessment of full blood count and presence of rhesus antibodies during pregnancy: further repeats if rhesus negative blood group, with Kleihauer test after delivery.
- Other tests may be taken if there is an existing disease (e.g. thyroid function tests, blood glucose monitoring, anti-epileptic drug levels) or if other conditions are suspected (e.g. sickle-cell anaemia, pre-eclampsia, thalassaemia, hepatitis B, hyperemesis gravidarum).
- Antenatal screening tests for fetal normality (e.g. alphafetoprotein).
- Cross-matching prior to blood transfusion, or group and save prior to operative delivery.

This is not an exhaustive list, but it does indicate that women are often asked to give blood specimens. Fear of needles or of fainting can be real fears; midwives should be sensitive to both the physical and psychological aspects of the skill. Care and time should be taken to gain an informed consent and measures used to improve the experience (see below) if the woman is very anxious.

Suitable sites

Blood is always taken from a vein, never an artery. Arterial blood is only ever sought by medical staff in specific circumstances (e.g. for blood gas analysis). The physiological additional blood volume during pregnancy and the general body warmth of the pregnant woman both create vasodilatation, making venepuncture easier than with many other groups of people. Being healthy, their veins are also often in a good condition. The midwife should appreciate the anatomy of the arm below the elbow. The basilic, median cubital and cephalic veins are all appropriately placed in the antecubital fossa and are suitable sites for effective venepuncture (Fig. 46.1). The skin should be free from infection, inflammation and bruising.

Choosing a vein

Clearly visible veins are often nearer to the skin surface but are often smaller and so are harder to obtain blood samples from. Both visual inspection and palpation should be used when choosing a vein. On palpation a vein can be assessed for its size, mobility and suitability. A vein that has been repeatedly used for venous access may be thrombosed and will not feel 'bouncy' and full. The veins in the antecubital fossa are often supported by subcutaneous tissue and so are less likely to roll when venepuncture is attempted. The application of a tourniquet that obstructs the venous return only (arterial pulse should still be felt) increases venous filling and so makes the choice of vein easier. Scales (2008) indicates that tourniquet use should be for a maximum of 1 minute. This means that it will be released while the other preparations are made and then reapplied once ready to puncture. The woman can also be asked to clench and unclench her fist a couple of times, but this isn't always necessary and can affect the results. Often women will know from past experience which are their 'good' veins. Palpating the vein also allows the midwife to avoid three other structures:

- valves, which are seen as 'nodules' within the vein and make specimen collection both very difficult and painful if venepuncture is attempted below the valve
- arteries, which have a palpable pulse
- nerves, which often run close to arteries.

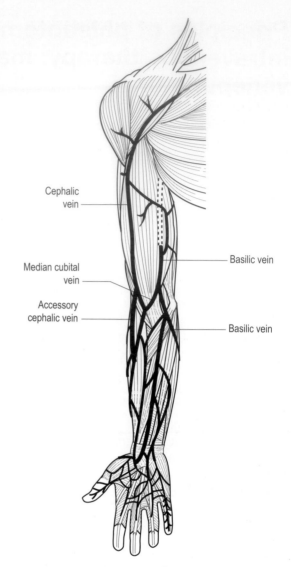

Figure 46.1 • Suitable veins for venepuncture (Adapted with kind permission from Williams 1995)

Pain relief

Many authors now advocate the 'cough' technique to decrease pain on venepuncture (Lavery & Ingham 2005). This involves asking the woman to look away and to cough, as she coughs the venepuncture is undertaken. It does require the midwife to be ready. The mechanism is unclear but success is reported. Other types of distraction may be employed and local anaesthetic creams may also be prescribed. If they are used it is necessary to wait for the required time in order for the full effect; this is 1–2 hours, depending on which one is used.

Asepsis and skin preparation

Venepuncture can introduce bacteria either locally at the site, or systemically. Asepsis should be maintained, all items being sterile, the midwife adhering to standard precaution and personal protective equipment use. Hand decontamination is important, especially between women and well fitting gloves should be worn. Non-sterile gloves are acceptable if a non-touch technique is used (see Chapter 10). Lavery & Ingram (2005) note that tourniquets can be a source of infection, disposable ones should be used. The skin should be cleansed with either a 70% alcohol-impregnated wipe or if taking blood for blood cultures, 2% chlorhexidine gluconate with 70% alcohol (Scales 2008). Cleansing using friction for at least 30 seconds (rather than swift wiping which only serves to disturb the skin bacteria) is indicated (Witt 2008). The skin should be given at least 30 seconds to air dry, this allows for the evaporation of the bacteria and a less painful puncture. The vein should not be repalpated.

Equipment

Equipment should be:

- sterile and used in such a way as to maintain asepsis (discussed above)
- ideally a closed vacuum system that also protects the midwife from contact with body fluids
- chosen according to the vein and the practitioner's competence.

Closed systems use a vacuum so that as the vein is punctured and the 'syringe'/bottle is applied to the system there is no leakage of blood. A 21-g needle should be used. Other equipment may be chosen (e.g. winged devices); the procedure is adapted according to the equipment used, midwives are advised to work within their local protocols. Syringes and needles increase the risk of contamination and needlestick injuries. Not all specimen bottles are standard in their colours and uses, local knowledge is necessary, along with knowledge regarding safe and swift transport and specimen request forms. Portable sharps boxes should be used correctly and a used needle should *never* be resheathed.

Possible complications

(adapted from Scales 2008)

- Pain: increased by poor choice of site, poor technique (hitting arteries, valves or nerves), wet skin cleanser and too large a needle. All of these complications can be avoided with a good choice of site, adequate preparation and competent technique.
- Bruising: this may be caused if the tourniquet is not released at the appropriate time, if the bleeding is not arrested and if the needle is advanced too far (puncturing the posterior wall of the vein). The application of an ice pack (after the bleeding has stopped) is indicated. Care should be taken with a woman with a known or suspected clotting disorder to ensure that haemorrhage does not occur after venepuncture.
- Accidental puncture of an artery: red oxygenated blood is seen, the needle should be removed and pressure applied for at least 5 minutes. Document the error. Avoid this with careful vein selection.

PROCEDURE: maternal venepuncture

- Gather equipment:
  - cleansed receiver
  - vacuumed system with 21-g needle (often green) or sterile alternative
  - appropriate specimen bottles
  - 70% alcohol-impregnated wipe
  - non-sterile gloves
  - antiseptic hand rub
  - sterile gauze
  - tourniquet
  - adhesive plaster (if not allergic)
  - specimen request form
  - portable sharps box.
- Gain informed consent; ensure correct specimen is being taken from correct woman. When the woman is comfortable, support her arm in an accessible position; good light is required.
- Wash hands.

- Apply the tourniquet approximately 5–7 cm above the antecubital fossa; encourage the woman to clench and unclench her fist a couple of times if necessary.
- Identify the chosen vein by palpation, retaining the site of entry in the 'mind's eye'. Release tourniquet.
- Apply hand rub and gloves.
- Cleanse the skin thoroughly (>30 seconds); wait for it to dry (>30 seconds).
- Assemble the needle/bottle/holder, reapply the tourniquet, gently unsheath the needle.
- Using the non-dominant hand, apply slight tension to the skin below the point of entry (this will anchor the vein).
- Insert the needle into the vein at a 30° angle; be decisive but not too firm.
- Fill the blood bottles according to system used.
- If blood does not appear the needle may be 'nudged' a little further in, or withdrawn a small amount (if no blood is seen, or the woman is in acute pain, remove the needle, collect new equipment and try another site).
- Release the tourniquet, withdraw the needle and immediately apply pressure (Witt 2008) to the puncture site using the gauze for the next minute (the woman should be encouraged to do this, if able). Keep arm horizontal.
- Apply plaster if required, once the bleeding has stopped.
- Dispose of sharps immediately into the sharps box, dispose of other equipment correctly.
- Remove gloves and wash hands.
- Label the specimen bottles and request form whilst with the woman; send the specimen to the laboratory. Ensure that the results are acted upon on return.
- Document and act accordingly.

ROLE AND RESPONSIBILITIES OF THE MIDWIFE

These can be summarised as:

- undertaking the procedure competently and safely
- education and support of the woman
- referral if necessary
- contemporaneous record keeping.

Summary

- Venepuncture is a skill that all midwives should be able to complete competently.
- Consider the 'cough' or other diversionary technique (see p 318).
- It is an aseptic procedure that ideally uses a closed vacuum system so that there is no contact with body fluids.
- Specimens should be in the correct bottles, labelled and dispatched, and the results acted upon accordingly.

SELF-ASSESSMENT EXERCISES

The answers to the following questions may be found in the text:

1. List the occasions when a woman may be asked to supply a blood specimen.
2. Describe how to locate a suitable vein for venepuncture.
3. Discuss the techniques that can be employed to make this a positive procedure for the woman.
4. What equipment is required to complete the technique safely?
5. Demonstrate how to undertake venepuncture correctly.
6. Discuss the possible complications that can occur, and the techniques used to reduce them.
7. Summarise the role and responsibilities of the midwife when undertaking venepuncture.

References

Lavery I, Ingram P: Venepuncture: best practice, *Nurs Stand* 19(49):55–65, 2005.

Scales K: A practical guide to venepuncture and blood sampling, *Nurs Stand* 22(29):29–36, 2008.

Williams PL, editor: *Gray's Anatomy*, ed 38, Edinburgh, 1995, Churchill Livingstone.

Witt B: Venepuncture. In Doughty L, Lister S, editors: *The Royal Marsden Hospital manual of clinical nursing procedures student edition*, ed 7, Oxford, 2008, Wiley Blackwell, pp 1055–1075.

Principles of phlebotomy and intravenous therapy: intravenous cannulation

47

CHAPTER CONTENTS

As one of the vascular access devices, peripheral intravenous cannulae (PIC) are commonly sited and utilised in midwifery care. A peripheral cannula is sited into a vein for the purposes of infusing fluids or administering medicines via the intravenous route. Performing the skill requires training, supervised practice and ongoing maintenance of the skill. Depending on local protocol, cannula insertion is often only undertaken by qualified staff. PICs feature highly in the nursing and midwifery literature partly because of the risks of localised and systemic infection from their incorrect insertion, use or removal. This chapter reviews the skills of siting and removing a PIC, along with the role and responsibilities of the midwife.

LEARNING OUTCOMES

Having read this chapter the reader should be able to:

- discuss the indications for cannulation
- describe how the site is selected and the equipment chosen
- describe a safe cannulation technique
- describe the correct removal of an intravenous cannula
- summarise the role and responsibilities of the midwife.

Considerations for the childbearing woman

The additional blood volume in pregnancy and higher body temperature usually mean that the veins are prominent and are therefore easier to gain access to. PICs should only be inserted when there is a clinical indication, and it should be removed as soon as that aspect of care is completed. Undertaking an assessment prior to insertion of a cannula aids the process and reduces the risks. This includes assessment of the woman – previous experiences, age, health, informed consent, suitable site, known allergies – as well as considerations regarding the nature of the medication to be administered and for how long (Lavery & Smith 2007).

Indications

- Fluid replacement or drug administration in an emergency.
- Administration of whole blood or blood products.
- For drugs requiring IV administration.
- In preparation for a potential complication or operative delivery, e.g. caesarean section, previous caesarean section in labour aiming for vaginal delivery, multiple or breech birth.
- Administration of patient-controlled analgesia.
- Fluid administration with epidural analgesia.

Choice of site

Correct choice of site considers:
- Structures to avoid:
  - the dominant arm
  - areas that are painful, bruised, tortuous, thrombosed, inflamed or with existing skin infection, e.g. eczema
  - areas with compromised circulation, oedema or fracture
  - joints, valves in the vein (seen as bulges), bone, ligaments, muscle, nerves or tendons
  - arteries, particularly those that run in unexpected directions.
- Try to choose:
  - a vein (identified by its lack of pulse and the ability to empty and fill by occluding and releasing it digitally)
  - a vein in good condition (often described as bouncy (Dougherty 2008a), that can be palpated in the lower half of the arm, e.g. dorsal venous network (back of the hand) and cephalic and basilic veins of the forearm (Fig. 47.1).

Preparation

Venous access is improved if the practitioner and woman are relaxed and if certain physical measures are undertaken. A tourniquet should be placed 7–8 cm above the chosen site, heat may be applied (heat pack or warm water), gravity or vein filling may be utilised (clenching/unclenching fist) and gentle tapping or stroking the vein may increase its

prominence (Dougherty 2008a). If indicated, topical analgesia may be used, but (depending on type chosen) needs 1–2 hours to be effective. A small amount of local anaesthetic such as lidocaine may be injected intradermally (see Chapter 20) at the proposed puncture site. This needs only 3–5 minutes to take effect.

Asepsis and use of standard precautions

Strict asepsis is indicated for the insertion and ongoing use of a peripheral intravenous cannula. All equipment should be sterile and for single use only, a sterile dressing pack and sterile gloves are used. Other personal protective equipment (PPE) includes the use of an apron. All sharps should be disposed of at the point of use in a portable sharps box. If continual use of a PIC is needed it should be renewed after 72–96 hours.

Skin cleansing should be undertaken using either 2% chlorhexidine or 70% alcohol (Dougherty 2008a). Gentle friction is necessary for at least 30 seconds, in a circular motion from centre to periphery. A rapid 'one wipe' of the skin merely disturbs the skin flora. The skin should then air dry for up to 1 minute, the vein should not be repalpated once the skin has been cleansed.

Choice of equipment

A cannula should be a suitable size for both the vein and the fluid that is to be infused. A large bore cannula should be used for the childbearing woman: sizes 14 or 16 gauge.

Cannulae may vary slightly according to the manufacturer, but generally consist of a polyurethane piece of tubing with a hub, into which there is a bevelled needle (stylet), also with a hub. Wings may be attached for ease of securing the cannula and there may or may not be a needleless injection port (Fig. 47.2). Once inserted a closed system is maintained. Any additional apparatus that needs connecting to the cannula should be done so aseptically and only if necessary. A transparent polyurethane dressing helps the cannula to stay in place, allows for observation of the site, permits the woman to bathe but does take skill to apply correctly (Lavery & Ingham 2006). A poorly dressed cannula increases the risks of leaking, extravasation, infection, air embolism and trauma.

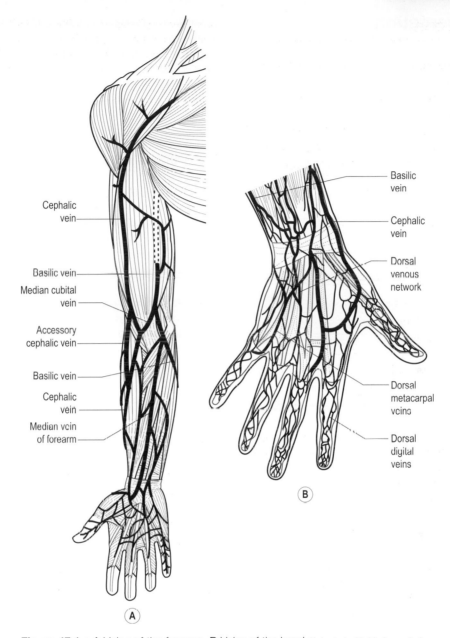

Cephalic
vein

Basilic vein

Median cubital
vein

Accessory
cephalic vein

Basilic vein

Cephalic
vein

Median vein
of forearm

Basilic
vein

Cephalic
vein

Dorsal
venous
network

Dorsal
metacarpal
veins

Dorsal
digital
veins

A

B

Figure 47.1 • A Veins of the forearm. B Veins of the hand (Adapted with kind permission from Williams 1995)

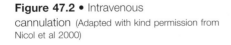

Figure 47.2 • Intravenous cannulation (Adapted with kind permission from Nicol et al 2000)

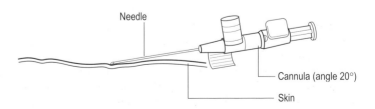

Needle

Cannula (angle 20°)

Skin

Documentation

As part of the overall strategy to reduce hospital acquired infections cannula care is subjected to standards of good practice principles, including documentation. Local arrangements may include specific forms for this (Morris & Tay 2008 have a good example), but the information should be clear in the woman's record. It should include:

- date and time of insertion (this should also be written on the dressing)
- clinical indication, cannula size and site chosen
- drugs administered including any local anaesthetic, flushing agent or bolus push
- name and signature of person siting it
- proposed plan, particularly removal time.

(Adapted from Lavery & Ingham 2006)

Ongoing care

Dougherty (2008a) is clear that a cannula should be flushed before and after use with 0.9% sodium chloride, using two techniques, pulsation and positive pressure. Pulsation involves a repeated push/pause action which disturbs any adhering substances and so lessens the infection risk (Lavery & Ingham 2006). Positive pressure requires that as the syringe is disconnected from the port pressure is maintained on the plunger so that blood does not flash into the tip. There is a less likelihood then of the cannula occluding. A cannula that is not in constant use should be flushed every 24 hours and examined at that time for any signs of possible complications.

Complications

On insertion of the PIC care should be taken to stabilize the vein by applying gentle traction to the skin. It is possible to cannulate alongside a vein rather than into it. Equally, veins can be punctured out through the back wall of the vein if the angle of insertion is too great. Pain and bruising will be experienced (Ingram & Lavery 2007). In the event of a failure to insert the cannula the circumstances may dictate whether one further attempt is made or whether a more senior colleague is called. Repeated failed attempts are distressing for the woman and reduce the number of suitable veins available.

Once inserted the midwife needs to be alert to several other possible complications:

- Phlebitis: inflammation of the vein may be caused by the presence of the cannula or its movement in the vein; by the drugs or fluids infused through it and by the presence of infection. The RCN (2007) cites Jackson's (1998) Phlebitis Scale, in which various criteria (e.g. redness, pain, swelling) are given a score. The extent to which these things are seen determines the action necessary. Infection can become systemic.
- Infiltration: if the PIC is dislodged non-vesicant (non-blistering) fluids are inadvertently administered into the surrounding tissue rather than the vein.
- Extravasation: vesicant (blistering) fluids are inadvertently administered into the surrounding tissue. Vesicant drugs can cause tissue necrosis and therefore significant morbidity (Dougherty 2008b). Examples include phenytoin, sodium bicarbonate, 50% dextrose, potassium and cefotaxime.
- Bleeding: this may be seen as haematoma formation or as obvious haemorrhage.

(Adapted from RCN 2007)

PROCEDURE: intravenous cannulation

If topical analgesia is to be used the vein would be selected, the cream applied and covered. The procedure would commence 1–2 hours later (depending on which medication was applied).

- Gain informed consent, ensure privacy.
- Wash hands, put on apron and gather equipment onto the bottom shelf of a dressings trolley (or suitable surface in the home):
  - appropriately sized (for vein and fluid) sterile cannula with needleless port
  - sterile dressing pack (tape may be needed if attempt fails)
  - semi-permeable occlusive dressing
  - cleansing solution
  - portable sharps box
  - tourniquet

- ○ sterile gloves and hand rub
- ○ 0.9% sodium chloride (with sterile needle and 10 mL syringe) for flushing
- ○ disposable sheet.
- Use hand rub, cleanse working surface with approved wipes and establish a sterile field (see Chapter 10), add the gloves, cannula and cleansing fluid.
- Position the arm so that it is supported, in a good light, with the disposable sheet beneath it.
- Apply the tourniquet approximately 7–8 cm above the intended site so that the veins can fill, but arterial flow is not obstructed; ask the woman to clench her fist a few times to encourage the veins to fill.
- Select the most likely vein by palpation; identify a marker (e.g. a freckle) to recall the intended puncture site. Release the tourniquet.
- Use hand rub and apply gloves.
- Cleanse the skin thoroughly for at least 30 seconds in a circular 'centre to periphery' action, allow it to air dry for 30–60 seconds, reapply the tourniquet.
- Immobilise the vein by supporting the skin below the insertion point, with slight tension, using the non-dominant hand.
- Insert the cannula at an angle of approximately 20°; as the vein is entered a flashback of blood is seen in the hub (this will vary according to the device used).
- Reduce the angle of insertion almost to skin level, advance the cannula slowly a few millimetres further, pause and withdraw the needle halfway; a second flashback will be seen along the cannula.
- Gradually advance the cannula into the vein, up to the hub, while simultaneously withdrawing the needle until almost withdrawn, remembering to remain at the same depth, following the direction of the vein. Release skin traction.
- Release the tourniquet, gently occlude the vein above the cannula and withdraw the needle completely. Dispose of needle into sharps box, cap off the cannula or attach the needleless port or intravenous infusion.
- Support it carefully while securing with the dressing.
- If required, blood specimens should be taken before flushing the cannula or adding the infusion line.
- Draw up the saline and flush the cannula through the port using the positive pressure and pulsation

techniques described above. An aseptic non-touch technique is maintained. Attach the infusion line if required.
- Ensure the woman is aware of ongoing care of the cannula, asking her to report any adverse effects.
- Dispose of the equipment correctly, remove gloves, apron and wash hands.
- Complete records and ensure ongoing care of the cannula and/or infusion (see Chapter 48).

Ingram & Lavery (2007) discuss the slightly alternative techniques that can be employed when siting a PIC. These depend upon the clarity of the vein and the dexterity of the midwife.

Removing a peripheral cannula

Cannula removal is much more pleasant for the woman than insertion. The midwife should ensure that it is clinically indicated before removing it. Asepsis is maintained, a sterile dressing should be applied to the puncture site following removal and observations for wound healing should be undertaken in the days following. The midwife adheres to PPE use and should wear an apron and sterile gloves.

PROCEDURE: removal of a peripheral intravenous cannula

- Gain informed consent and gather equipment:
  - ○ sterile gloves and apron
  - ○ sterile gauze and tape
  - ○ disposable sheet
  - ○ portable sharps box
  - ○ alcohol hand rub.
- Wash hands and apply apron.
- Position the arm so that it is supported, with the disposable sheet beneath it.
- Loosen the tape around the cannula.
- Open the gauze, apply hand rub and then gloves.
- Begin to withdraw the cannula from the vein; prepare to place the gauze immediately over the puncture site as the cannula is withdrawn.
- Apply continuous pressure to the puncture site for at least 1–2 minutes.
- Place the cannula into the sharps box.
- Secure the gauze with tape once satisfied that bleeding has stopped.

- Ensure the woman is comfortable.
- Dispose of remaining equipment correctly, remove gloves and apron, wash hands.
- Ask the woman to call if any signs of bleeding appear.
- Complete records.

ROLE AND RESPONSIBILITIES OF THE MIDWIFE

These can be summarised as:

- correct selection of site, use of equipment, insertion and removal of peripheral cannula
- appropriate training and maintenance of the skill
- education and support of the woman
- ongoing care and observation of the site
- correct documentation.

Summary

- Peripheral intravenous cannulation is an uncomfortable, invasive technique.
- The midwife should be appropriately trained and able to maintain the skill.

- It is an aseptic procedure, using the correct sized cannula for the vein and nature of the fluid.
- The site is chosen with care, avoiding arteries and joints but choosing the basilic or cephalic veins of the hand and forearm.
- Complications may arise both on insertion and in the following days. Vigilant care is needed to prevent them.

SELF-ASSESSMENT EXERCISES

The answers to the following questions may be found in the text:

1. Discuss the indications for cannula insertion.
2. Describe how to choose a suitable site for a PIC.
3. Discuss the type of equipment selected, with a rationale for each.
4. Describe and demonstrate how a cannula is inserted correctly.
5. Discuss the complications that may arise following cannula insertion.
6. Describe how to remove a cannula correctly.
7. Summarise the role and responsibilities of the midwife when inserting and removing a peripheral intravenous cannula.

References

Dougherty L: Peripheral cannulation, *Nurs Stand* 22(52):49–56, 2008a.

Dougherty L: IV therapy: recognizing the differences between infiltration and extravasation, *Br J Nurs* 17(14):896–901, 2008b.

Ingram P, Lavery I: Peripheral intravenous cannulation: safe insertion and removal technique, *Nurs Stand* 22(1):44–48, 2007.

Lavery I, Ingham P: Prevention of infection in peripheral intravenous devices, *Nurs Stand* 20(49):49–56, 2006.

Lavery I, Smith E: Peripheral vascular access devices: risk prevention and management, *Br J Nurs* 16 (22):1378–1383, 2007.

Morris W, Tay MH: Strategies for preventing peripheral intravenous cannula infection, *Br J Nurs*

(IV therapy supplement) 17(19):S14–S21, 2008.

Nicol M, Bavin C, Bedford-Turner S, et al: *Essential nursing skills*, ed 2, Edinburgh, 2000, Mosby.

RCN (Royal College of Nursing): *Standards for infusion therapy*, London, 2007, RCN.

Williams PL, editor: *Gray's anatomy*, ed 38, Edinburgh, 1995, Churchill Livingstone.

Principles of phlebotomy and intravenous therapy: intravenous infusion

48

CHAPTER CONTENTS

This chapter focuses on the skills involved with the setting up, monitoring and discontinuation of an intravenous infusion, including reference to the types of solution commonly used and the monitoring of fluid balance. These are skills primarily used in the hospital setting for the childbearing woman and the baby. For the woman, having an intravenous infusion in progress can be debilitating, affecting her mobility and independence. She may require assistance in caring for herself and for her baby. It can also alter her body image. There are associated risks with intravenous infusion therapy, ranging from phlebitis to death (Scales 2008).

LEARNING OUTCOMES

Having read this chapter the reader should be able to:

- discuss the indications for an intravenous infusion
- describe the different types of fluid solution commonly used for an intravenous infusion
- describe the formula for calculating the flow of an intravenous infusion
- discuss the midwife's role and responsibilities in relation to intravenous infusion therapy
- discuss how fluid balance is monitored and the significance of this.

Definition

An intravenous infusion is the introduction of sterile fluid into the blood circulation. When intravenous therapy is expected to be short term, access to the circulation is usually via the veins of the back of the hand, wrist or lower arm. If intravenous therapy is expected to be long term, lasting several days or weeks, the subclavian vein or internal jugular vein is the usual site of cannulation. The latter is rarely used in midwifery. Prior to commencing an intravenous infusion, cannulation is required (see Chapter 47). Due to the risk of infection it is important to use a non-touch technique throughout.

Indications

- Maintenance of fluid, electrolyte and nutrient balance when oral fluids or food are withheld or not tolerated, e.g. pre- and postoperatively.
- Hypovolaemia, e.g. haemorrhage, shock, dehydration.
- Administration of drugs, e.g. Syntocinon.

Equipment

Intravenous administration set

These are sterile prepacked sets consisting of a long piece of tubing with a drip chamber and trocar at the top end and a nozzle at the bottom end that connects to a cannula. Around the tubing is an adjustable roller clamp that alters the flow of fluid (Fig. 48.1); this should be positioned on the upper third of the tubing. It is important to reposition the clamp from time to time to prevent the tubing from kinking as it may then attempt to straighten out pushing the clamp open (Sarpal 2008). There are two main types used in midwifery – one for the administration of clear fluids and one for blood transfusion, the latter having a double chamber and a filter.

Burette sets or volume control devices are used when an infusion pump is unavailable, to obtain greater control over the flow rate. The drip chamber is calibrated, with a clamp above and below the chamber, and is filled with the amount of fluid to be infused during 1 hour. The flow rate is calculated according to the drop factor (varies according to manufacturer's instructions) and the amount prescribed. It will require refilling each hour. As it limits the amount of fluid transfused, it reduces the risk of the woman receiving too much fluid too quickly.

The use of a closed system of infusion will reduce the risk of infection; with each connection that is added to the infusion line, the infection risk increases (Dougherty et al 2008, NPSA 2007). For example, three-way taps used between the cannula and infusion line are difficult to keep clean and can act as a reservoir for microorganisms, which multiply in the warm, moist environment, increasing the risk of infection (Dougherty et al 2008).

Infusion pumps

A variety of infusion pumps are available that adjust the infusion flow electronically, administering a prescribed amount of fluid over a set time. The midwife should know how the infusion pump works and ensure it is properly cleaned and maintained.

Syringe pumps

Syringe pumps may also be used for the administration of drugs (e.g. insulin) and are useful when a

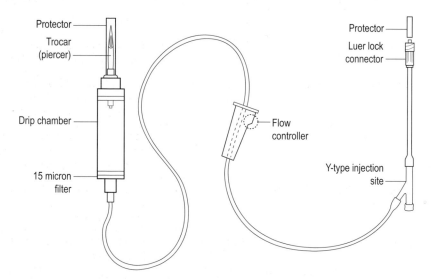

Figure 48.1 • An intravenous administration set (Adapted with kind permission from Jamieson et al 2002)

small volume of a highly concentrated drug is required (see Chapter 23).

Volumetric pumps

Volumetric pumps can accurately measure the volume of fluid to be infused; different pumps may require different administration sets.

Intravenous fluid

Intravenous fluid can be one of a variety of solutions (Table 48.1) with different types of containers used, for example, soft plastic bag, glass bottle, semi-rigid plastic (polyfusor). Glass containers have a rubber bung covered by a sterile seal that is removed and wiped with an alcohol-impregnated swab just prior to insertion of the trocar from the top end of the infusion set. To facilitate flow of the fluid, a sterile air inlet needle is inserted through the rubber bung to equalise the pressure within the bottle. Sterile scissors should be used with the semi-rigid container to cut off the end of the entry conduit. The trocar is inserted into this tube and twisted to ensure a good fit. Soft bags have an end that is twisted off or has two flaps that are

pulled apart and the trocar inserted as for the semi-rigid container. Soft and semi-rigid containers do not require venting.

Checking the infusion solution prior to administration

A doctor must prescribe the solution, which is checked by two people, one of whom should be a qualified midwife, nurse or doctor to ensure the correct infusion is given to the correct woman. The midwife should check:

- the woman's name and unit number
- the medicine administration chart – type of infusion fluid and amount to be infused, which should be accurately written up and signed
- the fluid is checked that it is the correct solution and volume and that it has not expired
- the fluid should be examined for signs of discoloration, cloudiness or sediment and the container examined for signs of contamination
- the flow rate should be calculated if an infusion pump is not available
- the batch number should be recorded on the medicine administration chart.

Table 48.1 Intravenous infusion solutions commonly used in midwifery

Solution	Example	Indication for use
Crystalloid: isotonic solutions (same tonicity as blood)	0.9% sodium chloride 5% dextrose	To compensate for fluid loss from diarrhoea and vomiting by expanding the circulating volume
Crystalloid: hypotonic solutions (lower particle concentration than plasma)	0.45% sodium chloride	To compensate for fluid loss by moving fluid into intracellular spaces Used if sodium intake restricted
Crystalloid: hypertonic solutions (higher tonicity than plasma)	20% dextrose	To compensate for fluid loss by moving fluid from intracellular to extracellular spaces Used to correct hypoglycaemia
Colloids: undissolved particles (protein, starch, sugar) too large to pass through capillary walls	5% or 25% albumin	Draws fluid from interstitial and intracellular spaces Used when crystalloid solutions are ineffective
Plasma expanders Colloid fluids	Dextran, gelofusine	To expand plasma volume by drawing fluid from interstitial spaces
Blood and blood products	Whole blood, packed cells	To maintain circulatory volume, increase particular blood components

Calculating the flow rate of the intravenous fluid

The midwife should refer to the administration set being used for details of the number of drops per millilitre, referred to as the drop factor. Commonly the drop factor is 20 for clear fluids and 15 for blood. It is important to ensure the fluid is infused over the correct period of time to prevent over- or under-infusion, both of which can have serious consequences. The following formula is used to calculate the number of drops per minute:

$$\frac{\text{Volume of solution (mL)} \times \text{number of drops/mL (drop factor)}}{\text{Required infusion time (minutes)}}$$

For example, if 500 mL Hartmann's solution is prescribed over a 4-hour period, using an administration set with a drop factor of 20, the flow rate will be:

$$\frac{500 \times 20}{240} = 41.67 = 42 \text{ drops per minute,} \\ \text{approximately}$$

Use of an infusion pump

This should be used according to the manufacturer's instructions. Generally the following formula can be used to calculate the rate (mL/hour):

$$\text{Rate (mL/hour)} = \frac{\text{Volume (mL)}}{\text{Time (hour)}}$$

For example, if an infusion pump is to be used to administer 500 mL Hartmann's solution over 4 hours, the rate should be set at:

$$\frac{500}{4} = 125 \text{ mL/hour}$$

PROCEDURE: commencing an intravenous infusion using a fluid bag

- Gain informed consent.
- Ensure a patent cannula is *in situ*.
- Gather equipment:
  - administration set
  - infusion solution
  - sterile or clean receiver
  - hand rub plus sterile or non-sterile gloves
  - infusion stand
  - infusion pump if required
  - dressing, if required; preferably a clear dressing to allow good visualisation of the cannulation site (must be sterile).
- Wash hands.
- Open the administration set and close the roller clamp below the drip chamber.
- Remove cover from the top end of the tubing and from the infusion bag, without touching either opening.
- Insert the trocar into the fluid bag.
- Suspend the fluid bag from an infusion stand.
- Gently compress the drip chamber to partially fill it.
- Remove the cover from the other end of the tubing and place over the receiver, taking care not to touch it.
- Slowly release the flow control clamp to fill the tubing with fluid.
- Remove any air bubbles by running the fluid into the receiver without touching the sides of the receiver.
- Close the roller clamp.
- Replace the cover on the end of the tubing until ready to connect to the cannula.
- Connect to infusion pump if being used.
- When required, apply hand rub and gloves, occlude the vein, remove the cover and connect the tubing to the cannula using a non-touch technique.
- Adjust the flow rate accordingly using the roller clamp.
- Apply dressing if required.
- Dispose of equipment correctly and wash hands.
- Commence a fluid balance record.
- Document and act accordingly.

Changing the administration set

Gillies et al (2005) suggest that the administration set can be changed every 96 hours as this is not associated with an increased risk of infection; however, the general consensus is that administration sets should be changed every 72 hours (Sarpal 2008,

Pratt et al 2007, RCN 2007). The exceptions to this are if a blood transfusion has been administered (change the tubing every 12 hours, McClelland 2007, RCN 2007), lipids have been administered (change the tubing every 24 hours) or the administration set has had a number of manipulations. Also, the tubing should be changed immediately if it becomes occluded or damaged, if it is disconnected from the cannula and each time the cannula is replaced (at least every 72 hours). The procedure is the same as above. It is useful to label the tubing with the date and time its use began so that it can be changed appropriately.

Changing the intravenous solution

Prior to the fluid bag emptying completely, the next solution should be checked ready for use. Speakman (1999) suggests this should be when there is less than 50 mL of fluid left to infuse. The fluid should be checked as discussed above. Before changing the solution, close the roller clamp, ensuring the drip chamber is half full. After hand washing and applying hand rub, the midwife should remove the tubing trocar from the fluid bag and insert it into the new solution. The roller clamp should be opened and the flow rate adjusted. Record keeping is completed as appropriate.

Ongoing care of the intravenous infusion

- The rate of flow should be closely observed to ensure the correct amount of fluid is being infused. The rate of flow can be influenced by the position of the arm or hand, particularly when the joint is flexed. The height of the infusion bag will also affect the rate; raising it increases the rate but it should not be more than 1.5 m above the infusion site (Sarpal 2008).
- The infusion site should be monitored at least once a day to ensure there are no complications, e.g. infection, phlebitis (RCN 2007), and the cannula is still *in situ* and patent.
- The cannula should be flushed regularly using pulsatile pressure (see p 324) at least every 24 hours or following administration of intravenous medication (Fuller 1998) with 0.9% sodium

chloride to reduce the risks of thrombus formation and colonisation from microorganisms. The syringe should be at least 10 mL to reduce the amount of pressure exerted on the vein (Lavery & Smith 2007). If the last 0.5 mL of the flushing solution is administered as the syringe is being withdrawn from the cannula port, a positive backflow of blood into the cannula is created; this is thought to prevent clotting at the site (Fuller 1998).
- The equipment should be monitored to ensure it is working properly.
- The woman should be assessed regularly to ensure there are no complications arising, including phlebitis, thrombophlebitis, infection, pain.

Monitoring fluid balance

To ensure the woman is tolerating the amount of fluid being infused a fluid balance chart should be commenced at the beginning of the infusion and maintained throughout. This is a method of measuring the amount of fluid taken into the body through the intravenous and oral routes, and comparing it with the amount of fluid lost from the body mainly in urine. Normally intake and output balance; however, if the amount of fluid taken in exceeds the amount excreted, water intoxication can result. Failure to excrete the excessive fluid load will result in rapid expansion of the body fluid compartments. Cardiac failure can ensue, characterised initially by increasing dyspnoea and peripheral oedema, unless fluid intake is restricted. A reduction in plasma osmolarity and oedematous cells can also result in convulsions and coma if the brain cells swell. If output exceeds intake, dehydration with shrinkage of cells and tissues can occur. An output of 500 mL daily is required to excrete the solutes that require elimination. Scales & Pilsworth (2008) suggest that the minimum urine output that is acceptable for someone with normal renal function is 0.5 mL/kg/hour.

A fluid balance chart is divided into two sections: intake and output. These are further divided into oral and intravenous fluids for intake. Output includes urine, vomit, diarrhoea, nasogastric drainage and loss from drains. Blood loss should also be recorded. The midwife should carefully measure the amount of fluid actually drunk by the woman and the amount of solution infused, keeping a cumulative total of the intake. All forms of fluid output should also be carefully measured and recorded, again with a cumulative total. This allows for a very quick assessment of the fluid balance status of the woman and any change such as decreasing urinary output should be notified to the doctor. It should be remembered that these charts do not take into account fluid obtained from food or insensible fluid loss. The midwife should total the intake and output at the end of a 24-hour period, document this in the appropriate records and act on the results accordingly.

Summary

- An intravenous infusion is a means of giving fluid or drugs directly into the circulation.
- It is not without risk and careful assessment of the woman is required during the procedure.
- It is debilitating for the woman who will require assistance in caring for herself and her baby.

ROLE AND RESPONSIBILITIES OF THE MIDWIFE

These can be summarised as:

- being responsible for commencing the intravenous infusion, using a non-touch technique to minimise the risk of infection
- ongoing care of the woman with an intravenous infusion, ensuring it is running correctly, replacing the infusion fluid according to the prescribed regimen, monitoring the condition of the woman for any adverse effects and assisting her with day-to-day activities
- recognising the significance of fluid balance and maintaining accurate fluid balance charts
- contemporaneous record keeping.

SELF-ASSESSMENT EXERCISES

The answers to the following questions may be found in the text:

1. What are the indications for an intravenous infusion?
2. Describe the main categories of infusion solutions used in midwifery.
3. How is an intravenous solution commenced, once cannulation has occurred?
4. What is the formula for calculating the flow rate of an intravenous infusion?
5. What are the responsibilities of the midwife during an intravenous infusion?
6. How is fluid balance recorded and why is this important?

References

Dougherty L, Farley A, Hopwood L, et al: Drug administration: general principles. In Dougherty L, Lister S, editors: *The Royal Marsden Hospital manual of clinical nursing procedures*, ed 7, Oxford, 2008, Blackwell Publishing, pp 202–253.

Fuller A: The management of peripheral IV lines, *Prof Nurse* 13(10):673, 677–678, 1998.

Gillies D, Wallen MM, Morrison AL, et al: Optimal timing for intravenous administration set replacement, *Cochrane Database Syst Rev* (4) CD003588. DOI: 10.1002/14651858.CD003588.pub2, 2005.

Jamieson EM, McCall JM, Whyte LA: *Clinical nursing practices*, ed 4, Edinburgh, 2002, Churchill Livingstone.

Lavery I, Smith E: Peripheral vascular access devices: risk prevention and management, *Br J Nurs* 16(22):1378–1382, 2007.

McClelland B: *Handbook of transfusion medicine*, ed 3, London, 2007, The Stationery Office.

NPSA (National Patient Safety Agency): *Promoting safer use of injectable medicines*, London, 2007, NPSA.

Pratt RJ, Pellowe CM, Wilson JA, et al: Epic2: National evidence-based guidelines for preventing healthcare-associated infections in NHS hospitals in England, *J Hosp Infect* 65(1) Suppl 1:S1–164, 2007.

RCN (Royal College of Nursing): *Standards for infusion therapy*, London, 2007, RCN.

Sarpal N: Drug administration: infusion devices. In Dougherty L, Lister S, editors: *The Royal Marsden Hospital manual of clinical nursing procedures*, ed 7, Oxford, 2008, Blackwell Publishing, pp 290–309.

Scales K: Intravenous therapy: a guide to good practice, *Br J Nurs* 17(19):S4–112, 2008.

Scales K, Pilsworth J: The importance of fluid balance in clinical practice, *Nurs Stand* 22(47):50–58, 2008.

Speakman E: Fluid, electrolyte and acid–base balances. In Potter PA, Perry AG, editors: *Fundamentals of nursing concepts, process and practice*, ed 4, St Louis, 1999, Mosby, pp 835–889.

Principles of phlebotomy and intravenous infusion: blood transfusion

49

CHAPTER CONTENTS

This chapter examines the safe administration of a blood transfusion for women (not babies) and the midwife's role and responsibilities. Blood grouping, the dangers of transfusion and suitable equipment are all discussed in detail.

LEARNING OUTCOMES

Having read this chapter the reader should be able to:

• define blood transfusion, listing its likely uses in the maternity care setting

• discuss why O Rhesus-negative blood is the universal donor and AB positive the universal recipient

• discuss in detail the role of the midwife when caring for a woman receiving a blood transfusion, citing the PACK mnemonic (Bradbury & Cruickshank 2000).

Definition

Whole blood or components of blood are introduced into the venous circulation, usually for the purposes of treating a clinical abnormality. Shortage of red blood cells results in hypoxia and the circulatory system needs to have sufficient blood within the vessels to sustain blood pressure, heart rate and all other circulatory functions. The Department of Health (DH 1994) recommends using whole blood quickly for the management of massive obstetric haemorrhage. Maternity units have two units of O Rhesus-negative blood available for immediate transfusion to any woman while awaiting cross-matched blood, such is the significance of blood transfusion in saving lives.

Blood transfusion can be a controversial treatment: it is the transfer of live tissue from one person to another – a transplant. Some people will refuse transfusion; Lewis (2005) includes guidelines for the management of obstetric haemorrhage in women who decline blood transfusion. Despite careful screening, there is the possibility of disease or antibody transmission and blood is an expensive treatment that varies in its availability.

Transfusion is a practice that is governed by various legal and local protocols. It is not a treatment that should be undertaken lightly or with complacency.

Each year serious errors are reported, these include deaths, serious morbidity and other 'near miss' reactions (SHOT 2007). There is a duty for UK Hospital Trusts to report transfusion incidents to the Medicines and Healthcare Products Regulatory Agency (MHRA). This should be done by the recognised person, often the transfusion practitioner; if in doubt the haematologist is the person to approach. The responsibility for safe and effective transfusion rests with the multidisciplinary team, but especially with those directly administering it (e.g. the midwife). The National Patient Safety Agency (NPSA 2006) Practice Notice (Right Patient, Right Blood) contains the competencies required by staff for taking the specimens and establishing the transfusion. It also considers other issues such as identification of the woman and how it might be improved.

Indications for maternal transfusion

Indications for transfusion include:

* hypovolaemia, e.g. after a significant haemorrhage
* low haemoglobin
* clotting disorders
* certain blood diseases.

Blood can be administered in different forms: whole blood, packed red cells (plasma removed), platelet concentration, fresh frozen plasma, white blood cells and cryoprecipitate (clotting factors). Other less common preparations are also available and other developments include the salvaging of one's own blood before a planned procedure and 'washing' and returning one's own cells in the event of an intraoperative haemorrhage (McClelland 2007). The midwife needs to keep updated on these and similar issues. The inappropriate use of blood has an effect in both human and financial terms. Where appropriate other measures (e.g. oral or intravenous iron therapy) may be utilised. The midwife has a responsibility in the provision of antenatal care, and in the management of obstetric haemorrhage emergencies to ensure that the need for a transfusion is minimised.

Blood groups

Blood groups are defined as A, B, AB or O Rhesus-negative or positive. The group is determined by the presence of an antigen on the red cell surface and an

Table 49.1 Antibodies/antigens of the blood groups

Group	Antigen	Antibody
A	A	B
B	B	A
AB	AB	None
O	None	AB

antibody in the serum. Individuals with group A, for example, have A antigens on their surface and B antibodies in the serum (Table 49.1).

An incompatible blood donation initiates the antigen–antibody reaction, causing red blood cells to agglutinate (clump together); this is a serious transfusion reaction, potentially leading to kidney failure and death. Blood group O is known as the universal donor (having no antigens for antibodies to fight), while group AB is known as the universal recipient (having no antibodies to fight foreign antigens). Eighty-five percent of the population have an additional antigen on their red cells, the Rhesus factor. If Rhesus-positive blood is introduced into a Rhesus-negative person, antibodies then form, with a haemolysing effect on the next introduction of Rhesus-positive blood. Therefore the true universal donor is O Rhesus-negative (Rh−) and the true universal recipient is AB Rhesus-positive (Rh+). It should be noted that the presence of maternal antibodies (e.g. anti-D, anti-Kell, etc.) means that cross-matching should be undertaken carefully to ensure a safe match. They can also have life-threatening consequences to the fetus and as such care must be taken to screen maternal blood before 12 weeks gestation to identify any potential problems (Anderson 2004).

Safe protocols

There are considerable dangers associated with blood transfusion (see below). SHOT (2007) indicate that many of the problems are associated with incorrect checking procedures. The British Committee for Standards in Haematology (BCSH 1999) task force has recommended national guidelines that cover all aspects of transfusion care. Bradbury and Cruickshank (2000) summarise these as PACK:

* **P**atient and pretransfusion checks
* **A**sepsis and apparatus
* **C**hecking and clerical procedures
* **K**eeping vigilant with accurate records.

Patient and pretransfusion checks

- A full history must be taken of any previous transfusions, transplants, pregnancies and current medication to identify any possible risk factors for this transfusion. Full information should be given, allowing the woman to make an informed decision for consent (where appropriate) prior to the blood being cross-matched.

- The woman must have identification attached to her (wrist band or other valid ID, e.g. photocard) that accurately shows her full name, date of birth, gender and ID number. In Wales her address is required too (Gray et al 2007).

- The initial blood sample should be taken from the woman after she has been verbally identified, as well as identified with her notes and, ideally, identity bracelet. The bottles should be filled and labelled in her presence (RCN 2006) with her full name, date of birth (DoB), gender, hospital number (ID) and signature of staff taking the sample. The request form is equally thorough, completed after the blood has been taken and dispatched with the sample immediately. Only one woman at a time should be bled (McClelland 2007).

- When ready, the blood is collected from the blood fridge within 30 minutes of commencement of transfusion (blood that has been out of the fridge for longer should be reported to the haematologist for their decision as to whether to proceed). A form is taken with the woman's identification details on it, it is checked thoroughly with the blood details. A record is made in the blood bank register of the woman's identification details, the blood donation number, date and time of removal and name and signature of person collecting it. The blood is handled carefully and transported correctly; some areas have a specific collection box. All staff that collect blood should be trained and fully aware of their responsibilities.

Asepsis and apparatus

- Strict asepsis is adhered to throughout the transfusion. Hand washing and the use of standard precautions and personal protective equipment is indicated according to local protocols.

- The midwife screens the blood visually before the transfusion, the expiry date is checked and blood with any colour changes, bubbles, leakage or clotting is not used. These may indicate bacterial contamination. The unit should be completed within 4 hours of leaving the cold storage facility. Longer than this increases the infection risk (McClelland 2007). Nothing should be added to a unit of blood. If other medication is required it is administered separately.

- A single lumen standard intravenous cannula can be used for blood unless a rapid transfusion is needed. A large bore cannula (14 g) would then be selected.

- Whilst similar to an intravenous giving set, blood transfusion sets have a double chamber that acts as a filter to debris (Fig. 49.1). The integral filter is a 170–200 micron filter. The giving set should be changed after 12 hours and on completion. It is not necessary to prime the giving set with normal saline and glucose should not be administered before or after a transfusion through the same cannula. Other blood products should be transfused through correct sterile giving sets and should not follow any other transfusion in the same giving set.

- The fragile nature of blood cells means that only a blood transfusion giving set and pump may be used, or a blood giving set where the rate is set manually. A blood administration set generally administers blood at 15 drops per mL (whereas standard intravenous administration sets are 20 drops per mL), but this should be confirmed on the packet. The infusion rate (drops per minute) is calculated accordingly:

$$\frac{\text{Amount to be transfused (mL)} \times 15 \text{ (i.e. drops in each mL)}}{\text{Hours for transfusion in minutes}}$$

e.g. if one unit of 500 mL is to transfuse over 4 hours, what is the infusion rate?

$$\frac{500 \times 15}{240}$$

Answer: 31 drops per minute approximately.

If a rapid transfusion is needed an approved rapid infusion device should be used. For transfusions of 4–6 units running 2- to 4-hourly, warming is not necessary. For rapid transfusions, exchange transfusions in neonates or administration through a central line, an approved blood warmer is used. Blood is never placed into hot water, microwaved or put on radiators.

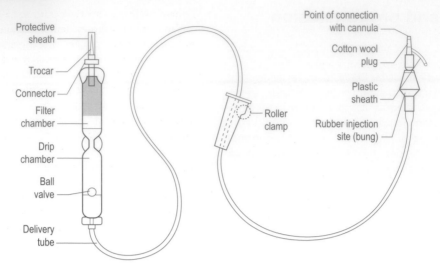

Figure 49.1 • Blood transfusion giving set; note the filter and double chambers (Adapted with kind permission from Jamieson et al 2002)

Checking and clerical procedures

Once the blood is obtained from the cold storage facility careful checking is undertaken prior to its transfusion. The medicine administration chart is scrutinized as for any other medication (see Chapter 18), noting any special requirements. Local protocols will dictate whether it is one midwife plus one other, or a midwife alone who checks the details and therefore administers the transfusion. This should be in accordance with the Nursing and Midwifery Council Guidelines Standards for Medicines Management (NMC 2008). Two practitioners are advised if the woman is unable to communicate verbally (for whatever reason):

- Checking must be meticulous: begin by asking the woman to state her full name and date of birth. Check that this information corresponds with her identity band.

- Establish that all identifiers on the blood compatibility label agree with the blood component, including the blood group and donation number and that all details relating to the woman's identity agree. Any discrepancies whatsoever should be referred to the haematologist before the transfusion is commenced. The checking should be uninterrupted and at the bedside.

Keeping vigilant with accurate records

- The dangers of blood transfusion are discussed below; the midwife must be vigilant in observing for signs and symptoms throughout. Ideally the woman is positioned where she is easily seen and transfusion at night is avoided unless absolutely necessary.

- Where applicable the woman is encouraged to notify the midwife of any unexpected reactions: anxiety, pain, breathlessness, shivering or flushing. Ensure there is a call bell to hand.

- There is little evidence as to the frequency of observations while a blood transfusion is running. However, given that serious reactions can occur within the first 10–15 minutes, it is prudent to:

  ○ undertake a full set of baseline observations *before* the transfusion commences including temperature, pulse, respiration and blood pressure

  ○ repeat these after 15 minutes, with the transfusion running slowly for that time

  ○ observe the woman carefully and to repeat the observations at any time that she may complain of any changes in how she is looking or feeling

  ○ repeat them frequently if any changes in vital signs are noted

○ complete a full set of observations on completion of the unit

○ treat each new unit in this way.

- An unconscious woman will not be able to report any changes and so additional vigilance is needed, including urine output.

- Vigilance is needed to ensure that the unit runs to time.

- Records must be thorough. Document the time commenced on the medicine administration chart along with the donation number of the unit (sometimes an adhesive label). Ensure that ongoing observations and fluid balance are maintained, and any other documentation, e.g. traceability records, are completed as per local protocol.

- Once completed the time is recorded with the observations, the next unit may be commenced or the transfusion discontinued if no further blood is needed.

- If there have not been any reactions observed the blood bag is disposed of into the clinical waste.

- Haematological screening is completed the following day, e.g. full blood count and urea and electrolytes.

Dangers of blood transfusion

- Transfusion incompatibility: signs of haemolytic reactions include fever, flushing, shivering, rigors, loin pain, headache, chest pain, tachycardia, tachypnoea, hypotension, haematuria, haemorrhage, oliguria, anxiety and possible death. Usually a rapid reaction, within a few mL of transfusion. *Action*: stop transfusion, maintain venous access with normal saline, call medical aid urgently, resuscitate the woman.

- Circulatory overload: women have an increased blood volume in pregnancy (1.5 L extra) making it easier to overload their circulatory system if they are not hypovolaemic; fluid gathers in the lungs (pulmonary oedema) resulting in dyspnoea, hypertension, tachycardia, cough and raised central venous pressure. May be seen during or after transfusion. *Action*: stop transfusion, call medical aid, administer oxygen and diuretic.

- Febrile reaction: as much as possible, white cells are removed from donated blood, but after a large transfusion women can have a significant febrile reaction. This includes hyperpyrexia,

rigors, sweating and tachycardia. Onset is often within 30–90 minutes and it can mimic a haemolytic reaction. *Action*: stop transfusion, call medical aid, exclude haemolytic reaction. If transfusion is to continue, antihistamines and steroids may be needed. A mild febrile reaction (temperature rise of up to 1.5 °C) is often seen, antipyretics may be given, care should always be taken to ensure that a 'mild' reaction is not the onset of a major reaction.

- Allergic reaction: the severest type of reaction is anaphylaxis (see Chapter 18); it can occur within 30 minutes, exhibiting rash, wheezing, shortness of breath and hypotension. *Action*: stop transfusion, call medical aid (urgently if clearly anaphylaxis), resuscitate using adrenaline (epinephrine) and steroids.

- Thrombophlebitis, air embolism, iron overload, hypothermia, excess potassium and reduced calcium are other dangers that can occur, either with or following the transfusion. For any untoward sign medical aid is called.

Slow-running transfusion

The infusion may stop if the vein goes into spasm from the cold blood. A warm compress may dilate the vein and encourage blood flow. Occlusion of the cannula may be overcome with gentle flushing using 0.9% sodium chloride. However, if time has elapsed the blood may have clotted in the tubing and a new administration set will be required.

PROCEDURE: administering a blood transfusion

This procedure applies to transfusions of 4–6 unit size. (Massive transfusions of larger numbers incur some different issues such as warming, rapid transfusion and central venous pressure (CVP) monitoring):

- Gain informed consent, collect blood from the blood fridge. A flushed cannula should already be in place. Wash hands and apply apron.

- Approach the woman with her records, the blood and all equipment needed. Confirm identity and undertake the thorough checking procedure as discussed above.

- Complete and record baseline vital sign observations (see above).

- Prime a blood administration set: close the clamp, pull back the tabs to expose the entry portal and insert the giving set. Turn the bag upside down, open the clamp, squeeze the blood through the first chamber and a third of the way through the second chamber. Close the clamp. Re-invert the bag, hang up, open the clamp and run through so that blood comes to the end of the line (Atterbury & Wilkinson 2000). Use hand rub, apply non-sterile gloves and aseptically attach the tubing to the cannula.
- Establish that the woman is comfortable and the call bell is within reach.
- Transfuse the first 50 mL over the next 10–15 minutes, observing the woman closely.
- Complete all documentation.
- After 15 minutes complete a full set of observations and adjust the flow rate.
- Observe the woman throughout and call the obstetrician if anything untoward occurs; complete observations as necessary (see above).
- Complete a full set of vital sign observations on completion of the unit.
- Commence the second unit (if prescribed) by removing the first bag and replacing it with the new one. Undertake all observations and adjustments to flow rate as for the first unit.
- When the transfusion is complete, wash hands, apply non-sterile gloves, remove the administration set (dispose of it correctly) and either commence an intravenous infusion, cap off the cannula or remove the cannula, depending on the treatment protocol. The blood bag is disposed of into the clinical waste.
- Complete records, ensuring all details of the transfusion are in the woman's notes.
- Repeat blood tests are taken the following day.

ROLE AND RESPONSIBILITIES OF THE MIDWIFE

These can be summarised as:

- undertaking the procedure competently, maintaining up-to-date knowledge in the whole procedure of blood transfusion, including the reporting of untoward incidents if necessary
- contemporaneous record keeping
- instigating referral when necessary.

Summary

- Blood transfusion is valuable in saving lives; blood should be correctly cross-matched and checked to avoid incompatible transfusions and should be stored and transfused correctly.
- There are dangers associated with blood transfusion; the midwife should maintain careful observation of the woman throughout.

SELF-ASSESSMENT EXERCISES

The answers to the following questions may be found in the text:

1. What is a blood transfusion?
2. When may a blood transfusion be necessary?
3. Which blood group and Rhesus factor is the universal donor? Why is this?
4. Describe the process that protects the woman from receiving an incompatible transfusion.
5. Describe how the midwife would recognise that haemolysis was occurring.
6. If a unit of blood containing 420 mL were to be transfused over 3 hours how many drops per minute would it flow at?
7. When does the midwife assess vital sign observations during a transfusion?

References

Anderson T: Blood transfusion: the hidden dangers, *Pract Midwife* 7(3):12–16, 2004.

Atterbury C, Wilkinson J: Blood transfusion, *Nurs Stand* 14(34): 47–52, 2000.

BCSH (British Committee for Standards in Haematology, Blood Transfusion Task Force): The administration of blood and blood components and the management of transfused patients, *Transfus Med* 9:227–238, 1999.

Bradbury M, Cruickshank JP: Blood transfusion: crucial steps in maintaining safe practice, *Br J Nurs* 9(3):134–138, 2000.

DH (Department of Health): *Report on confidential enquiries into maternal deaths in the United Kingdom 1988–1990*, London, 1994, HMSO.

Gray A, Hearnshaw K, Izatt C, et al: Safe transfusion of blood and blood components, *Nurs Stand* 21(51): 40–47, 2007.

Jamieson EM, McCall JM, Whyte LA: *Clinical nursing practices*, ed 4, Edinburgh, 2002, Churchill Livingstone.

Lewis G, editor: *The Confidential Enquiry into Maternal and Child Health (CEMACH)*, Why Mothers Die 2000–2002 Report on confidential enquiries into maternal deaths in the United Kingdom. London, 2005, RCOG Press.

McClelland DBL: *Handbook of transfusion medicine*, London, 2007, TSO.

NMC (Nursing and Midwifery Council): Standards for Medicines Management, London, 2008, NMC.

NPSA (National Patient Safety Agency): *Safer Practice Notice 14 Right Patient, Right Blood*, 2006. Online. Available: http://www.npsa.nhs.uk, February 2009.

RCN (Royal College of Nursing): *Right blood, right patient, right time*, London, 2006, RCN.

SHOT (Serious Hazards of Transfusion initiative): Annual report 2007. Online. Available: http://www.shotuk.org, 7 April 2009.

Principles of moving and handling

50

CHAPTER CONTENTS

Manual handling accidents have far-reaching implications, not only for the midwife who is unable to work in both the short and sometimes the long term and who may suffer pain and disability, but also for employers, in terms of time lost from work and large financial compensation packages paid out to employees (Barnes 2007, Cowell 1998, RCN 2004, Rinds 2007a, Smedley et al 2005, Stevens 2004, White 1998). In 1998 a nursery nurse was awarded £78 000 in compensation following a lifting injury that resulted in severe damage to her back and an inability to work for 4 years (Tolley 2000). In 2004 the Royal College of Nursing

obtained £4 million compensation for members who were injured at work (Nursing Standard 2007). Staff requiring time off from work to recover from a back injury and who experience a recurrence are likely to require longer periods of time off to recover than they needed initially (Wasiak et al 2006).

Injuries can occur through the use of incorrect lifting techniques, inappropriate lifting and moving as well as adopting poor posture for procedures such as delivery and assisting with breastfeeding. This chapter focuses on the principles of moving and handling, considering how the risk of injury can be minimised, and employers' and employees' responsibility in relation to this. Relevant anatomy of the spine is discussed and related to both lifting and posture, and how injury can occur. There is a vast amount of literature and legislation relating to manual handling which is added to regularly; hence it is not possible to cover this in detail. This chapter provides an overview of manual handling and the reader is advised to read other texts and visit the Health and Safety Executive website (www.hse.gov.uk) for further information.

LEARNING OUTCOMES

Having read this chapter the reader should be able to:

* discuss the responsibilities of both the employer and employee in reducing the risk of injury occurring when moving or handling
* describe the anatomy of the spine and related structures, relating this to the mechanics of moving and handling

- identify situations that place the midwife at increased risk from a moving and handling injury
- discuss how lifting should occur, should it be required
- describe how a good posture can be achieved.

Back injuries appear to be more common in newly qualified and very senior staff. Blue (1996) suggests this may be due to acute trauma in newly qualified staff, but could be a result of the cumulative effect of smaller traumatic episodes, combined with reduced physical fitness, for older, more senior staff. Both employers and employees have a responsibility to make every effort to reduce the risk of injury occurring. For employees this could include maintaining their own fitness levels; Blue (1996) suggests back injuries occur less frequently in people who are physically fit and undertake high-energy activities on a regular basis such as swimming and running.

Anatomy of the spine

The spine, or vertebral column, is responsible for maintaining the upright posture of the body, provides flexibility of movement and protects the spinal cord. The spine consists of 33 separate bones or vertebrae: 24 moveable and 9 fused vertebrae (Fig. 50.1):

- seven cervical vertebrae: C1–C7 (the neck)
- twelve thoracic vertebrae: T1–T12 (the upper trunk)
- five lumbar vertebrae: L1–L5 (the lower trunk)
- five fused sacral vertebrae: S1–S5 (the sacrum)
- four fused coccygeal vertebrae (the coccyx).

The vertebrae articulate with their immediate neighbours, with muscles attached, and the thoracic vertebrae meet with the ribs. The coccyx articulates with the sacrum at the sacrococcygeal joint. Each vertebra has a main body, situated anteriorly, that acts as a shock absorber as the posture changes. The size of the vertebral body varies throughout the vertebral column, beginning small with the cervical vertebrae, increasing in size to the lumbar vertebrae. Behind the body is the vertebral foramen, a large central cavity that contains the spinal cord, with nerves and blood vessels passing out through spaces between the vertebrae.

A flexible intervertebral disc connects the vertebral bodies to each other. These discs, which have a

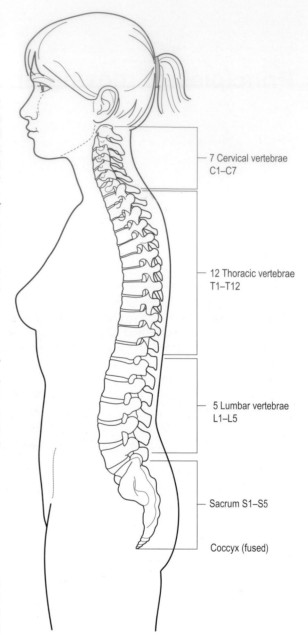

Figure 50.1 • Vertebral column-bones and curves (Adapted with kind permission from Wilson & Waugh 1996)

fibrocartilage outer layer surrounding an inner semi-solid centre, assist with absorbing shock from movement and affect the flexibility of the spine. The vertebrae and discs are supported by ligaments that help to maintain the vertebrae in position and limit the amount of stress transmitted to the spine by restricting excessive movement. The ligaments do not produce as much support for the lumbar vertebrae, creating an inherent weakness in this area. The lumbar vertebrae experience higher levels of stress when the back is bent and the knees kept straight while lifting than when keeping the back straight and the knees bent (Kroemer & Grandjean 1997). This stress increases significantly if the back is twisted, as can occur when leaning over a bed.

The vertebral column is not straight, but has four curves (see Fig. 50.1):

- cervical curve (convex curve anteriorly)
- thoracic curve (concave curve anteriorly)
- lumbar curve (convex curve anteriorly)
- sacral curve (concave curve anteriorly).

The first three curves are important in relation to posture; when they meet in a midline centre of balance, weight distribution is balanced and a healthy posture ensues, protecting the supporting structures from injury (Blue 1996).

Considerations for moving and lifting

There are four important categories that should be considered in relation to moving and lifting, as these can affect the likelihood of an injury occurring (HSE 1992):

1. the task
2. the load
3. the working environment
4. the individual.

The task

Does the task involve:

- holding an object or load away from the trunk?
- twisting or stooping?
- reaching upwards?
- using large vertical movements?
- carrying an object for a long distance?
- strenuous pushing or pulling?
- repetitive handling?
- insufficient rest or recovery?
- unpredictable movement of an object, e.g. carrying fluids?

The load

Is the load or object:

- heavy?
- bulky?
- difficult to hold?
- unstable, e.g. fluid?
- intrinsically harmful, e.g. sharp?

The working environment

Within the environment, are there:

- constraints on posture?
- poor or slippery floors?
- variations in levels?
- poor lighting conditions?

The individual

Does the job:

- require an unusual capability, e.g. in relation to weight of load?
- cause a hazard to anyone with a health problem?
- cause a hazard to anyone who is pregnant, or who has had a baby within the past 2 years?
- require special information or training?

A positive answer to any of these questions indicates that a risk assessment should be undertaken prior to any moving or lifting activities, with the aim of reducing the risk of injury as far as possible. The risk assessment involves identifying hazards and risks, which includes the potential to cause harm not only to the midwife but also the woman and the likelihood and severity of harm resulting (Rinds 2007b).

Principles of lifting

It is inevitable that some lifting will occur, mainly relating to equipment; lifting people is not usually part of the midwife's role. There are variations in the maximum weight an individual can lift. Women generally have lower lifting strength than men and an individual's physical capability is affected by age and health (HSE 1998). Lifting strength increases until a person's early twenties, with a gradual decline thereafter. The HSE (1998) suggests this becomes more significant from the mid-forties, with the risk of manual handling injury being highest 'for employees in their teens and fifties and sixties'. The maximum weight one should lift is also affected by whether the individual is standing or sitting, with the latter lifting a significantly lower weight than the former. It is also influenced by whether the elbows are bent or straight and the position of the object to be lifted – higher weights are more permissible if at waist height than if at head or feet height. Pregnancy will also affect the maximum weight a woman should attempt to lift (Tolley 2000). It is therefore important to take these factors into account when undertaking a risk assessment.

Rinds (2007b) and Stevens (2004) point out, however, that no-lift policies imposed by employers are, in several circumstances, illegal. For example, the midwife has a duty of care to manually lift an immobile woman away from danger such as fire if this is the only method of removal available, or to move the woman if she is unable to relieve pressure on her body and is at increased risk of pressure-ulcer formation (see Chapter 53). To reduce the risk of injury, the midwife needs to understand the principles involved. However, women should be encouraged to be mobile and independently move themselves rather than be reliant on midwifery staff wherever possible (Barnes 2007).

The normal adult has an imaginary 'centre of gravity' that is close to the base of the spine when standing in an upright symmetrical position. The feet form the base, and a vertical line drawn through the centre of gravity will reach the floor halfway between the feet, between the balls and heels (the baseline). This determines the person's balance and how far the position can be altered by leaning or reaching before balance is lost (Pheasant 1991). A body that experiences prolonged periods of imbalance may suffer stress and strain to the muscles of the trunk and abdomen, and – if not relieved – injury and pain (Jamieson et al 2002). Imbalance can be reduced by keeping the centre of gravity within the baseline, achieved by widening the foot stance – the feet should be shoulder distance apart. This also creates a circle of stability and moving out of this circle places the individual at risk of injury.

The vertebral column supports the weight of the head, neck, arms, hands and upper trunk. As the weight of the upper body increases so does the force placed on the spine. If an object is being carried, the spine is compressed further. The acts of walking, bending and twisting the trunk also increase the force placed on the spinal column, particularly the intervertebral discs. So, when moving an object that also requires the midwife to walk, bend or twist, considerable force is placed on the intervertebral discs. It is important that when moving whilst lifting, the feet are pointing in the direction of movement; this will also help to reduce the risk of twisting.

To minimise the risk of injury when lifting a load, the spine should be straightened, in alignment with the head (which should be raised), the knees relaxed, abdominal muscles tightened and the base widened. The load should be held as near to the body as possible (Fig. 50.2). When lifting with a rounded back, curvature of the lumbar spine results, applying asymmetrical pressure on the intervertebral discs. If continued, the pressure can result in the disc eroding, resulting in a 'slipped' disc. This is where the outer layer ruptures and the centre of the disc herniates through the gap to press on the spinal nerves or their roots. Damage to the surrounding tissues can also occur. In severe cases, the prolapsed discs can compress the spinal column.

It is also important to ensure that the object being lifted is kept as close to the body as possible by keeping the elbows tucked in close to the body and avoid reaching. The compression forces increase with both the weight of the object and the further away from the body it is held, and directly affects the amount of stress placed on the lumbar spine (Kroemer & Grandjean 1997). Movements should be smooth throughout the lifting episode.

The safe biomechanical principles used when moving people or objects, discussed above are:

- stand in a stable position
- avoid twisting
- bend the knees
- keep the elbows tucked in
- tighten the abdominal muscles
- keep the head up
- move smoothly.

Blue (1996) recommends using the entire hand when lifting as this encourages a better grip on the object and reduces the need for unnecessary movements to readjust the grip. The use of handles can also encourage a better grip on an object.

Within the maternity setting most women are mobile, with a very small minority requiring assistance with mobility, although Mander (1999) suggests immobility and impaired mobility will increase due to changes in obstetric practice (e.g. epidural

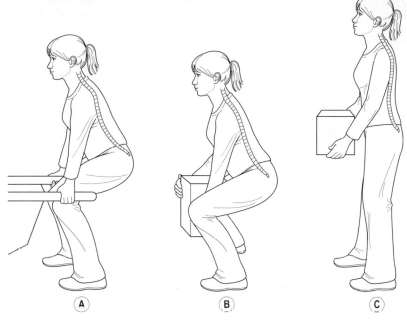

Figure 50.2 • Position of spine when lifting a load

analgesia, increasing caesarean section rates). Mobility should be encouraged as far as possible, as this not only reduces the incidence of injury to the midwife, but also promotes physical wellbeing in the mother. This can be facilitated with the use of electrical profiling beds (Rinds 2007b). Profiling beds allow for variable positioning by having sections under the mattress that raise and lower by pressing a button – thus allowing women to raise the head of their bed to bring them to a sitting position or provide a knee break to stop them sliding down the bed (Fernandes 2007).

When this is not possible, the use of appropriate moving and handling equipment is important. For women who need assistance to move up the bed, devices such as monkey poles and sliding sheets are useful. The woman should be reminded to bend her knees and flex her head towards her chest to reduce the shearing effect when lifting herself. The midwife can press against the woman's feet to prevent them slipping while she is moving up the bed. It is useful to discuss this with the woman prior to surgery whenever possible and to watch her practise moving herself up the bed following these principles. When women need to be moved from one bed to another (e.g. following caesarean section), sliding devices should be used. These are slid underneath the woman and allow her to slide

between the two surfaces with minimal effort from the midwives (Fig. 50.3). The woman can also be advised to turn on her side and push herself upright with her hand, using the elbow nearest the bed as a prop. Once sitting upright, it will be easier for the woman to get up from the bed unaided, particularly if the bed is lowered so that her feet are placed on the floor.

When a woman is being moved using a hoist, sling or sliding device, it is important to ensure her dignity is maintained and that she feels safe. The importance of maintaining communication throughout the procedure is emphasised as this will also encourage cooperation from the woman and ensure all members of the team are working together (Blood 2005, Pellatt 2005).

Therefore, when lifting or moving is unavoidable, the midwife should ensure that:

- mechanical aids are used whenever possible
- the feet are widened to maintain balance
- the back is straight to prevent unnecessary pressure on the intervertebral discs
- the knees are bent to reduce the pressure on the vertebral column
- the object being lifted is kept close to the body, grasping the object between the knees if being lifted from the floor

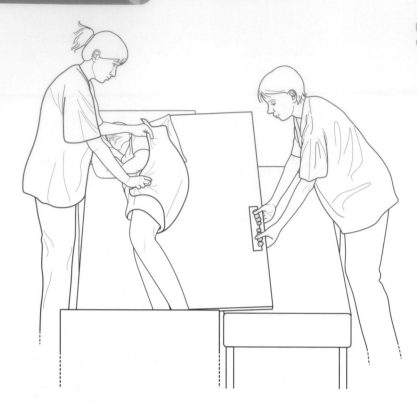

Figure 50.3 • Slide placed underneath woman

- the body is not twisted or rotated when lifting or lowering the object
- sufficient numbers of people are involved to ensure the maximum load per person is not exceeded. These people must understand the correct technique and be able to work as a team, with one member acting as the coordinator and directing the proceedings.

Correct posture

The midwife may also sustain injury through bad posture, particularly if prolonged, when strain is placed on the muscles of the back. Situations where this can occur include:

- sitting for long periods (including driving)
- supporting a labouring woman
- delivery
- perineal suturing
- assisting with breastfeeding
- making beds.

Sitting

When sitting with the back straight, the pelvis is tilted forward and the posture is maintained by the muscles, which can tire quickly. The pressure on the intervertebral discs is increased compared with a standing position. To reduce the need for muscle effort, slouching can occur. This allows the pelvis to rotate backwards and the posture and weight of the trunk are maintained more by the ligaments than the muscles. While this is effective in reducing the workload on the muscles, it doubles the force placed on the intervertebral discs, compared with the upright position (Pheasant 1991). The pressure can be reduced by using a chair with a good back rest; the pelvis rotates backwards, as for the slouched position, but the spine flexes again when it comes into contact with the back of the chair. This results in less pressure being placed on the intervertebral discs, which can be reduced further by the use of a pad in the lumbar region, possibly to a pressure that is 30–40% lower than when in a standing position (Pheasant 1991).

Stooped posture

The midwife may have a stooped posture, where the trunk is inclined forward in situations such as delivery and assisting with breastfeeding. In this situation the weight of the upper body is supported by post-vertebral muscles. Contraction of these muscles can result in the intervertebral discs becoming compressed.

Asymmetric posture

The midwife may adopt an asymmetric posture involving side bending when delivering a woman in an alternative position, particularly if she is upright or on all fours and the midwife is on the floor. This again increases the pressure on the spine and predisposes to injury. Whenever the midwife is required to adopt an unusual position, careful consideration should be given to maintaining a symmetric posture and not to maintain the position for long periods to avoid undue pressure on the muscles and ligaments.

Employers' responsibilities

The Manual Handling Operations Regulations 1992 (HSE 1992) require employers, as far as is reasonably practicable, to remove the need for employees to undertake manual handling where there is a risk of injury. Employers are required to undertake a risk assessment for any situation in which manual handling may be required. This should take place before the situation arises to give the employer sufficient time to take measures to reduce the risk of injury to employees (e.g. use of appropriate equipment). Each employer should have a safer patient handling policy (most but not all UK hospitals have a manual handling policy, Smedley et al 2005). Manual lifting should be avoided and manual handling should only occur if it does not involve lifting most or all of a person's weight (RCN 1996).

Employees' responsibility

In relation to risks at work, employees have a duty to cooperate with their employers in relation to safe manual handling and be familiar with the manual handling policy. They should inform their managers of any situations that could be considered to put them at risk of injury. They also have a responsibility to ensure they make full use of equipment provided for manual handling. Employees must know how to use the equipment properly, attending appropriate training sessions to update and maintain their knowledge and skills.

ROLE AND RESPONSIBILITIES OF THE MIDWIFE

These can be summarised as:

- being familiar with the manual handling policy and attending regular training sessions
- informing the employer of any situations in which a risk assessment should be undertaken
- using moving and handling equipment correctly
- knowing how to lift a load correctly
- being able to achieve a good posture in whichever position is undertaken
- recognising the situations in which the midwife is at risk of injury from poor posture and taking steps to reduce the risk of injury.

Summary

- Incorrect moving and handling techniques can cause serious damage to the physical health of the midwife.
- The midwife should not be involved in lifting another person, but should use appropriate equipment for this purpose.
- Incorrect or inappropriate moving and handling techniques can result in physical and psychological harm to the person being moved/handled.
- The midwife is at risk of physical injury when adopting a poor posture.

SELF-ASSESSMENT EXERCISES

The answers to the following questions may be found in the text:

1. What are the responsibilities of the midwife and the employer in relation to moving and handling?
2. Describe the anatomy of the spine and associated structures that are involved in the mechanics of moving and handling.
3. Identify five situations from clinical practice that place the midwife at increased risk from a manual handling injury and discuss how the midwife can reduce the risk.
4. When lifting a load, how can the risk of injury be reduced?
5. How can the midwife achieve a good posture and what is the significance of a poor posture?

References

Barnes AF: Moving and handling. Erasing the word 'lift' from nurses' vocabulary when handling patients, *Br J Nurs* 16(18):1144–1147, 2007.

Blood R: Safe moving and handling of individuals, *Nurs Residential Care* 7(10):439–441, 2005.

Blue CL: Preventing back injury among nurses, *Orthop Nurs* 15(6):9–19, 1996.

Cowell R: Equipment for moving and handling patients, *Prof Nurse* 14(2):123–127, 129–130, 1998.

Fernandes T: Suitable moving and handling equipment: a guide, *Int J Ther Rehabil* 14(4):187–191, 2007.

HSE (Health and Safety Executive): *Manual handling guidance on regulations; manual handling operations regulations*, London, 1992, HMSO.

HSE (Health and Safety Executive): *Manual handling. Manual handling operations regulations 1992; guidance on regulations*, Norwich, 1998, HMSO.

Jamieson EM, McCall JM, Whyte LA: *Clinical nursing practices*, ed 4, Edinburgh, 2002, Churchill Livingstone.

Kroemer KHE, Grandjean E: *Fitting the task to the human: a textbook of occupational ergonomics*, ed 5, London, 1997, Taylor and Francis.

Mander R: Manual handling and the immobile mother, *Br J Midwifery* 7(8):485–487, 1999.

Nursing Standard News: HCAs bear brunt of workplace injuries, *Nurs Stand* 22(14–16):9, 2007.

Pellatt GC: Safe handling. The safety and dignity of patients and nurses during patient handling, *Br J Nurs* 14(21):1150–1156, 2005.

Pheasant S: *Ergonomics, work and health*, Basingstoke, 1991, Macmillan.

RCN (Royal College of Nursing): *Introducing a safer handling policy*, London, 1996, RCN.

RCN (Royal College of Nursing): *Safer patient handling*, London, 2004, RCN.

Rinds G: Moving and handling: part one, *Nurs Residential Care* 9(6):260–262, 2007a.

Rinds G: Moving and handling, part two: risk management, *Nurs Residential Care* 9(7):306–309, 2007b.

Smedley J, Poole J, Waclawski E, et al: Assessing investment in manual handling risk controls: a scoring system for use in observational studies, *Occup Environ Med* 62(1):63–65, 2005.

Stevens DR: Manual handling and the lawfulness of no-lift policies, *Nurs Stand* 18(21):39–43, 2004.

Tolley: *Health and safety at work handbook 2000*, ed 13, Croydon, 2000, Tolley.

Wasiak R, Kim J, Pransky G: Work disability and costs caused by recurrence of low back pain: longer and more costly than in first episodes, *Spine* 31(2):219–225, 2006.

White C: How to prevent injury caused by moving and handling, *Nurs Times* 94(34):57–60, 1998.

Wilson KJW, Waugh A: *Ross and Wilson anatomy and physiology in health and illness*, ed 8, Edinburgh, 1996, Churchill Livingstone.

Principles of perioperative skills

51

CHAPTER CONTENTS

Caesarean section (CS) rates continue to rise within the UK with some hospitals delivering over 30% of babies by caesarean section (BirthChoiceUK 2009). Women can also attend theatre for procedures such as manual removal of placenta, perineal repair, abscess drainage and cervical suture removal. NICE (2004) lists the estimates of risks and benefits of CS, for which there are few benefits listed, and unfortunately surgery may result in fatality. The midwife has a significant role in caring safely for the woman before, during and after surgery.

This chapter considers care prior to elective and emergency surgery, intraoperative care and postoperative recovery care. It focuses largely upon caesarean section, but the principles may be applied to other types of surgery.

Care in theatre is specialised care, requiring cooperative teamwork between all the professional groups involved. The midwife may take on a number of different roles (e.g. pre- or postoperative care, theatre scrub nurse or runner, recovery care).

LEARNING OUTCOMES

Having read this chapter the reader should be able to:

- discuss thorough preoperative care prior to elective and emergency CS
- summarise the general principles of intraoperative care
- discuss recovery and post CS care
- summarise the midwife's responsibilities in each role.

Reducing rates of caesarean section

Reducing the risks of surgery is a significant aspect of care. If, however, the need for surgery itself can be reduced, this is highly advantageous. NICE

(2004) recommend an increase in homebirth, external cephalic version for a singleton breech, continuous labour support, partogram use, availability of fetal blood sampling for suspected fetal distress, induction of labour post maturity and consultation with a consultant prior to surgery.

Preparation for surgery

Delivery by CS is very different from vaginal delivery, but is still nevertheless the precious birth of someone's child. Some women may anticipate operative delivery to be useful in helping them to avoid the pain of labour and so psychologically prepare for surgery and the recovery afterwards. Other women may feel cheated of a labour experience and feel deeply distressed at being delivered by caesarean section, particularly if it is an emergency. Emergency surgery can also be a frightening experience in which the woman may fear for her life or that of her baby. Psychological care before, during and afterwards are all vital components of care (Wiklund et al 2008).

Physical preparation for elective surgery

Many of the physical complications that occur during or after surgery can be reduced or eradicated by careful preoperative preparation. The National Patient Safety Agency (NPSA) (2009) has adapted the World Health Organization (WHO) surgical safety checklist for use with all operative procedures across England and Wales (online copies are available from the NPSA).

Consultations with obstetrician and anaesthetist

Elective CS should be undertaken after 39 weeks gestation to reduce the baby's risks of respiratory disorder. Each woman should be seen by an obstetrician (see above) and anaesthetist prior to surgery. Other members of the multidisciplinary team may also be included (e.g. theatre nurse, physiotherapist). The woman's health, reason for surgery and suitability for chosen anaesthetic are all assessed (ASA 2007, AAGBI & OAA 2005). NICE (2004) recommend offering all women regional anaesthesia (spinal or epidural), the risks being less than with a general anaesthetic although Afolabi et al (2006) found no clear evidence to support regional over general anaesthesia and suggest the type of anaesthesia chosen will be dependent on whether the woman wishes to be asleep or awake for the procedure. Equally, all women should give both verbal and written consent; clearly this can only be after thorough discussions of the risks and benefits of the CS. Women who seek CS for social and not clinical reasons may be denied their request or referred for a second opinion.

A full blood count will confirm the haemoglobin level. Other haematology screening is not routinely required (NICE 2004) for healthy women with uncomplicated pregnancies but is considered on an individual basis. Usually blood is taken to be grouped and saved and if indicated (e.g. major placenta praevia) crossmatched prior to surgery. High risk CS (e.g. placenta praevia) must take place where blood transfusion services are readily available. Other investigations may be ordered as indicated (e.g. chest X-ray). The midwife will undertake an antenatal assessment and baseline vital sign observations. Allergies (e.g. to latex, antibiotics, etc.) should be carefully documented. It is helpful to discuss what is likely to happen on the day of surgery, the surgery itself, postoperative care and analgesia. Ideally this will occur prior to the elective surgery date so that the woman arrives on the day with all of the preparations completed.

Care of the gastrointestinal tract

Fasting prior to surgery is indicated so that the risk of aspiration is reduced; however, it is advisable to continue to take prescribed medication with clear fluid unless contraindicated (Crenshaw & Winslow 2006). It takes approximately 6–8 hours for the stomach to be empty from food, and 2–3 hours for fluids (ASA 2007, Scott et al 1999). However, pregnancy, labour, some drugs (e.g. pethidine) and anxiety can all delay gastric emptying; nevertheless starvation for periods of longer than 6 hours is unnecessary and distressing for the woman. Antacid therapy or H_2 antagonists are given so that the gastric acid will be less acidic and reduced in volume, respectively – the woman should have received these to take at home the night before and/or the day of surgery. An antiemetic may also be included to reduce nausea. The ASA (2007) recommend metoclopramide due to its efficacy in reducing intrapartum nausea and vomiting. An intravenous (I.V.) infusion will be sited prior to the surgery, particularly if preloading is required for regional anaesthesia to reduce the risk of hypotension (ASA 2007). Good hydration also reduces the risks of thromboembolism.

Premedication

Premedication are drugs administered prior to surgery in preparation for, or as part of, the anaesthetic. They may be prescribed in any form according to need – relaxant, antiemetic, analgesic, etc. The most likely premedication in the maternity setting are the antacid/H_2 antagonists and/or antiemetics described above. Other drugs would be administered with caution, anticipating their transfer across the placenta. It becomes important therefore that a premedication is given at the prescribed time, and that the anaesthetist is informed if for some reason the surgery is then delayed.

Skin preparation

In an attempt to reduce postoperative wound infections, preoperative skin preparation is indicated. This is discussed in Chapter 52 but remains a largely inconclusive science. The woman, as a minimal requirement, should take a shower. She will wear a gown, without any underwear, particularly noting that bras may reduce chest expansion and have metal components that may interact with other theatre equipment. She is asked not to use deodorant or talcum powder, both of which may be flammable. All make-up is removed, so that the actual colour of her nail beds and mucous membranes may be seen in order to recognise any cyanosis. Hair removal from the wound site remains controversial; shaving is technically contraindicated due to the abrasions of the skin and the likely increase of wound infection. Hair may be clipped or a depilatory cream used, but often a small number of pubic hairs are shaved immediately below the site for incision, as close to the surgery time as possible (see Chapter 52 for a fuller discussion).

Care of bladder and bowels

Constipation may be a problem postoperatively after fasting and being immobolised; it is therefore better for the bowel to be emptied preoperatively. Glycerin suppositories may be administered the evening before surgery if necessary (see Chapter 22). An indwelling catheter is used to prevent any trauma or overdistension to the bladder during surgery and is sometimes inserted prior to transfer to theatre, or at the time of surgery (see Chapter 14).

Thromboembolic prophylaxis

Death from pulmonary embolism (following deep vein thrombosis (DVT)) is a serious risk for childbearing women who have experienced surgery or any period of immobility. This is discussed in detail in Chapter 54, but correctly sized compression stockings should be applied prior to surgery, particularly for women with higher risk factors (e.g. obesity or varicose veins). Early mobilisation and a subcutaneous heparin regimen will be commenced postoperatively.

Identity and removal of prosthesis

All prostheses are removed prior to surgery (e.g. contact lenses, false limbs, dentures). Hearing aids may be retained depending on the surgeon/anaesthetist. Capped teeth are noted if general anaesthesia is to be administered due to the risk of being dislodged and inhaled. Metallic jewellery is removed, but wedding rings can be taped securely in place. Identity bands are worn; some hospitals require two identity bands for surgical cases, one on the wrist, one on the ankle. It is important to use allergy alert bands should an allergy be present.

Observations

On the day of surgery a baseline set of observations should be undertaken, to include temperature, pulse, blood pressure, respirations and auscultation of the fetal heart, reporting any deviations to the obstetric surgeon and anaesthetist.

Record keeping

The midwife will ensure that all of the physical and psychological preparation is recorded contemporaneously, including the theatre checklist.

Emergency surgery

Preparation for emergency surgery should include all of the above, but is often carried out much more quickly. Fasting, for example, is not possible.

Antacids and antiemetics are administered, and if necessary, i.e. before general anaesthetic, the stomach contents may be removed using a wide-bore nasogastric tube. I.V. sodium citrate raises the pH of gastric contents quickly without increasing the volume significantly (Farman 2004). The reader will appreciate that the speed required means that the preparation may be seen to be less thorough than for elective surgery, and therefore there are higher intraoperative and postoperative risks from emergency surgery.

Intraoperative care

The midwife's role will vary in this setting depending upon which of the roles is undertaken. Theatre care is very detailed; general principles are summarised below, but the reader is encouraged to consider other literary sources. The following general principles should be upheld in theatre:

The most important person present is the woman. Her dignity and safety should be maintained whether awake or anaesthetised. Her safety is paramount, whether that is her internal safety:

- Maintenance of her airway and respirations: with a general anaesthetic this includes using preoxygenation, a cuffed endotracheal (ET) tube, cricoid pressure (see Fig. 55.1, p 386), rapid sequence induction and mechanical ventilation. A protocol will exist should intubation fail; the anaesthetist and operating departmental practitioner (ODP) will instigate this.
- Pulse oximetry monitoring is used throughout to detect any hypoxia regardless of type of anaesthesia (see Chapter 6).
- The theatre table should have a tilt of 15° to avoid aortocaval occlusion.
- Blood pressure is monitored throughout and maintained by adjusting the fluid volume; fluid balance is essential.
- Asepsis is maintained throughout to reduce the risk of infection; I.V. antibiotics are offered routinely (cephalosporin or ampicillin) to reduce postoperative infection (NICE 2004). Costantine et al (2008) recommended this is undertaken prior to skin incision and not following cord clamping to reduce the incidence of infection (with no detrimental effect on the baby); Gould (2007) recommends antibiotics are given 30 minutes prior to the induction of anaesthesia to achieve high levels of antibiotics within the blood and tissues as this reduces the number of resident microorganisms.

- Maintenance of normothermia: recording the woman's temperature every 30 minutes during surgery, use of fluid warming devices and if required forced warm air (Patientsafetyfirst 2009).
- Known allergies should be accommodated; a latex-free trolley should be available in theatre for affected women.

Or her external safety, that is, care of the immobile or unconscious woman: safety upon the operating table, care of numb limbs and pressure areas (see Chapter 53), attention to temperature maintenance, prevention of burns from diathermy equipment, care of infusion lines, monitors, etc.

Theatre work is teamwork, for which all members of the team should be able to recognise their limitations and call in more senior or expert help if needed. The Department of Health (DH 1998) indicates that often consultant level expertise is either not called or called too late, and that sometimes the severity of the situation is not recognised by junior staff. Anaesthetists should be supported by skilled help (e.g. ODP). Communication should be good between all team members, especially if laboratory or haematology support is required (DH 1998).

Theatre is a sterile environment in which strict surgical asepsis is maintained. Scrubbed persons wear sterile gowns and gloves, all of which are applied after scrupulous hand hygiene (see Chapter 9). The rear of the gown is handled at the edges by the person fastening it, but the front remains totally sterile. Disposable drapes are used to establish a sterile field; these are only touched by a scrubbed person. All items within the sterile field should be sterile and are opened and transferred in such a way as to retain their sterility. Everyone in the theatre environment moves around in such as way as to maintain the integrity of the sterile field. The air is scavenged and – as a restricted area – only people wearing theatre clothing and footwear are permitted. External sources of potential infection (e.g. shoes) are prohibited.

Theatre should also be appropriately stocked with all necessary equipment: drugs and anaesthetic gases, anaesthetic machine, monitors, resuscitation equipment, I.V. fluids and infant resuscitaire, amongst other things.

Staff should also protect themselves, working under the protection of the health and safety legislation, use of extensive standard precautions (e.g. masks with visors, aprons, wellingtons) and moving and handling requirements. Those with close patient contact may choose to double glove.

Swabs, needles and instruments are all counted initially with the circulating midwife and the number of needles and swabs are recorded on a board where the scrub midwife can see them. Any additional items opened during the surgery are added to the information on the board. As the wound is closed swabs, needles and instruments are checked and counted; the scrub midwife uses the circulating midwife again to establish that the final count equates with the original one. This ensures that nothing has been retained inside the wound and the skin should not be closed until the final count is completed and correct. Contemporaneous records should be completed; these may include a theatre register or anaesthetic record.

CS under regional anaesthesia means that the woman will be able to appreciate fully all that's happening. She and her partner's wishes can be respected, e.g. silence may be requested so that the mother's voice is the first one heard by the baby, immediate skin-to-skin contact may be possible and early breastfeeding should not be ruled out (Coggins 2003). Equally, being awake can be a time of heightened anxiety. Care should include preparing her for the environment and the sensations (pushing and pulling, but not pain) that she may experience.

For the woman having a general anaesthetic, there is a heightened sensitivity to sound as the anaesthetic is administered. She will also require repeated and ongoing reassurance as she recovers, drifting in and out of sleep.

Specific guidance is given within the NICE guidelines (NICE 2004) as to the surgical techniques that reduce pain, haemorrhage and infection. These include issues such as transverse abdominal incision using the Joel Cohen incision (Mathai & Hofmeyr 2007): a straight skin incision undertaken 3 cm above the symphysis pubis, blunt incision of the uterus and other layers (using scissors, not a knife, to extend if required), avoiding forceps, use of I.V. oxytocin and controlled cord traction for placental delivery (Anorlu et al 2008), uterine suturing in two layers within the abdomen, non-suturing of the visceral or parietal peritoneums or

subcutaneous tissue (unless >2 cm) and avoidance of superficial or routine wound drains (Gates & Anderson 2005).

Care of the baby: resuscitation equipment and personnel should be on hand if there has been a general anaesthetic or fetal compromise. Care should be taken to label the infant and maintain body temperature.

The placenta and membranes are assessed as for any other delivery.

Cord blood is taken if the woman is Rhesus negative and an umbilical artery and venous pH is performed if there was fetal compromise.

Postoperative care

This should be completed in a recovery area where there is immediate access to oxygen, suction, resuscitation equipment, monitors, emergency call bells and appropriately skilled one-to-one staff.

After a general anaesthetic an airway is usually inserted following extubation by the anaesthetist; the woman removes this spontaneously as she regains consciousness.

Postoperative care, particularly that given during the recovery period, encompasses all of the following, whichever type of anaesthetic has been administered:

- maintenance of the airway, with or without oxygen therapy
- assessment of respirations, heart rate, blood pressure and temperature
- use of pulse oximetry for oxygen saturation with assessment of colour
- correct positioning, care of numb limbs and pressure areas
- assessment of consciousness
- assessment of levels of pain, administering analgesia as indicated, care of patient-controlled analgesia (PCA; see Chapter 23)
- care of I.V. infusion/blood transfusion and fluid balance
- care of wound (and drain if appropriate)
- observation of loss *per vaginam*
- care of urinary catheter/urinary output
- return of sensation following regional anaesthesia
- time with the baby and opportunities to feed
- administration of subcutaneous heparin at a time decided by the anaesthetist.

Observations

All vital sign observations should be completed at 5-minute intervals initially. As time passes and observations remain within normal limits the frequency of observations may be reduced to every 15 minutes, 30 minutes, etc. They should be half hourly for at least 2 hours and hourly thereafter until satisfactory (NICE 2004). After approximately 1 hour the woman should be conscious, comfortable, semi-recumbent if appropriate and able to tolerate sips of water. She will remain in the recovery area until the anaesthetist and midwife are satisfied that she may be transferred to the ward area. All of the care listed above is ongoing throughout recovery care. Record keeping is particularly important, and the midwife should have access to calling the anaesthetist and/or obstetrician at any time if any deviations from the norm are noted.

The baby

The baby is cared for accordingly, noting that babies born in theatre:

- are often cooler
- need to be fed as soon as possible
- should be labelled before leaving theatre
- are more likely to experience respiratory distress.

Other issues

Consideration is given to the partner and their needs. Birth registers, etc. are completed as for any other birth.

Ongoing care

Psychologically, there is relief and enjoyment of the new baby, but it may be tinged by pain, immobility, distress (if rapid emergency or major complications were present) and frustration that progress appears slow. In the days following the surgery the woman will appreciate sensitive and individualised midwifery care and should have the opportunity to review her care and future pregnancies with her obstetric team.

Postoperative care, while individualised, will probably include attention to hygiene and oral care, thromboembolic prophylaxis (see above), vital sign observations, pressure area care, urinary output and analgesia.

For analgesia, NICE (2004) recommend diamorphine as the initial analgesic of choice, noting that PCA offers the woman good pain relief. Non-steroidal anti-inflammatory drugs can also be given concurrently and continued after the opioids have stopped. Where diamorphine or morphine has been given intrathecally, the midwife will need to assess respirations hourly for 24 and 12 hours, respectively (NICE 2004). Opioids given epidurally or via PCA require hourly respiration rate observations throughout the treatment and for 2 hours after discontinuation. Good pain relief is essential to the woman's recovery.

Sips of water are given within the first hour of surgery. Thereafter the woman may eat or drink as she wishes (NICE 2004). Intravenous infusion is discontinued when appropriate, usually when the woman is tolerating fluids although the venflon may be left *in situ* until the woman is mobile (often the following day but it will require flushing to maintain patency; see Chapter 47). The urinary catheter is removed when appropriate and voiding encouraged (see Chapter 14); this should be at least 12 hours after the last regional analgesia. Early mobilisation is encouraged and naturally the woman will require support and care with her baby, particularly to establish breastfeeding. While this is often a motivating factor for the woman after CS, the midwife should ensure that the woman is having sufficient rest and is not over-tired.

The wound may be uncovered after showering, after 24 hours, and will be cared for as discussed in Chapter 52. Haemoglobin estimation may be completed on the third postoperative day after postnatal diuresis has occurred. The midwife should be sensitive to the woman's emotional state, noting that she has undergone two significant life experiences: having a baby and major surgery. Standard postnatal assessment is a part of each day's care in conjunction with specific postoperative needs.

Debriefing is recommended prior to leaving hospital so that women can discuss the reasons why the caesarean section took place and the implications for future childbearing (Baxter 2007, NICE 2004).

Discharge from hospital will depend upon the woman's progress and social support; it may be from 24 hours to 3–4 days. Postsurgery advice includes pain management, importance of rest and nutrition, what to do should complications arise, avoiding lifting – Gould (2007) advises the amount lifted in the first 6 weeks should be no more than the weight of a full kettle – and driving until free of discomfort, effective contraception for at least 1 year and attendance for assessment (often with the obstetrician) at the end of the puerperium.

Audit of CS care is recommended in order that units can both provide quality care and reduce the CS rate.

ROLE AND RESPONSIBILITIES OF THE MIDWIFE

These can be summarised as:

- evidence-based practice throughout
- preoperative care to reduce intra- and postoperative complications
- skilled care within theatre and recovery
- comprehensive postoperative care
- effective multidisciplinary teamwork and recognition of limitations where appropriate
- referral when indicated
- contemporaneous record keeping.

Summary

- Theatre care is detailed and specialised; childbearing women have increased risk factors including aspiration, aortocaval occlusion and thromboembolism.
- Preoperative preparation should include consent, identity, care of the gastrointestinal and urinary tracts, skin preparation, removal of prostheses,

thromboprophylaxis and psychological support; good preoperative care can reduce the intra- and postoperative risks.

- Intraoperative care considers the woman to be the highest priority for maintaining her internal and external safety. This comprises many aspects of care.
- Postoperative care focuses on vital sign observations, airway and consciousness, pain relief, assessment of wound and haemorrhage, care of infusions, bladder care, adaptation to parenthood, feeding and psychological support.

SELF-ASSESSMENT EXERCISES

The answers to the following questions may be found in the text:

1. Discuss the requirements and rationale for preoperative preparation prior to emergency caesarean section. Compare and contrast this with preparation for elective surgery.
2. Summarise the general principles of conduct and care in the theatre environment.
3. Discuss the midwife's role and responsibilities to the woman before, during and following caesarean section.
4. Describe the care that the midwife gives to a woman in the immediate and ongoing recovery period after a caesarean section under regional anaesthesia.
5. List other occasions when it may be necessary for childbearing women to undergo surgery.

References

AAGBI, OAA (The Association of Anaesthetists of Great Britain and Ireland and Obstetric Anaesthetists' Association): *OAA/AAGBI Guidelines for Obstetric Anaesthetic Services*, rev ed 3, London, 2005, AAGBI and OAA.

Afolabi BB, Lesi AFE, Merah NA: Regional versus general anaesthesia for caesarean section, *Cochrane Database Syst Rev* (4) CD004350. DOI: 10.1002/14651858. CD004350.pub2, 2006.

Anorlu RI, Maholwana B, Hofmeyr GJ: Methods of delivering the placenta at caesarean section, *Cochrane Database Syst Rev* (3) CD004737. DOI: 10.1002/

14651858.CD004737. pub2, 2008.

ASA (American Society of Anesthetists): Practice guidelines for obstetric anesthesia, *Anesthesiology* 106:843–863, 2007.

Baxter J: Do women understand the reasons given for their caesarian [sic] sections? *Br J Midwifery* 15(9): 536–538, 2007.

BirthChoiceUK: *Hospitals with highest and lowest caesarean section rates*, 2009, Online. Available, www. birthchoiceuk.com/Professionals/ CSHistory, 31 January 2009.

Coggins J: Caesarean birth: a birth none-the-less! 2009, *MIDIRS Midwifery Dig* 13(1):76–79, 2003.

Costantine MM, Rahman M, Ghulmiyah L, et al: Timing of perioperative antibiotics for cesarean delivery: a metaanalysis, *Am J Obstet Gynecol* 199(3):1–6, 2008.

Crenshaw JT, Winslow EH: Actual versus instructed fasting times and associated discomforts in women having scheduled cesarean birth, *J Obstet Gynecol Neonatal Nurs* 35(2):257–264, 2006.

DH (Department of Health): *Why mothers die. Report on confidential enquiries into maternal deaths in the United Kingdom 1994–1996*, London, 1998, The Stationery Office.

Farman J: Acid aspiration syndrome, *Br J Perioper Nurs* 14(6):266–272, 2004.

Gates S, Anderson ER: Wound drainage for caesarean section, *Cochrane Database Syst Rev* (1) CD004549. DOI: 10.1002/14651858. CD004549.pub2, 2005.

Gould D: Caesarean section, surgical site infection and wound management, *Nurs Stand* 21(32):57–66, 2007.

Mathai M, Hofmeyr GJ: Abdominal surgical incisions for caesarean section, *Cochrane Database Syst Rev* (1) CD004453. DOI: 10.1002/14651858.CD004453.pub2, 2007.

NICE (National Institute for Clinical Excellence): *Caesarean section: Clinical Guideline 13*, London, 2004, NICE.

NPSA (National Patient Safety Agency): *WHO Surgical Safety Checklist*, 2009. Online. Available: http://www.npsa.nhs.uk/nrls/alerts-and-directives/alerts/safer-surgery-alert/, 31 January 2009.

Patientsafetyfirst: *Reducing harm in perioperative care*, 2009. Online. Available: www.patientsafetyfirst. nhs.uk/Content.aspx?path=/interventions/Perioperativecare/, 31 January 2009.

Scott E, Earl C, Leaper D, et al: Understanding peri-operative nursing, *Nurs Stand* 13(49):49–54, 1999.

Wiklund I, Edman G, Ryding EL, et al: Expectation and experiences of childbirth in primiparae with caesarean section, *Br J Obstet Gynaecol* 115(3):324–331, 2008.

Principles of wound management: healing and care

52

A wound is any break in the skin and underlying tissues. Wound classifications mainly consider the extent, depth and causative factor. Midwives will be familiar with clean contaminated wounds (caesarean section (CS)), lacerations (perineal tears or trauma to nipples) and punctures (cannulation, venepuncture, capillary sampling). Wound care is underpinned by an appreciation of the physiology of wound healing. This chapter considers wound healing and the factors that influence it, the care of caesarean section wounds and the removal of wound closures. Wound drains are considered briefly. The reader will gain a holistic understanding

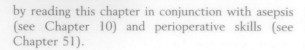

by reading this chapter in conjunction with asepsis (see Chapter 10) and perioperative skills (see Chapter 51).

LEARNING OUTCOMES

Having read this chapter the reader should be able to:

- describe the process of wound healing, identifying the factors that can affect it
- discuss the current evidence which underpins the care of surgical wounds
- describe an aseptic procedure and apply the principles to the dressing of wounds and drains and the removal of wound closures.

Physiology of wound healing

Healing of wounds begins following any injury to the body; an intact skin provides an efficient first line of defence against invading organisms. Wounds whose edges are in apposition (e.g. surgical wounds) heal quickly by first intention. Deeper, gaping wounds take longer to heal by secondary or tertiary intention.

There are four phases of wound healing:

1. haemostasis
2. inflammation
3. proliferation
4. maturation.

The length of time to progress through these phases varies for each wound and can be influenced by factors such as wound size, suturing, the clinical condition of the person and infection.

Haemostasis

This vascular phase begins immediately there is tissue damage. Vasoconstriction occurs to minimise bleeding and assist with initiating the coagulation process. A fibrin clot forms, temporarily closing the wound. While the clot is forming, blood or serous fluid may exude from the wound as the body tries to cleanse the wound naturally.

Inflammation

The blood vessels around the wound dilate, causing localised erythema, oedema, heat, discomfort, throbbing and sometimes functional disturbance.

Macrophages clear the wound of debris in preparation for new tissue growth. A small necrotic area forms around the wound margin where the blood supply was interrupted. Epithelial cells from the wound margin move under the base of the clot, the surrounding epithelium thickens and a thin layer of epithelial tissue forms over the wound. As the clinical signs of the inflammation phase are similar to those of infection (see below) it is important the midwife can distinguish between a wound that is healing normally and one that is infected. Provided the wound is clean, this phase lasts between 1–3 days, but is prolonged in the presence of infection or necrosis (South et al 2008).

Proliferation

This phase involves the growth of new tissue through three processes:

- granulation
- wound contraction
- epithelialisation.

During granulation, capillaries from the surrounding vessels grow into the wound bed. At the same time, fibroblasts produce collagen fibres, providing the framework for new connective tissue formation. Collagen increases the tensile strength and structural integrity of the wound. Healthy granulation tissue has a bright red, moist, shiny appearance, a 'pebbled' looking base and does not bleed easily.

Once the wound is filled with connective tissue, fibroblasts collect around the edges of the wound and contract, pulling the edges together. A firmer, fibrous epithelial scar forms as the fibroblasts and collagen fibres begin to shrink, resulting in contraction of the area and obliteration of some of the capillaries. This only occurs with healthy tissue that has not been sutured.

During epithelialisation new epithelial cells grow over the wound surface to form a new outer layer, recognised by the whitish-pink, translucent appearance of the wound. The process is enhanced in a moist, clean environment.

Maturation

Once epithelialisation is complete, the new tissue undergoes a time of maturation when it is 're-modelled' to increase the tensile strength of the scar tissue. In lightly pigmented skin, the scar initially appears red and raised, and then with time changes to a paler, smoother, flatter appearance. Scar tissue in darkly pigmented skin has a lighter appearance initially when compared with lightly pigmented skin. Mature scar tissue is avascular and contains no sweat or sebaceous glands or hairs. This phase can take up to 2 years to complete and may be the reason why some wounds that appear to have healed suddenly break down (Keast & Orsted 1998).

This healing process also occurs around sutures. When the sutures are removed, the epithelial cells can be dislodged and may be visible on the sutures as debris.

Wound healing by secondary intention occurs with deeper, wider wounds, whose edges cannot be brought into apposition. Inflammation may be chronic, with more granulation tissue forming at the expense of collagen during proliferation. Granulation tissue gradually fills the wound with re-epithelialisation beginning at the edges. Healing by secondary intention takes longer, resulting in more scar tissue forming.

Factors affecting wound healing

Temperature

A fall or a rise (above 30°C) both cause vasoconstriction and so impair wound healing.

Infection

Infection causes increased inflammation and necrosis, which delays wound healing. Poor surgical techniques (with an increased risk of haematoma; Olsen et al 2008), poor dressing techniques, a larger number of people in theatre (Reilly 2002), inadequate or mistimed antibiotic prophylaxis (for lower segment CS; Kaimal et al 2008) and wounds that are too dry or too wet predispose to colonisation or infection. A wound that is critically colonised has sufficient bacteria competing for oxygen and nutrients at the expense of healthy cells. It may not appear infected but will fail to heal.

Nutritional status

An adequate intake of protein, carbohydrate, fats, vitamins A, B, C and E, copper, zinc and iron are required. Proteins supply amino acids, essential for tissue repair and regeneration. Vitamins A and B and zinc are required for epithelialisation, and vitamin C and zinc are necessary for collagen synthesis and capillary integrity. Iron is required for the synthesis of haemoglobin which combines reversibly with oxygen to transport oxygen around the body.

Psycho-social factors

Good management of pain will reduce the woman's anxiety, improve her acceptance of the wound and so reduce stress. Anxiety, isolation and altered body image all reduce wound healing (South et al 2008).

Increasing age

This affects all phases of wound healing due to impaired circulation and coagulation, slower inflammatory response and decreased fibroblast activity.

Medical disorders

Medical disorders, and particularly those that impair circulation or tissue perfusion, can delay wound healing. Diabetes mellitus includes the additional risk of hyperglycaemia, this can inhibit phagocytosis and predispose to fungal and yeast infection. Malignancy and the need for chemotherapy were also shown to have an adverse influence on wound infection rates (Reilly 2002).

Drugs

Anti-inflammatory drugs suppress protein synthesis, inflammation, wound contraction and epithelialisation. Corticosteroids (from stress, steroid therapy or disease) delay both the inflammatory and immune responses.

Impaired oxygenation

A low arterial oxygen tension may alter collagen synthesis and inhibit epithelialisation. Poor tissue perfusion may occur in the presence of hypovolaemia, anaemia, obese tissue, smoking, poor mobility and alcohol. Oxygen is necessary for fibroblast activity. Johnson et al (2006), Olsen et al (2008) and the Joint Commission Perspectives on Patient Safety (JCPPS) (2008) all relate obesity with an increased risk of wound infection.

Surgery-related care

NICE (2004) suggest specific surgical techniques for caesarean section surgery. Failure to undertake these procedures increases the risk of poor healing post surgery.

Wound stress

Prolonged or violent vomiting, abdominal distension or laboured respirations may cause sudden tension on the wound, inhibiting the formation of collagen networks and connective tissue.

Summary

The factors listed above are sometimes categorised as either intrinsic or extrinsic factors. These refer to the internal issues that relate to the woman, for example, age, health, smoking, out-of-normal parameters for body mass index, presurgical rupture of membranes and those that relate to the external issues such as surgical technique, wound care, environmental hygiene, planned surgery and antibiotic prophylaxis. It becomes clear that the factors affecting wound management are considerable, significant and multidisciplinary.

Complications of wound healing

Haemorrhage

Haemostasis usually occurs within several minutes of an acute wound occurring. However, bleeding may occur if a bleeding point is not tied off, as a result of the clot or suture dislodging or infection, and may occur internally and externally. Internal bleeding can lead to haematoma formation.

Infection

Infection usually appears within 2–3 days of a traumatic injury or 4–5 days of a surgical wound. The wound site will appear red (often a spreading or tracking cellulitis), swollen and painful. There may also be weeping from the wound, usually a yellow, green or brown discharge (depending on the infecting organism); it may also be malodorous. The woman may have a pyrexia, tachycardia, a raised white cell count and a general malaise (Boyle 2006).

Dehiscence

If an acute wound does not heal properly the layers of skin and tissue can separate, usually during the proliferation phase. Separation can be partial or complete. It occurs more commonly where there is greater strain on the wound and decreased vasoconstriction (e.g. obesity), and particularly with abdominal wounds, if a sudden strain is placed on the wound (e.g. coughing, sitting up).

Evisceration

This is a rare medical emergency that occurs when the visceral organs begin to protrude through the separated wound layers.

Fistula

This may occur as a result of poor wound healing, possibly resulting from infection.

Wound management

Wound management aims to promote healing of the tissue and also to prevent any of the possible complications. Infection is one of the most common and costly complications. Ward et al (2008) found that post-discharge surveillance revealed that after caesarean section a greater number of women experienced morbidity from wound infection than was previously thought.

Preoperative considerations

Childbearing women who are healthy and enter hospital only a short time before their planned surgery have a lesser risk of wound healing complications than those who are unwell, anaemic, have a longer hospital admission, emergency surgery or presurgical rupture of the membranes. Measures that can optimise health before surgery should be taken; these include blood glucose levels within the norm, screening for and treating existing infections, reducing obesity and smoking cessation (JCPPS 2008).

Preoperative skin preparation has no researched base on which to practise. Showering is considered preferable to bathing. Grewal & Mann (2008) recommend showering as close to the planned surgical time as possible, the joint commission (JCPPS

2008) recommend the use of chlorhexidine the night before surgery and again on the day. Hair can harbour bacteria, become caught in the wound closure and may make dressing removal very uncomfortable. Hair removal also remains an unresolved issue. Simmons (1998) suggests that hair should be retained unless in the way, but also recognises that if removal is required, shaving is the most harmful way of doing it. Grewal & Mann (2008) recommend the use of depilatory creams the day before or the use of clippers in the anaesthetic room, the Joint Commission (JCPPS 2008) recognise that many people experience skin reactions with depilatory creams and so recommend the use of clippers only. These should only be used by someone who is correctly trained; clippers can also cause skin abrasions into which microorganisms can migrate.

Intraoperative care

Strict surgical asepsis should be maintained, with all standard precautions and personal protective equipment used as per the local protocol. Now well supported, including NICE (2004), is the use of a single dose of prophylatic cephalosporin antibiotics. Kaimal et al (2008) indicate the significance of it being administered before the skin incision is made. The skin of the operative site is cleansed; it is inconclusive as to the nature of the lotion that should be used. Cruse & Foord (1980) found little difference in the infection rate with the use of soap and alcohol-based products compared to povidone-iodine or chlorhexidine.

Chapter 51 highlights some of the other specific issues at surgery which can reduce the incidence of healing complications, e.g. avoidance of superficial wound drains, nature and positioning of incision, secured haemostasis to prevent haematoma formation.

Wound closure

Closure of the wound aims to bring the skin edges in neat apposition so that healing may begin by first intention. Mangram et al (1999) highlighted that a monofilament suture carried less infection risk than a multifilamented one. Reilly (2002) found that if sutures were left in place for longer than 10 days infection rates were greater. Wetter et al (1991) and Johnson et al (2006) both recommend the use of subcuticular suturing. Ward et al (2008) found

that wound infection was higher with staples than with a continuous suture, Olsen et al (2008) also found a slightly higher incidence of wound infection with the use of staples. Gould (2007a) recommends that for a transverse wound the sutures or staples can be removed after 4 or 5 days, once the new epithelium has become intact. Seven to 10 days is the recommended length of time for removal from a vertical incision. NICE (2004) indicate that superficial wound drains should be avoided for caesarean section wounds. If one is used it should be removed as soon as drainage ceases, ideally the next day (Gould 2007a).

Wound dressings

The wound dressing protects the wound from injury and external infection (until natural healing has begun), whilst absorbing any wound secretions. The dressing of choice is a non-adherent one with an absorbent pad and protective cover that also maintains humidity (Dale 1997, Reilly 2002).

Postoperative wound care

Cleaning and dressing wounds

A carefully sutured incision that has achieved haemostasis will be sealed by fibrin within 24 hours (Reilly 2002). At this point the dressing may be removed and the wound assessed. A risk assessment should take place to appreciate whether an aseptic (or a modified aseptic; Gilmour 1999) dressing technique is then necessary. Any signs of impaired healing or infection would indicate the need for an aseptic dressing technique.

Aseptic dressing technique

Chapter 10 discusses the principles of asepsis which are then applied to each situation. Wounds that need an aseptic dressing usually require cleansing. This removes bacteria, exudate and debris, amongst other things. However, unnecessary cleaning may disturb the healing process. Historically a variety of lotions have been used to clean wounds, current theory (South et al 2008) suggests the use of 0.9% sodium chloride, at body temperature. Either gloved hands or forceps may be used; proponents of forceps argue that hands offer greater contamination risks, while proponents of hands suggest that a lighter touch is achieved. Irrigation of the wound, using a sterile syringe, may also be undertaken.

The question of when a wound dressing should be changed remains unanswered. It would appear sensible to make a daily assessment, but not to disturb the wound by cleaning or redressing it unless necessary.

Longer term care

Gould (2007a) indicates that women need to be aware that wound healing involves several layers of tissue and that it takes time for the maturation phase to be completed (12 months). In both the short and long term women need to be aware of what constitutes impairment or complications for wound healing and so seek appropriate referral.

Caesarean section wounds: summary

For a woman with a lower segment caesarean section (LSCS) wound, the following principles are suggested, but the reader is encouraged to be aware of the evolving audits and evidence:

- The theatre dressing can be removed after 24–48 hours.
- The woman should shower daily, the wound being gently patted dry. A dry dressing may be applied to offer protection against clothing rubbing against the wound, otherwise it may be left uncovered.
- The wound should be assessed at every postoperative/postnatal assessment.
- Suture/clip/staple removal is planned for the correct day.
- If the wound is exuding fluid or shows any other signs of potential complications it should be swabbed (see Chapter 11 for technique), cleansed and redressed (non-adherent dressing that retains moisture). Referral may be necessary for antibiotic therapy.
- If a wound requires cleansing and redressing an aseptic technique is used. A risk assessment may determine that a clean technique is suitable if there are no signs of dehiscence. 0.9% sodium chloride (at body temperature) is used to cleanse the wound with either gloved hands or forceps, gauze swabs or syringe irrigation.

Perineal wounds

This chapter is focused upon surgical wounds but a word is necessary to highlight good practice when facilitating perineal wound healing. A perineal wound heals by first intention providing that the skin edges are in apposition. Not being a wound that is covered with a sterile dressing means that the potential for complications is greater than a surgical clean contaminated wound. The midwife should appreciate the appearance of the perineum post delivery and continue (largely by detailed discussion) to assess the healing and wellbeing through the postnatal period (Bick et al 2009). Oral/P.R. analgesia may be prescribed; the use of ice packs is commonly advocated but the effects of cooling on wound healing means that they should only be used for short periods of time and not after 24–48 hours (Boyle 2006).

Steen (2007) reiterates the factors that affect wound healing and notes that personal hygiene, good nutrition and reduced stress all contribute to promote wound healing. Gould (2007b) supports the view that scrupulous perineal hygiene is necessary, particularly after bathing, voiding and bowel movements. Pads should be changed 3 hourly and should not be touched before touching the wound (Gould 2007b). Chapter 12 considers the methods suitable for vulval toilet.

PROCEDURE: aseptic dressing technique

- Gain informed consent and establish that redressing is indicated.
- Collect the equipment on the lower shelf of a clean dressings trolley/utilise a clean surface in the home:
  - hand rub and sterile gloves
  - apron
  - sachet of 0.9% sodium chloride at body temperature
  - sterile dressing pack (in date) (should contain disposable bag and suitable dressing)
  - 10 mL syringe.
- Position the woman appropriately, maintaining privacy and dignity.
- Wash hands, apply apron, loosen the existing dressing, but keep the wound covered.

- Use hand rub, wipe the top of the trolley with an alcohol wipe.
- Open the outer layer of the pack, dropping it carefully onto the trolley.
- Open the inner wrapper of the pack touching only the edges of the paper; slide the other sterile items onto the sterile field (see Chapter 10), pour the saline into the gallipot.
- Loosen the existing dressing, place the disposable bag over the hand and remove the dressing (Nicol et al 2008).
- Invert the bag, with the dressing inside, and attach it to the side of the trolley as a refuse bag.
- Use hand rub and apply gloves.
- Assess the wound; if irrigation is indicated draw up the saline in the syringe.
- Cleanse the skin around the wound with gauze.
- Then either (depending on local protocol):
  - clean the wound with gauze and gloved hands or forceps, passing the swab from the 'clean hand' to the 'dirty hand' (see p 82); wipe with the 'dirty hand', using each swab to wipe once only, wiping from areas of discharge outwards. Discard the swab, repeat as necessary; *or*
  - hold a piece of gauze at the dirtier end of the wound and irrigate with the syringe, from clean to dirty, catching the fluid in the gauze (this is the preferable method).
- Dry the surrounding skin.
- Apply and secure the dressing.
- Ensure the woman is comfortable; discuss findings and ongoing care with her.
- Dispose of equipment correctly
- Remove apron, gloves and wash hands.
- Return the trolley to the clean area, washing it down if required.
- Document findings and act accordingly.

Removal of sutures, clips or staples

The decision to remove sutures, clips or staples is taken according to the assessment of healing of the wound. Removal is often 4–5 days after the surgery. Sutures that are retained for too long increase the infection risk and delay wound healing. Suture removal is an aseptic procedure, a receptacle is required to place clips or staples in so that they can be disposed of correctly in the sharps bin. If the wound gapes after any of the sutures have been removed the midwife will refer the woman before removing them all, and may apply an adhesive suture and sterile dressing in the meantime. Obviously, only non-absorbable sutures need to be removed.

Removing sutures

The aim of correct suture removal is to ensure that no part of the external suture is taken through internally:

- Lift and hold the external part of the suture with forceps using the non-dominant hand.
- Cut beneath the knot as near to the skin as possible using scissors or stitch cutter in the dominant hand (Fig. 52.1A).
- Remove the suture by pulling it gently through the skin.

This principle applies whether the sutures are interrupted, continuous or subcuticular. A continuous suture requires the midwife to lift, cut and pull through repeatedly, until the end of the suture is removed. Subcuticular suturing that is held in place with a bead should have the bead removed at the distal end of the wound so that on removal the suture is pulled from the end nearest to the midwife. The removal should be smooth; the woman may experience the pulling sensation rather than discomfort.

Removing staples

- Hold the staple remover as if a pair of scissors.
- Insert the lower blade directly under the staple.
- Squeeze the handles together; the staple will be lifted from the skin as it concertinas (Fig. 52.1B).
- Lift clear.

Removing Michel clips

- Hold the clip remover as if a pair of scissors.
- Insert the narrow blade under the clip.
- Squeeze the handles together; the clip will be lifted from the skin as it concertinas (Fig. 52.1C).

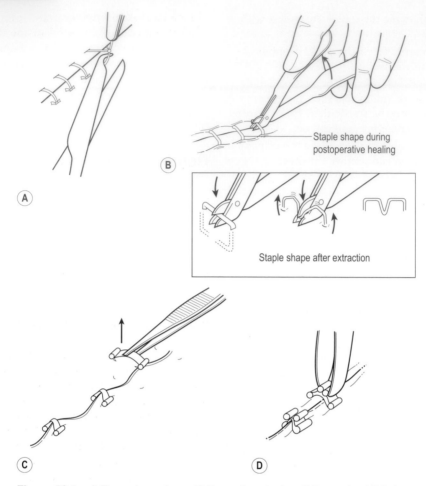

Staple shape during
postoperative healing

Staple shape after extraction

Figure 52.1 • A Removing sutures. B Removing staples. C Removing Michel
clips. D Removing Kifa clips (Fig. 52.1A and D adapted with kind permission from Jamieson
et al 1997; Fig. 52.1B adapted with kind permission from Lammon et al 1995; Fig 52.1C adapted
with kind permission from Jamieson et al 2002)

Removing Kifa clips

- Place the forceps over the wings of the clip.
- Squeeze the wings together.
- The clip will be lifted from the skin as it
  concertinas (Fig. 52.1D).

PROCEDURE: removing sutures, clips and staples

- Gain informed consent and gather equipment:
  - sterile gloves, plastic apron and hand rub

- suture removal pack/dressing pack with
  scissors, stitch cutter, staple or clip remover
  (includes receiver to place clips or staples in)
- portable sharps box.
- Position the woman to expose the wound,
  maintaining privacy and dignity.
- Apply apron and wash hands.
- Open the pack and establish a sterile field as
  described for aseptic procedure above. Open
  cutter/remover.
- Use hand rub and apply gloves.
- Assess the wound; if healing is evident
  remove the suture(s), clips or staples

as described above, placing sutures into the refuse bag, clips or staples into receiver. If in doubt as to wound healing, consider removing every other suture. Refer early in the procedure if it is clear that healing is not complete.

- Assist the woman to be comfortable.
- Dispose of equipment correctly, including all sharps directly into the sharps box.
- Remove apron, gloves and wash hands.
- Document findings and act accordingly.

Care of wound drains

A wound drain reduces the dead space and decreases the likelihood of haematoma formation, but can increase the risk of wound infection by supplying a route for microorganisms to track deeply into the tissue (Briggs 1997). A wound may be drained by using either an open or a closed drainage system; a closed system is usually vacuumed (which 'pulls' the exudate from the tissues) whereas an open drain drains with gravity. The nature of the surgery determines whether a drain is inserted, and if so, which type.

Postoperatively, wound drains are observed for their drainage and must be kept positioned so that they are able to drain correctly and do not pull or fall to the floor. Any drainage from the wound drain should be recorded on the fluid balance chart. Briggs (1997) suggests that the optimal time for removal is after 24 hours although this will also depend on how much is draining.

Emptying a wound drain

Care should be taken to maintain the integrity of the closed drainage system to reduce infection risks; however, the drain should be emptied if the vacuum is reduced or lost, or if the drain is to be retained for longer than 24 hours.

Drains vary; the midwife will need to be familiar with individual types. Most drains have the vacuum mechanism integral to them, usually by compressing the drain. The principles of emptying a wound drain are:

- It is an aseptic procedure in which the midwife wears sterile gloves, cleanses the emptying port with an alcohol-impregnated wipe before and after emptying the drain, and empties it into a sterile receiver.
- Once the drain is emptied the vacuum is achieved and the drain sealed.
- There is minimal disruption for the woman.
- The procedure and volume are documented.

Dressing a wound drain

If required for longer than 24 hours, the drain may require re-dressing. Asepsis is required; the area is cleansed with 0.9% sodium chloride and a hole is cut (with sterile scissors) into the non-adherent dressing so that it sits snugly around the drain (Fig. 52.2) and is secured with tape.

Removal of a wound drain

Asepsis is indicated as there will be a small open wound when the drain has been removed. The drain should have its vacuum released before it is removed, and the woman should be aware that removal is a slightly uncomfortable procedure. After removing the stitch, one hand supports the skin gently, while the other removes the drain. The area is cleansed and an appropriate dressing is applied. The amount that has drained is recorded on the

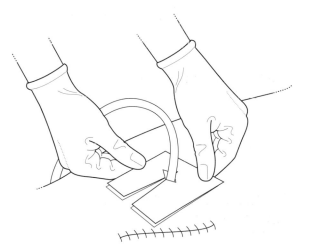

Figure 52.2 • Dressing a wound drain (Adapted with kind permission from Jamieson et al 1997)

fluid balance chart and the drain is disposed of in the clinical waste. The tip of the drain may be sent for laboratory investigation if required. The woman may require analgesia before or after the procedure. The site will need assessing the following day.

ROLE AND RESPONSIBILITIES OF THE MIDWIFE

These can be summarised as:

- understanding the physiology of wound healing and application of this to practice
- application of evidence-based care with regard to wound healing
- undertaking all procedures correctly with an aseptic technique when indicated
- referral if indicated
- contemporaneous record keeping.

Summary

- Surgical wounds heal mainly by primary intention; the four phases of wound healing can be affected by various factors.
- Evidence-based perioperative and wound care aim to reduce the possible

complications, infection being one of the biggest risks.
- Asepsis is required if a wound or drain needs dressing and for wound closure removal.
- There are still aspects of wound care that are ritualistic and not researched.

SELF-ASSESSMENT EXERCISES

The answers to the following questions may be found in the text:

1. Describe the four phases of wound healing.
2. How would the midwife distinguish between a wound that is healing normally and one that is infected?
3. Discuss the factors that enhance or impair wound healing.
4. Describe the management of the wound following caesarean section.
5. Describe how to remove sutures correctly. Compare and contrast the removal of clips and staples with sutures.
6. What complications are associated with wound healing?
7. Describe how to empty, dress and remove a wound drain.

References

Bick D, MacArthur C, Winter H: *Postnatal care evidence and guidelines for management*, ed 2, Edinburgh, 2009, Elsevier, pp 19–40.

Boyle M: *Wound healing in midwifery*, Oxford, 2006, Radcliffe, pp 36 & 75.

Briggs M: Principles of closed surgical wound care, *J Wound Care* 6(6): 288–292, 1997.

Cruse P, Foord R: The epidemiology of wound infection, *Surg Clin North Am* 6(1):27–40, 1980.

Dale J: Wound dressings, *Prof Nurse Study* Suppl 12(12):S12–S14, 1997.

Gilmour D: Redefining aseptic technique, *J Community Nurs* 13(7):22–26, 1999.

Gould D: Caesarean section, surgical site infection and wound management, *Nurs Stand* 21(32):57–66, 2007a.

Gould D: Perineal tears and episiotomy, *Nurs Stand* 21(52):41–46, 2007b.

Grewal JK, Mann N: Perioperative care. In Doughty L, Lister S, editors: *The Royal Marsden Hospital manual of clinical nursing procedures student edition*, Oxford, 2008, Wiley Blackwell, pp 783–825.

Jamieson EM, McCall JM, Blythe R, et al: *Clinical nursing practices*, ed 3, Edinburgh, 1997, Churchill Livingstone.

Jamieson EM, McCall JM, Whyte AW: *Clinical nursing practices*, ed 4, Edinburgh, 2002, Churchill Livingstone.

JCPPS (Joint Commission Perspectives on Patient Safety): Preventing surgical site infections (SSI), *Jt Comm Perspect Patient Saf* 8(9):8–11, 2008.

Johnson A, Young D, Reilly J: Caesarean section surgical site infection surveillance, *J Hosp Infect* 64(1):30–35, 2006.

Kaimal AJ, Zlantnik MG, Cheng YW, et al: Effect of a change in policy regarding the timing of prophylactic antibiotics on the rate of postcaesarean delivery surgical site infections, *Am J Obstet Gynaecol* 199(3):310.e1–310.e5, 2008.

Keast DH, Orsted H: The basic principles of wound care, *Ostomy Wound Manage* 44(8):24–31, 1998.

Lammon CB, Foote AW, Leli PG, et al: *Clinical nursing skills*, Philadelphia, 1995, W B Saunders.

Mangram AJ, Horan TC, Pearson ML, et al: Guideline for prevention of surgical site infection, *Am J Infect Control* 27(2):97–134, 1999.

NICE (National Institute for Clinical Excellence): *Caesarean section: Clinical Guideline 13*, London, 2004, NICE.

Nicol M, Bavin C, Cronin P, et al: *Essential nursing skills*, ed 3, Edinburgh, 2008, Elsevier.

Olsen MA, Butler AM, Willers DM, et al: Risk factors for surgical site infection after low transverse cesarean section, *Infect Control Hosp Epidemiol* 29(6):477–484, 2008.

Reilly J: Evidence based surgical wound care on surgical wound infection, *Br J Nurs* (Suppl) 11(16): S4–S12, 2002.

Simmons M: Preoperative skin preparation, *Prof Nurse* 13(7): 446–447, 1998.

South C, Tanay AM, Tinne N: Wound management. In Doughty L, Lister S, editors: *The Royal Marsden Hospital manual of clinical nursing procedures student edition*, Oxford, 2008, Wiley Blackwell, pp 1097–1162.

Steen M: Perineal tears and episiotomy: how do wounds heal? *Br J Midwifery* 15(5):273–280, 2007.

Ward VP, Charlett A, Fagan J, Crawshaw SC: Enhanced surgical site infection surveillance following caesarean section: experience of a multicentre collaborative post-discharge system, *J Hosp Infect* 70:166–173, 2008.

Wetter LA, Dinneen MD, Levitt MD, Motson RW: Controlled trial of polyglycolic acid versus catgut and nylon for appendicectomy wound closure, *Br J Surg* 78(8):985–987, 1991.

Principles of restricted mobility management: pressure area care

53

Women may have restricted mobility for many reasons – bed rest due to antepartum haemorrhage, pre-eclampsia, during and following epidural anaesthesia, general anaesthetic, following a postpartum haemorrhage or postoperatively, etc. – making them vulnerable to or at an accelerated risk of pressure ulcer formation. Babies who are unwell, particularly the very preterm babies, are also vulnerable to or have an elevated risk of developing pressure ulcers. Damage to skin and underlying fatty tissues from pressure ulcers causes pain. If the ulcer becomes infected, septicaemia and/or bone infection can ensue; muscle or bone may be destroyed in severe cases. These complications of restricted mobility, although they are not commonly seen within the midwifery setting, do occur (Butcher 2004, Hughes 2001), increase morbidity and mortality and are often avoidable; it is important that the midwife develops the knowledge and skills to reduce their incidence. The Royal College of Nursing and the National Institute for Health and Clinical Excellence (RCN & NICE 2004) recommend that all healthcare professionals undergo relevant training and education in the assessment and prevention of pressure ulcers.

This chapter focuses on the principles of pressure area care including a discussion of the aetiology and classification of pressure ulcers. The factors that influence the development of pressure ulcers are given, followed by a discussion of the assessment of skin integrity.

LEARNING OUTCOMES

Having read this chapter the reader should be able to:

- discuss why pressure ulcers occur
- identify factors that increase the risk of pressure ulcer formation
- describe the four stages of pressure ulcer formation
- undertake assessment of the skin, recognising normal and abnormal changes resulting from pressure
- discuss the principles of pressure area care.

Pressure-area care

This is undertaken to reduce the incidence of pressure ulcer formation. A pressure ulcer is a skin ulceration that forms due to localised tissue necrosis, commonly found on the parts of the body that have received unrelieved pressure or friction, or both. It has previously been referred to as a 'decubitus ulcer', 'pressure sore' or (less commonly) a 'bedsore'.

A variety of risk assessment tools are available for use in the clinical setting (e.g. the remodified Norton Scale, Braden Scale, RAPS scale) with varying degrees of success. Their use does not appear to prevent pressure ulcers worsening or from further ones developing [European Pressure Ulcer Advisory Panel (EPUAP) 2009a, RCN & NICE 2005] but the presence of a grade 1 pressure ulcer should be considered a significant risk factor for the development of a more severe form of pressure ulcer. The RCN & NICE (2004) recommend these should not replace clinical judgement, but should be used only as an aide-mémoire. Moore & Cowman (2008) reviewed the studies of risk assessment tools compared to the use of clinical judgement for assessing the risk of pressure ulcer development, but found no randomised trials had been undertaken and were unable to form a conclusion as to their value. However, of the tools available, Pancorbo-Hidalgo et al (2006) found the Braden Scale offered the best balance between specificity and sensitivity and the best risk estimate for pressure ulcer formation and concluded that both this scale and the Norton Scale were more accurate than nurses' judgement in predicting the risk of pressure ulcer formation.

It is important to identify individuals at risk of developing pressure ulcers (EPUAP 2009a) by considering the woman or baby's general medical condition, undertaking an assessment of their skin, mobility, moistness (including level of continence), nutrition and pain levels. For those identified as being at increased risk, appropriate intervention should be utilised.

Aetiology of pressure ulcers

Pressure ulcers develop as a result of two processes, occurring either separately or together:

1. unrelieved pressure
2. shearing and friction.

Unrelieved pressure

Pressure within the capillaries varies from 35 mmHg (arterial) to 16 mmHg (venous) (South et al 2008). External pressures above this will result in occlusion of the capillaries. If the pressure is prolonged, even with low-intensity pressure, the resulting anoxia causes tissue ischaemia and necrosis. Necrosis may begin in the muscle that lies over the bone. The length of time the pressure needs to be applied for damage to occur will vary from person to person.

Healthy lightly pigmented skin with a good circulation blanches when blood flow is restricted (e.g. fingertip pressure). The skin whitens, replacing the usual red/darker skin tones. The effects of pressure can be seen when the pressure is removed and a sudden, large increase in blood flow occurs, up to 30 times the normal resting value. This results in a normal 'reactive hyperaemia', when blanching is replaced by a bright red flush, lasting usually less than 1 hour. Providing the lymphatic vessels are not damaged and excess interstitial fluid is removed, there is no permanent damage. However, if there is lymphatic vessel damage, tissue changes occur and large amounts of interstitial fluid are squeezed out. The cells rub together and the cell membranes rupture, releasing toxic intracellular material and normal skin colour is not restored. A deep pressure ulcer can arise when the lymphatic vessels and muscle fibres tear. In the healthy adult with full sensation, this will result in pain causing the individual to move (Benbow 2008). Where sensation is impaired (e.g. epidural anaesthesia) the change of position does not occur spontaneously.

Abnormal reactive hyperaemia and induration can occur with excessive pressure, causing the affected area to appear darker than the surrounding skin. Absence of blanching with a fingertip may also be seen. These effects can last for more than 1 hour after the pressure has been removed, possibly up to 2 weeks (Ayello 1999).

Darkly pigmented skin does not blanch or change colour when pressure is applied, making it more difficult to recognise impending tissue damage.

Shearing and friction

A shearing force is the pressure exerted against the skin in a direction parallel to the body's surface, occurring when the body moves up or down the bed while in an upright position. As the layers of muscle and bone slide in the direction of the body movement, the skin and subcutaneous layers stick to the bed surface, causing the bone to slide down into the skin, with a force exerted onto the skin.

A shearing force results at the junction of the deep and superficial tissues. The microcirculation is compressed and damaged, causing microscopic haemorrhage and necrosis deep within the tissues. This is compounded by the decreased capillary blood flow resulting from the external pressure pressing against the skin. Eventually, a channel opens through the skin and the necrotic area drains through this. The areas commonly affected by shearing forces are the sacrum and coccygeus. Benbow (2008) suggests the effects of shearing are exacerbated by moisture, highlighting the importance of ensuring the sheets underneath the woman are dry. Shearing forces can be reduced if the head is kept below 30° (Ayello 1999), i.e. place the chin on the chest when moving.

Friction is the mechanical force that is exerted when the skin is dragged across a coarse surface (e.g. bedding). The epidermis is rubbed away, giving the appearance of a shallow abrasion injury, often on the elbows and heels. The effects of friction are exacerbated by moisture (as for shearing) (Benbow 2008).

Common sites for pressure ulcer formation

Although pressure ulcers can form on any part of the body, the commoner sites are the heels, toes, knees, buttocks (sacral and coccygeal area, ischial tuberosities and greater trochanters), shoulders, elbows and ears (Fig. 53.1). Preterm babies can develop friction injuries when their delicate, immature skin rubs against bedding. The elbows and knees are primary sites for this to occur. Pressure may also occur from drainage tubes, indwelling catheters (against labia), nasogastric tubes (nasal passages), nasal oxygen cannulae and antiembolic stockings.

Classification of pressure ulcers

There are four recognised stages of pressure ulcer formation related to the depth of tissue damage and recognisable by changes seen to the skin and underlying tissues (EPUAP 2009b):

- Grade 1: intact skin showing non-blanchable erythema – the early sign of potential ulcer

formation. The skin may also be warm, discoloured, show signs of oedema, induration or hardness. The EPUAP (2009a) suggests these can be used as indicators of pressure ulcer development particularly for people with darker skin.
- Grade 2: partial-thickness skin loss of epidermis and/or dermis – a superficial ulcer that presents as an abrasion, blister or shallow crater.
- Grade 3: full-thickness skin loss and damage/necrosis of subcutaneous tissue which does not extend through the underlying fascia – presents as a deep crater that can also undermine adjacent tissue.
- Grade 4: damage/necrosis to underlying tissue, muscle, bone or supporting structures, e.g. tendon with or without full thickness skin loss.

In addition to these four stages, the National Pressure Ulcer Advisory Panel (2007) suggests another two, ungraded, stages:

- Suspected deep tissue injury: localised area of purplish/maroon discoloured skin or a blood-filled blister. Prior to this being seen, pain may be felt and the area can appear firm, soft, warmer or cooler than the adjacent tissue. Darkly pigmented skin may present with a thin blister over a darker wound bed. This stage occurs before the appearance of a grade 1 pressure ulcer.
- Unstageable: there is full-thickness tissue loss with the ulcer base covered by slough (ranging in colour from yellow, tan, grey to green or brown) which may or may not have a scab over the top of it. The depth and grade of the pressure ulcer cannot be determined until the wound has been debrided.

Factors influencing development

- Impaired sensory input: an altered sensory perception resulting in decreased or no experience of pressure and pain, with no awareness of the need to move, e.g. epidural or spinal analgesia.
- Impaired motor function produces an inability to move despite the presence of pain or pressure, e.g. epidural analgesia.
- Immobility, e.g. bed rest/reduced mobility.

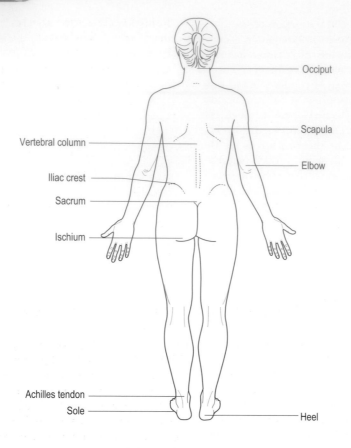

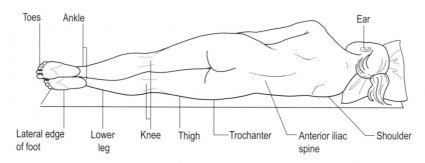

Figure 53.1 • Pressure area sites

- Decreased circulation.
- Altering levels of consciousness.
- Severe/chronic illness.
- Previous history of pressure damage.
- Oedema: reduces blood circulation in affected tissues and impairs clearage of waste products.
- Anaemia.
- Poor posture.
- Infection.

- Obesity may accelerate the development; adipose tissue may have an inadequate blood supply and be more susceptible to ischaemia.
- Inadequate dietary intake of protein, carbohydrate, fat, vitamins and trace elements, all of which are necessary for collagen synthesis and maturation, promoting healthy skin and wound healing. May also influence amount of subcutaneous fat which acts as padding between bone and skin.

- Excessive moisture on the skin (e.g. urine, sweat, liquor, wound exudate, faeces): decreases skin's resistance to physical factors such as shearing forces and pressure.
- Temperature changes.
- Immunosuppression.
- Increasing age resulting in loss of subcutaneous fat and skin elasticity and generalised skin atrophy.
- Use of equipment that provides no pressure relief, e.g. lithotomy straps.

Pregnant women are also considered to be at risk of developing pressure ulcers (RCN & NICE 2005) although this is possibly due to a combination of some of the factors listed above rather than pregnancy *per se*.

Assessment of skin integrity

The midwife, using good (preferably natural) lighting, should inspect the skin and potential pressure ulcer sites. The frequency is determined by individual needs and influenced by the presence of risk factors. For those women who are willing and able, the midwife can show them how to inspect their own skin and that of their baby. The condition of the skin, particularly over the bony prominences (e.g. sacrum, heels, hips, ankles, elbows, occiput) should be assessed initially to determine whether it is intact, dry, oedematous, red, indurated or cracking (EPUAP 2009a).

The presence of hyperaemia should be noted when it first appears and steps taken to minimise pressure on the affected area. The area should be rechecked after 1 hour to determine if hyperaemia is still present. The midwife should look for persistent erythema and the absence of blanching on fingertip pressure in lightly pigmented skin by depressing the skin firmly but gently with a clean fingertip. When the pressure is removed the colour of the skin is noted. In darkly pigmented skin the colour should be observed; purplish/bluish discoloration that is darker than the surrounding skin is abnormal. The location, size and colour of the affected area should be recorded; Ayello (1999) recommends using a marker pen to outline the area to make reassessment easier and more accurate.

The skin is also assessed for other signs of potential damage:

- localised heat over the affected area; with further tissue damage this heat is replaced by coolness, a sign of tissue devitalization
- localised oedema: the area will feel spongy and the skin may appear shiny and taut
- localised induration
- break in the skin integrity, e.g. blister, pimple.

Where signs of pressure ulcer formation are seen, it is important the midwife documents:

- the cause (if known)
- site/location
- dimension (measured with a ruler/tape measure)
- grade of pressure ulcer
- amount and type of exudate
- signs of local infection seen
- wound appearance
- pain score
- description of surrounding skin and any odour emitted.

The Tissue Viability Nurse must also be involved (RCN & NICE 2005). Photographs or tracing of the pressure ulcer with a ruler by the side of it may be required to enable accurate assessment of how the pressure ulcer is changing.

Appropriate strategies should be put into place to prevent any deterioration in the condition and number of pressure ulcers (e.g. using high-specification foam mattresses and pressure-relieving devices, positioning and repositioning regimen). Young & Clark (2003) are currently undertaking a review of the studies addressing positioning and whether certain positions or particular frequencies of changing positions affect the incidence and severity of pressure ulcer. Their results will be published on the Cochrane database and the reader is advised to review their findings when published.

Principles of pressure area care

The aim is to prevent the development of pressure ulcers by:

- identifying those who are either vulnerable to or at an elevated risk of pressure ulcer development and undertake a risk assessment within 6 hours (RCN & NICE 2005)
- regular assessment of the skin, noting the colour, integrity, presence of blanching, oedema or heat

- relieving pressure by assisting the woman or baby to change position on a regular basis (depending on the condition of the individual and the duration of hypoxia; with lightly pigmented skin the duration of redness is approximately half that of the duration of hypoxia). A turning chart may be used to record the time of turning and the positions used
- use of high specification foam mattresses with pressure-relieving properties for women and babies at elevated risk (McInnes et al 2008, RCN & NICE 2004)
- raising the bedclothes from the body, e.g. bedding should be loosened at the end of the bed or left untucked, or using a bed cradle
- placing a pillow between the knees of the woman when lying laterally to reduce the pressure from the top leg
- removing all creases, crumbs, etc. from the bedding as these can exert unnecessary pressure
- increasing circulation by passive or active exercises (see Chapter 54)
- ensuring the woman or baby is adequately hydrated; a fluid balance chart may be required
- ensuring the diet is well balanced, referring to the dietician if there are any difficulties
- ensuring the woman has her head below 30° if she is moving up or down the bed to reduce the shearing forces
- use of appropriate equipment for manual handling to prevent friction and shearing
- good hygiene, especially if incontinent or sweating profusely, but avoiding soap as it is usually alkaline and can dry the skin; after washing, the skin should be dried with gentle patting motions
- use of moisturisers for dry skin areas

- use of soft cotton bedding in preference to synthetic fibres.

ROLE AND RESPONSIBILITIES OF THE MIDWIFE

These can be summarised as:

- identifying women and babies who are vulnerable to and at elevated risk of developing pressure ulcers
- assisting the woman and baby with measures to reduce pressure ulcer formation
- referral as appropriate
- correct documentation.

Summary

- Pressure ulcers develop as a result of unrelieved pressure, and shearing and friction.
- They are avoidable; the midwife needs to be aware of who is vulnerable or at elevated risk and to assess the skin condition regularly.
- There are a number of measures that can be taken to reduce the likelihood of pressure ulcer formation; the midwife should be familiar with these.

SELF-ASSESSMENT EXERCISES

The answers to the following questions may be found in the text:

1. How do pressure ulcers arise?
2. What factors predispose to pressure ulcer formation?
3. Describe the different stages of pressure ulcer formation and how these are recognised.
4. What is the midwife looking for when an assessment of the skin is undertaken?
5. How can the midwife provide pressure area care to reduce the risks of pressure ulcers forming?

References

Ayello EA: Skin integrity and wound care. In Potter PA, Perry AG, editors: *Basic nursing: a critical thinking approach*, ed 4, St Louis, 1999, Mosby, ch 38.

Benbow M: Pressure ulcer prevention and pressure-relieving surfaces, *Br J Nurs* 17(13):830–835, 2008.

Butcher M: Risk of pressure damage for women using maternity services, *Nurs Times* 100(41):46–47, 2004.

EPUAP (European Pressure Ulcer Advisory Panel): *Pressure Ulcer Prevention Guidelines*, 2009a. Online. Available: http://www.

epuap.org/glprevention.html, 29 March 2009.

EPUAP (European Pressure Ulcer Advisory Panel): *Pressure Ulcer Treatment Guidelines*, 2009b. Online. Available: www.epuap.org/gltreatment.html, 29 March 2009.

Hughes C: Obstetric care. Is there a risk of pressure damage after epidural anaesthesia, *J Tissue Viability* 11(2):56–58, 2001.

McInnes E, Bell-Syer SEM, Dumville JC, et al: Support surfaces for pressure ulcer prevention, *Cochrane Database Syst Rev* (4): CD001735. DOI: 10.1002/14651858.CD001735.pub3, 2008.

Moore ZEH, Cowman S: Risk assessment tools for the prevention of pressure ulcers, *Cochrane Database Syst Rev* (3): CD006471. DOI: 10.1002/14651858.CD006471.pub2, 2008.

National Pressure Ulcer Advisory Panel: *Pressure Ulcer Stages Revised by NPUAP*, 2007. Online. Available: www.npuap.org/pr2, 29 March 2009.

Pancorbo-Hidalgo PL, Garcia-Fernandez IM, Lopez-Medina IM, et al: Risk assessment scales for pressure ulcer prevention: a systematic review, *J Adv Nurs* 54(1):94–110, 2006.

RCN (Royal College of Nursing), NICE (National Institute of Clinical Excellence): *The use of pressure-relieving devices (beds, mattresses and overlays) for the prevention of pressure ulcers in primary and secondary care*, 2004. Online. Available: www.nice.org.uk/nicemedia/pdf/cg007fullguideline.pdf, 29 March 2009.

RCN (Royal College of Nursing), NICE (National Institute of Clinical Excellence): *Pressure ulcer management: The management of pressure ulcers in primary and secondary care. A Clinical Practice Guideline*, London, 2005, NICE.

South C, Tanay MA, Tinne N: Wound management. In Dougherty L, Lister SE, editors: *The Royal Marsden Hospital manual of clinical nursing procedures*, ed 7, Oxford, 2008, Blackwell Publishing, pp 955–960.

Young T, Clark M: Re-positioning for pressure ulcer prevention, *Cochrane Database Syst Rev* (4): CD004836. DOI: 10.1002/14651858.CD004836, 2003.

Principles of restricted mobility management: prevention of thromboembolism

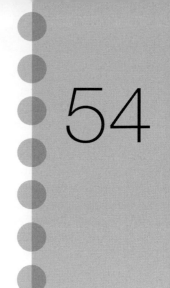

54

This chapter focuses on the principles of preventing the formation of thromboembolism. Venous thromboembolism (VTE) remains a significant cause of maternal mortality (Lewis 2007). Restricted mobility is one of several risk factors that affect its incidence. Complications such as thromboembolism affect physical, psychological and social aspects of the woman's care at a time when she should be preparing for/enjoying motherhood. As well as life threatening, the implications may also be both short and long term. The current risk factors are highlighted, prophylactic measures (exercises, deep breathing, anticoagulation and graduated compression stockings) are discussed and the role and responsibilities of the midwife are summarised.

LEARNING OUTCOMES

Having read this chapter the reader should be able to:

- discuss the risk factors for VTE in childbearing women

- describe the leg and breathing exercises that can be undertaken during any periods of immobility
- discuss briefly when and how anticoagulation therapy may be prescribed
- discuss how graduated compression stockings are correctly applied and worn
- highlight the midwife's role and responsibility in relation to the prevention of VTE.

Thrombus formation

There is a higher risk of blood clot formation (thrombus) if there is stasis in blood flow, greater coagulation of the blood and damage to vessel walls (Elliott & Pavord 2008). Child bearing, with changes in blood chemistry, pressure from the gravid uterus and relaxation of the vessel walls, has all three of these risks physiologically. It is suggested that pregnancy increases the risk of VTE 10-fold, the puerperium 25-fold (McColl et al 1997). The risks in pregnancy are immediate; 10 women died from pulmonary embolism (migration of the thrombus from leg or abdominal veins to the lungs) in their first trimester in the period 2003–2005 (Drife 2007).

Midwives need to be alert to additional risk factors that women may have:

- previous venous thromboembolism or family history
- increasing age, over 35 years
- existing or acquired haematological abnormalities, e.g. clotting disorders, sickle-cell disease, lupus anticoagulant
- obesity (particularly morbidly obese women), where body mass index is >30 at booking

- dehydration
- parity 4 or higher
- gross varicosities
- medical illness (particularly inflammatory disorders), paralysis of lower limbs
- pregnancy-related disorders: pre-eclampsia, hyperemesis, ante- or postpartum haemorrhage, prolonged labour
- surgery in pregnancy or puerperium
- delivery by midcavity forceps
- significant infection, e.g. pyelonephritis
- immobility more than 4 days, particularly after delivery
- ovarian hyperstimulation syndrome.

(Adapted from Drife 2007)

The greater the number of risks, the higher the possibility of thrombus formation. It should also be noted that as situations change, the need for risk assessment is ongoing.

Prophylaxis

For all childbearing women immobolisation should be kept to a minimum and dehydration avoided (RCOG 2004). This means that all women should be encouraged to remain active, but if for whatever reason there are longer periods of inactivity then specific exercises to aid venous blood flow should be undertaken. The midwife can utilise the skills of an obstetric physiotherapist, particularly for a woman in high dependency care or on long-term bed rest.

Exercises

Passive and active exercises are movements of the muscles and joints through their normal range, undertaken with the aim of promoting circulation, maintaining and improving muscle tone and preventing the development of joint contracture. Passive exercises are undertaken by the midwife (e.g. if the woman is unconscious) until such times when the woman can do them herself. As well as encouraging circulation the exercises can also reduce oedema. Oedematous legs can be raised slightly, provided they are well supported. Women with restricted mobility should be actively discouraged from crossing their legs (knees or ankles), as this can also impede circulation. Exercises should be undertaken with caution in the woman with pre-eclampsia, in consultation with the obstetric team.

- Foot exercises: the woman should sit or lie with her knees straight, then flex and extend her ankles by moving her feet towards and away from her body at least 10 times (Fig. 54.1). She should then circle her ankles by moving her feet in a clockwise direction at least 10 times, then in an anticlockwise direction, keeping her hips and knees still (Fig. 54.2). These exercises are particularly important for the postoperative woman (Brayshaw & Wright 1994).

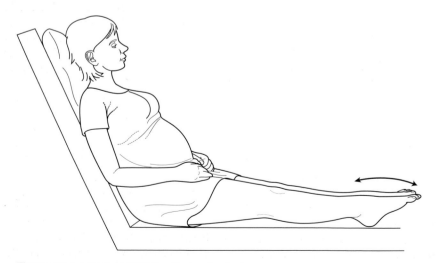

Figure 54.1 • Foot exercises – flexing the feet

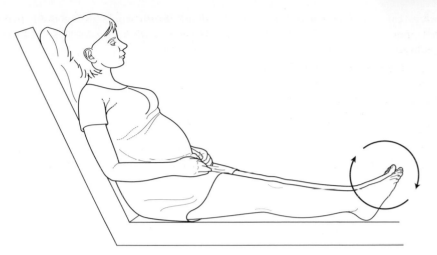

Figure 54.2 • Circling the ankles

- Leg tightening: the woman should sit or lie on the bed with her legs straight. As she pulls her toes towards her legs, the back of her knees should press down towards the bed and the position held for 4 seconds, then relaxed. This exercise should be repeated five times (Brayshaw & Wright 1994).

Deep breathing exercises

Inflating the lungs well assists venous return from the legs as well as avoiding stasis of secretions in the lungs. Following a general anaesthetic breathing exercises should be undertaken to assist with the removal of anaesthetic gases as well as promoting venous return.

The woman should preferably be sitting and take two to three deep breaths to improve ventilation and repeat frequently. The woman should also be encouraged to follow the deep breathing with short forced expirations, referred to as 'huffing', to loosen secretions. This reduces the risk of a chest infection developing.

Anticoagulation

Based on individual risk assessment (three or more risk factors; see pp 377–378) women may be given low molecular weight heparin prophylactically. This is a subcutaneous injection, once or twice a day depending on dose, usually administered into the abdomen (see Chapter 20). It is commenced as early in the antenatal period as possible and may continue postnatally depending on the risks (RCOG 2004). It can be self-administered following instruction; if care is carried out at home a sharps box should be supplied. As with any anticoagulation therapy the woman should be alert to signs of haemorrhage and know who to contact if this occurs.

Graduated compression stockings

Specific prophylaxis often includes the wearing of graduated compression (e.g. TED) stockings alongside anticoagulation therapy. (If a thrombus is suspected or confirmed, both of these treatments are required.) Graduated compression stockings deliver a gradient of compression which reduces the cross-sectional area of the lower limb. This increases the velocity of blood flow in the veins and reduces the risk of venous stasis (Walker & Lamont 2008). Graduated compression stockings are often made of nylon with elastane or lycra (other mixes are available) in two main lengths: full length and below knee. The gradient of compression means that 18 mmHg is delivered at the ankle, 14 mmHg mid-calf and 8–10 mmHg at the thigh. Whilst there is some debate about the use of full or below-knee stockings it is clear that whichever sort is used they should be fitted and worn correctly.

The midwife is required to measure the woman's legs. This is undertaken in the morning ideally, before the effects of oedema are evident. The woman should stand with her feet flat on the floor; both legs should be measured as size differences between the legs can occur and a different sized stocking may be required for each leg. The leg measurements should also be reviewed on a regular basis as changes may occur (e.g. occurrence of or disappearance of oedema). The measurements should be documented in the woman's records, along with the size of stockings issued.

If below-knee stockings are used, three measurements are required (Fig. 54.3A):

1. the narrowest point around the ankle, above the ankle bone
2. from the base of the heel to just below the knee
3. the widest part of the calf.

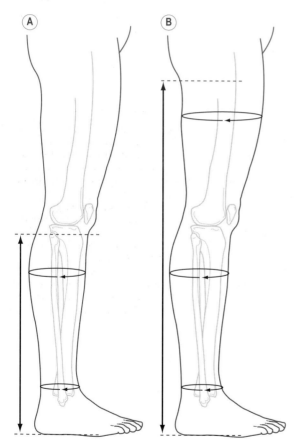

Figure 54.3 • A Measuring the leg for below-knee stockings – just above the ankle bone, the widest part of the calf and the distance from base of heel to just below the knee. B Measuring the leg for full-length stockings – just above the ankle bone, the widest part of the calf, the widest part of the thigh and the distance from the base of the heel to the gluteal fold

If full-length stockings are used, two further measurements are necessary (Fig. 54.3B):

4. the widest part of the thigh
5. from the base of the heel to the gluteal fold.

If the legs are not measured, the graduated compression stockings are unlikely to be a good fit. If too loose, compression will not be applied and they are likely to roll down. If too tight, they can be uncomfortable and cause trauma, possibly increasing the risk of thrombus formation.

It is important that the stockings are applied correctly, ensuring there are no wrinkles and that the bands over the feet and at the top are not so tight as to apply excessive pressure. They should be put on first thing in the morning before getting out of bed to dry legs and feet. To apply the stockings:

- a hand is inserted into the stocking up to the seamed heel
- the heel is held between the forefinger and thumb and the stocking turned inside out, until the heel pocket is seen
- the stocking is placed over the foot, with the heel pocket positioned over the heel
- the stocking is pulled over the foot and up the leg.

If the stockings are difficult to apply, moisturising the legs before putting the stockings on may help. Wearing examination gloves may make it easier to grip the stocking. As pregnancy progresses, the woman may find it increasingly difficult to apply the stockings herself and may require assistance with this. Graduated compression stockings should be washed and dried according to the manufacturer's instructions.

It should be clear to the woman when the wearing of the stockings should cease (often 6 weeks after caesarean section), but this may also be an individualised assessment. Post-thrombotic syndrome (the valves of the leg veins are less competent with pain, cellulitis, oedema and ulceration being persistent problems) can occur several years after a thrombosis and so wearing of the stockings is then indicated for some time.

ROLE AND RESPONSIBILITIES OF THE MIDWIFE

These can be summarised as:

- application of evidence-based best practice to prevent VTE in childbearing women
- advice, care, education and support of women with potential risk factors

- undertaking competent clinical care particularly in relation to anticoagulation prophylaxis and the application of graduated compression stockings
- referral as appropriate
- contemporaneous documentation.

Summary

- Thromboembolism is a major cause of maternal mortality; pregnancy alone is a risk factor, other risks include previous VTE, obesity and increased parity.
- Gentle foot and leg exercises, deep breathing, anticoagulation prophylaxis and the use of graduated compression stockings can all contribute to reducing the risk of VTE.

- Immobility and dehydration should be avoided whenever possible.
- Graduated compression stockings must be fitted and worn correctly to be effective.

SELF-ASSESSMENT EXERCISES

The answers to the following questions may be found in the text:

1. What measures can be taken to promote venous circulation?
2. Identify the women most at risk of VTE.
3. How would the midwife ensure that a below-knee compression stocking is the correct size?
4. Describe to a woman the correct way to undertake leg and breathing exercises.
5. What are the role and responsibilities of the midwife in relation to the prevention of thromboembolism in a woman with restricted mobility?

References

Brayshaw E, Wright P: *Teaching physical skills for the childbearing year*, Hale, 1994, Books for Midwives.

Drife J: Thrombosis and thromboembolism. In Lewis G, editor: *The confidential enquiry into maternal and child health (CEMACH) Savings mothers' lives: reviewing maternal deaths to make motherhood safer – 2003–2005*, The seventh report on confidential enquiries into maternal deaths in the United Kingdom, London, 2007, CEMACH, pp 55–69.

Elliott D, Pavord S: Thrombo-embolic disorders. In Robson E, Waugh J, editors: *Medical disorders in pregnancy*, Oxford, 2008, Blackwell Publishing, ch 15.

Lewis G, editor: *The confidential enquiry into maternal and child health (CEMACH). Savings mothers' lives: reviewing maternal deaths to make motherhood safer 2003–2005*, The seventh report on confidential enquiries into maternal deaths in the United Kingdom, London, 2007, CEMACH.

McColl M, Ramsay J, Tait R, et al: Risk factors for pregnancy associated venous thromboembolism, *Thromb Haemost* 78(4):1183–1188, 1997.

RCOG (Royal College of Obstetricians and Gynaecologists). *Thromboprophylaxis during pregnancy, labour and after vaginal delivery*, 2004, Guideline No. 37. Online Available: http://www.rcog.org.uk/, 1 April 2009.

Walker L, Lamont S: Graduated compression stockings to prevent deep vein thrombosis, *Nurs Stand* 22(40):35–38, 2008.

Principles of cardiopulmonary resuscitation: maternal resuscitation

CHAPTER CONTENTS

Maternal collapse is fortunately a rare but potentially catastrophic and fatal emergency. This chapter considers effective cardiopulmonary resuscitation for a childbearing woman. The reader is encouraged to read this chapter in conjunction with Chapter 56 (neonatal resuscitation) to compare and contrast the resuscitation skills.

LEARNING OUTCOMES

Having read this chapter the reader should be able to:

- discuss in detail the role and responsibilities of the midwife when resuscitating a pregnant woman
- describe the equipment and how it is used
- demonstrate/simulate a maternal resuscitation technique.

Resuscitation is the means by which life is supported in the event of sudden apnoea or cardiac arrest; cardiac is the most likely cause of arrest in the adult. In the absence of asphyxia, the level of oxygen within the blood is high and it is essential that the circulation is restored quickly and takes precedence over ventilation (Handley 2005). It is now recognised that resuscitation can be effective when high quality cardiac compressions are maintained with minimal delay or interruptions, even when respiratory assistance is not given, thus if the midwife is unable or unwilling to give rescue/ventilation breaths resuscitation can still be successful and cardiac compressions should be commenced as soon as possible.

In a maternity setting where women are healthy and undergoing a physiological process, collapse is both rare and unexpected. The potential for complications does exist, some of which can be life threatening or fatal (CEMD 2004); Lewis (2007) highlights the importance for all staff to have regular audited training to enable them to recognise and manage impending maternal collapse and improve their basic, immediate and advanced life support skills, as poor resuscitation skills were noted to be a feature in a high number of maternal deaths. There are two implications for the midwife:

- the skills of managing maternal cardiopulmonary resuscitation are rarely used
- the need to maintain these skills for use at a moment's notice remains a priority, wherever the arrest may occur (Nolan 1998).

Considerations for child bearing

Whilst resuscitation techniques are modified for the childbearing woman to accommodate the physiological body changes (Table 55.1) the principles are the same as for any other resuscitation. The crucial difference is that the fetus is also compromised, but the presence of the fetus with its additional circulation may further compromise the mother and make resuscitation more difficult. Successful resuscitation of the mother becomes the priority, such that an emergency caesarean section may be carried out swiftly in order to improve the success of the resuscitation, whatever the gestation of pregnancy (Mitchell 1995).

A fewer number of modifications will be required for a newly delivered woman, but some of the physiological changes will remain. Silent regurgitation of the stomach contents is still a possibility until progesterone levels have returned to their prepregnant state. Cricoid pressure (gentle downward pressure on the cricoid cartilage to occlude the oesophagus) or intubation is a valuable means of preventing regurgitation of the stomach contents and should be considered for a childbearing woman from the moment of collapse (Fig. 55.1).

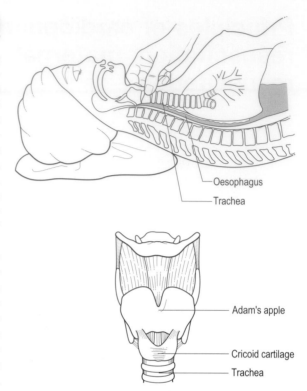

Oesophagus
Trachea

Adam's apple

Cricoid cartilage
Trachea

Figure 55.1 • Application of cricoid pressure (Adapted from Fraser & Cooper 2003)

Table 55.1 Pregnancy physiological differences and adaptation for resuscitation	
Physiological difference	**Resuscitation modification**
Gravid uterus: potential for massive internal concealed haemorrhage	Observations to detect haemorrhage. Prompt infusion using at least two wide bore cannulae, rapid request for cross-matched blood, stat. infusion I.V. fluid up to 2 L, but with careful fluid balance. Use of CVP monitoring
Additional circulation (maternal and fetal) causing increased cardiac workload	Caesarean section within 5 minutes if resuscitation not successful. Replace blood loss immediately
Aortocaval occlusion when supine	Wedge firmly to the left and manual displacement of the uterus
Splinting of diaphragm	May be harder to ventilate the lungs, requiring higher ventilatory pressures
Relaxation of cardiac sphincter of the stomach, silent regurgitation and aspiration of stomach contents a possibility	Application of cricoid pressure, use cuffed ET tube when intubated
Oedema of glottis, neck obesity, larger breasts	More difficult to intubate, call a skilled anaesthetist who is likely to be successful on the first attempt
Increased oxygen requirements	Begin resuscitation quickly using 100% oxygen

Anticipation and recognition of collapse

The midwife should be aware of the potential situations when apnoea and/or cardiac arrest may occur. These include:

- pulmonary embolism
- amniotic fluid embolism (anaphylactoid syndrome of pregnancy)
- massive ante- or postpartum haemorrhage
- eclampsia
- existing medical disorder, e.g. cardiac disorder, epilepsy
- trauma, e.g. road traffic accident
- drug toxicity, e.g. drug abuse, use of epidural or spinal analgesics, use of magnesium sulphate, general anaesthesia.

This is not an exhaustive list. Arrest can sometimes be averted by administering 100% oxygen, repositioning into a left lateral position, giving a bolus of intravenous (I.V.) fluid and then calling medical assistance.

Recognition of collapse

In the event of collapse, the midwife will make an assessment initially based on colour, movement, breathing and heart rate. There may be some variations according to the cause of the arrest, but generally the following features will be noted:

- colour: pale, cyanosed (heavily so if amniotic fluid embolism), clammy
- movement: no response to stimulation; midwife may have observed seizure or twitching immediately prior to arrest; woman will be slumped as if fainted
- breathing: absent, no rise and fall of the chest, no breath sounds heard or felt
- heart rate: absent (use major pulse, e.g. carotid (see p 38)).

Equipment

While some basic equipment is desirable, it is possible to complete a successful resuscitation without any equipment; however, the midwife usually has access to some equipment. Wherever the setting, protection from contact with body fluids is indicated by using facemasks rather than undertaking mouth-to-mouth resuscitation. Equipment should be checked regularly to ensure that it is present and working effectively. Cleaning and maintaining equipment is indicated according to manufacturers' instructions. A wedge is required for the pregnant woman; this should be firm enough to permit effective chest compression. Adaptations may be made in the home using books, files or other appropriate items.

Standard equipment includes:

- oxygen
- suction apparatus
- bag and facemask for ventilation (with oxygen reservoir) or pocket mask
- wedge
- Guedel airways, sizes 2 and 3
- resuscitation drugs
- stethoscope
- laryngoscope
- cuffed endotracheal (ET) tubes size 7–9 mm and 10 mL syringe
- introducer
- laryngeal mask airway
- connectors and bag for ventilator
- CVP line
- cannulae, I.V. lines and blood bottles
- defibrillator and cardiac monitor.

In hospital the equipment is usually stored on a trolley in an accessible place. The defibrillator should be plugged in so that it is always on charge but it has to be unplugged before the trolley can be moved! Defibrillation is only required to correct certain cardiac arrhythmias. In the event of it being used all personnel must stand away from the woman in order that they also do not receive an electric shock. Care must be taken if the defibrillator is used in a wet environment (e.g. a bathroom).

Initial assessment and actions

On finding a collapsed woman, the midwife should quickly assess the area to ensure there are no dangers to the midwife or to the woman (e.g. wet floor, wires from equipment). The midwife should approach the woman from the side and establish whether she is conscious by asking her if she is alright and firmly touching her shoulders. This should evoke a response; if none is forthcoming help should be sought immediately and resuscitative measures commenced.

An emergency call is sent instantly upon recognising that cardiac or respiratory arrest has occurred. The midwife should always be familiar with the quickest way to summon help: in the hospital setting, 2222 should be the specific emergency number (Soar & Spearpoint 2005); in the community it may be to telephone 999 (or 112 by mobile) and request paramedic assistance. The call should indicate where the arrest has occurred, including the name of the ward and specific location (e.g. first side room) or, if at home, the room the woman is in. It is important that the obstetric resuscitation team can gain entrance to the ward area; if the door is locked, ensure someone is ready to open the doors for them on their arrival. This applies equally in the community setting, where the front door should be left unlocked to enable the paramedic team to enter. The obstetric resuscitation team includes the obstetricians, anaesthetist, paediatricians, resuscitation officers, midwives and often porters (to transport equipment).

The woman should be turned onto her back, pillows removed (if present) and, if pregnant, a wedge positioned under the woman's right hip to displace the gravid uterus and minimise the risk of aortocaval compression. If a wedge is not available, a rolled up blanket or pillow can be used. This is easier to do with two people; however, if the midwife is on her own, Madams (2008) recommends placing both hands at the front and back of the woman's right knee, moving the knee forward and down to pull her hip forward. This creates space where the wedge, blanket or pillow can be placed so the woman's hip is held at an angle of 15–45° from the supine position. If additional staff are available, Kundra et al (2007) further advise manually displacing the uterus as both manoeuvres together effectively reduce the compression effect of the uterus.

Airway

Madams (2008) advises that the tongue is the main airway obstruction in collapsed or unconscious women during the intrapartum period. Opening the airway may be sufficient for the woman to re-establish respiration and prevent further compromise. Tilting the head backwards by applying pressure on the forehead with one hand and supporting the chin in position will facilitate this by positioning the head into a neutral position although a jaw thrust may be required (Madams 2008). Any obvious obstructions

seen within the mouth should be removed by suction, a finger sweep of the mouth should only be undertaken if there is an obvious obstruction seen that can be removed and no suction or Magill forceps are available. A finger sweep should not be undertaken blindly and inspection of the mouth should not take more than a few seconds. If there is concern about regurgitation of stomach contents in the pregnant unconscious woman, cricoid pressure should be applied when she is supine and maintained throughout the procedure or until intubation has occurred. Whilst there are three options for keeping the airway open, Madams (2008) recommends using a combination of chin support and jaw thrust with the head tilt, suggesting this is more effective in opening the pregnant woman's airway.

- Chin support: the midwife should place two/three fingers over the bony part of the tip of the chin, avoiding pressure on the soft tissues, and hold the chin in position.
- Jaw thrust: using both hands, the midwife should place two/three fingers either side of the bony part of the lower jaw to lift the lower jaw forwards. Avoid pressure on the soft tissues as this can occlude the airway.
- Use of oropharyngeal (Guedel) airway: if there is difficulty maintaining the chin support/jaw thrust while undertaking other resuscitation manoeuvres an appropriately sized airway (usually 2 or 3) inserted into the oropharynx will maintain the patency of the airway by pushing the tongue forwards, negating further manual assistance.

Airway size is assessed by holding the flange of the airway against the mid-point of the woman's lips, with the airway held horizontally so that the curved part of the airway curves around the woman's jaw; it should end at the angle of the jaw.

To insert the airway, the woman's head should be tilted backwards and the airway held in the inverted position, i.e. the opposite way up to its final position within the oropharynx, to allow the curved part of the airway to depress the tongue, preventing it from being pushed backwards. The airway is inserted following the curve of the woman's airway. As it reaches the junction of the hard and soft palate, the airway should be rotated 180° to turn it to the correct position while continuing to move it further into the mouth. When the airway is lying in the oropharynx the flange should sit between the woman's teeth. The tilted, neutral head position should be maintained and chin support given as required. The position of the airway should be assessed intermittently to ensure it has not been dislodged. If the woman begins to breathe, oxygen should be administered.

Breathing

When the airway is clear, breathing may follow spontaneously. To assess whether the woman is breathing, the midwife's head should be positioned close to the woman's head. This will ensure the midwife's eyeline is in line with the woman's chest so that chest movement can be looked and felt for. The midwife may also feel the woman's breath on her face when this close to the woman's nose and mouth. If the midwife is experienced in palpating the carotid pulse, this can be undertaken at the same time as assessing for breathing and should not take longer than 10 seconds.

If no effective breathing is seen cardiac compressions should be commenced before commencing ventilating the lungs (Handley 2005). However, if no-one has responded to the request for help, the midwife should summon help before moving on to cardiac compression. This may involve her leaving the woman to make a phone call or ring the emergency buzzer. As cardiac compressions are very tiring and can quickly lead to exhaustion on the part of the resuscitator, it is important that help is on its way. Frequent swapping of staff (every 2 minutes)

undertaking cardiac compression is recommended to avoid fatigue and maintain a high level of perfusion for the woman (Soar & Spearpoint 2005).

Circulation: cardiac compression

The hands should be placed in the middle of the lower half of the sternum with one hand placed over the other and the fingers interlocked (Fig. 55.2). With both arms straight, the midwife should lean over the woman from the left side, depress the sternum 4–5 cm towards her spine and then release the pressure (maintaining the hand position over the sternum). This is repeated until 30 chest compressions are completed and is then followed by two ventilation breaths. The compression and release of the chest should take the same length of time and the midwife should aim to achieve 100 compressions per minute. Chest compression and ventilation are continued at a rate of 30 : 2. If ventilation breaths cannot be given, cardiac compressions should continue uninterrupted (Handley 2005). Stringer et al (2007), whilst discussing the American Heart Association resuscitation guidelines, advise that uninterrupted cardiac compressions should be 'hard and fast' to get the correct depth and rate as over 50% of cardiac compressions undertaken are too shallow and do not deliver sufficient blood to the vital organs. Furthermore if compressions are interrupted, blood flow stops completely.

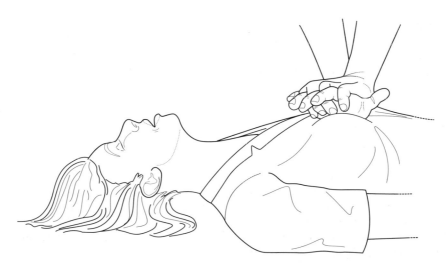

Figure 55.2 • Cardiac compression (Adapted with kind permission from Peattie & Walker 1995)

Ventilation breaths

Ventilation of the lungs is achieved by the use of a facemask which should have a deformable rim that fits snugly around the woman's mouth and nose when even pressure is applied to form an airtight seal. The correct size should be used so that it does not extend over the end of the chin or into the eye sockets. Fingertips are used to support the jaw and seal off the mask (grasping under the chin will also occlude the airway). An airtight seal is essential to ensure adequate ventilation, and the head should be maintained in the neutral position.

The facemask can be attached to a self inflating bag–valve–mask (BVM) system and oxygen attached as soon as possible (Madams 2008). If using a BVM, the blow-off valve should be tested before use by occluding the outlet and squeezing the bag. As the pressure rises, the blow-off valve makes a noise that confirms it is working and is safe for use. A good seal is needed from the mask; the bag is squeezed for one second (the valve will begin to blow when the correct pressure is reached) and the chest should rise as air enters the lungs (Soar & Spearpoint 2005). It can be difficult to see the chest rise with some pregnant women particularly in the latter weeks of pregnancy. In this instance the midwife should look for lateral chest and/or breast movement as an indication of lung inflation. The bag is then released to refill and the process repeated until two ventilation breaths have been given. Stinger et al (2007) suggest that prolonged ventilation breaths increase the likelihood of gastric inflation whilst taking valuable time that is needed for cardiac compressions.

This technique can be difficult for one person to manage as keeping the head and mask in position while squeezing the bag can be complex and requires practice. Ideally one person will hold the mask and head while another squeezes the bag (Fig. 55.3). The person supporting the airway should ensure that the chest rises with each inflation (see above).

A pocket mask can also be used and should be placed over the nose and mouth with the head in the neutral position and the jaw pulled upwards and forwards. The midwife blows through the opening on the pocket mask to inflate the lungs (a normal expiratory breath of approximately 400–600 mL) (Fig. 55.4).

Alternatively, mouth-to-mouth resuscitation can be undertaken if no other equipment is available and the midwife is comfortable doing this; however, this increases the risk of coming into contact with bodily fluids. The nose should be pinched with the thumb and forefinger to prevent air escaping through the nasal passages. The midwife should then place her mouth over the woman's mouth with a good seal and blow into her lungs as for the pocket mask. If mouth-to-mouth is not undertaken and no other means of inflating the lungs are present, the midwife should continue with cardiac compressions until help arrives with additional equipment.

If no chest movement is seen, the head and mask position should be checked and corrected, obvious

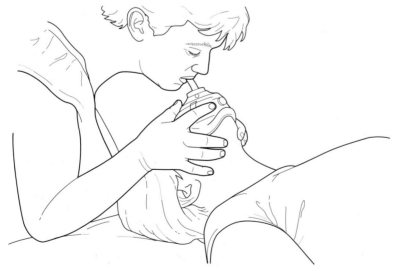

Figure 55.3 • Bag–valve–mask ventilation using two resuscitators

Figure 55.4 • Using a Laerdal pocket mask

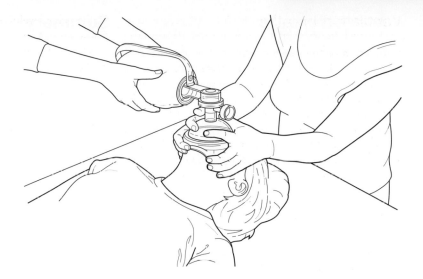

obstructions removed and the two ventilation breaths reattempted after the next set of cardiac compressions.

Additional measures

As further personnel and equipment arrive to assist with the resuscitation, a senior member of the emergency team will take overall control of the resuscitation and will make the decisions, usually the anaesthetist. The Shock Advisory Defibrillator (AED) should be attached whilst cardiac compressions continue and the verbal instructions followed (Davies 2005). If defibrillation occurs it is important everyone stands clear from the woman to avoid unnecessary shocks to themselves.

Other personnel can be usefully deployed to cannulate and commence fluid boluses of crystalloids or colloids. Drugs will be administered as requested; adrenaline (epinephrine) is often the drug of choice, but sodium bicarbonate and atropine may also be used. Such drugs are usually issued in a 'ready to administer' form. The midwife must be familiar with these and their dosages, mode of action and side effects.

At this point the midwife becomes less involved with the active resuscitation but has an important role to play in the care of the woman's family, preparation for theatre and documenting the events and times, drugs, etc.

If the woman is pregnant an emergency caesarean section is usually undertaken quickly to increase the chances of successful resuscitation (Stringer et al 2007); resuscitation should continue while surgery is happening. Castle (2009) advises that the equipment should be brought to where the woman is to undertake the caesarean section to save time rather than transferring her to the operating theatre and that the sterility adhered to within the theatre setting will not be possible.

If successful it is likely that the woman will be cared for in an intensive care unit until such time as she is able to be transferred back to maternity care. If unsuccessful, the senior member of the resuscitation team will decide at which point the resuscitation is abandoned. This is often in consultation with other members of the team.

PROCEDURE: maternal resuscitation

- Recognise the arrest and assess the situation for any potential dangers.
- Assess the level of responsiveness.
- If unresponsive, call for emergency assistance.
- Turn the woman on her back with a wedge under her right side and tilt her head back to the neutral position.
- Ensure the airway is open, using chin support, jaw thrust and/or an oropharyngeal airway as necessary, and remove obvious obstructions.
- Apply cricoid pressure until intubation has occurred (see Fig. 55.1) if required.

- Assess breathing and carotid pulse (if practised in this technique) taking no more than 10 seconds.
- If not breathing, commence cardiac compression at a rate of 100 beats per minute (bpm).
- After every 30 cardiac compressions, undertake two ventilation breaths where possible and maintain the rate at 30 : 2.
- Continue with resuscitation until spontaneous respiration or movement seen, or until told to stop by the senior person present (or if too exhausted to continue and there is no one to take over from you).
- If after 5 minutes there is minimal success, preparation should begin for caesarean section (if pregnant).
- Participate within the multidisciplinary team.
- Maintain detailed records of all actions taken.

Summary

- The skills of maternal resuscitation are rarely needed, but are skills that should be practised and adapted according to venue and available equipment.
- Cardiac compressions are the most important component of resuscitation and should be uninterrupted. Whilst two ventilation breaths are given after 30 compressions, this is not essential.
- Adaptations are required when resuscitating a pregnant woman due to the physiological changes of pregnancy that make resuscitation more difficult: a wedge and/or manual displacement of the uterus, cricoid pressure and preparation for caesarean section within 5 minutes.

ROLE AND RESPONSIBILITIES OF THE MIDWIFE

These can be summarised as:

- responses to avert the collapse if possible
- swift recognition and response in the event of arrest
- familiarization with resuscitation techniques, including adaptations for the pregnant woman
- familiarization with equipment, its use and maintenance
- awareness of other aspects of care, e.g. care of the family
- appropriate team work
- consultation with others, e.g. risk manager, supervisor of midwives, especially if resuscitation is unsuccessful
- detailed contemporaneous records.

SELF-ASSESSMENT EXERCISES

The answers to the following questions may be found in the text:

1. State a rationale for each of the necessary adaptations when resuscitating a pregnant woman.
2. List the essential equipment required and indicate how and when each piece would be used.
3. Describe, in order, the actions taken when finding a woman in a state of collapse.
4. Draw a diagram to indicate the correct positioning of the hands for chest compression and discuss how this is undertaken in practice.
5. Discuss how effective lung ventilation may be achieved.
6. Summarise the role and responsibilities of the midwife when resuscitating a pregnant woman.

References

Castle N: Neonatal and maternal resuscitation. In Chapman V, Charles C, editors: *The midwife's labour and birth handbook*, ed 2, Oxford, 2009, Blackwell Publishing Ltd.

CEMD: *Why mothers die. The Confidential Enquiries into Maternal Deaths in the United Kingdom 2000–2004*, London, 2004, RCOG Press.

Davies S: Resuscitation Council (UK) Guidelines, 2005: In *The use of automated external defibrillators*, 2005. Online. Available: http://www.resus.org.uk/pages/aed.pdf, 6 April 2009.

Fraser DM, Cooper MA, editors: *Myles textbook for midwives*, ed 14, Edinburgh, 2003, Churchill Livingstone.

Handley A: Resuscitation Council (UK) Guidelines, 2005: In *Adult Basic Life Support*, 2005. Online. Available: http://www.resus.org.uk/pages/bls.pdf, 6 April 2009.

Kundra P, Khanna S, Habeebullah S, et al: Manual displacement of the uterus during caesarean section, *Anaesthesia* 62(5):460–465, 2007.

Lewis G, editor: *The confidential enquiry into maternal and child health (CEMACH), Saving mothers' lives: reviewing maternal deaths to make motherhood safer – 2003–2005*, The seventh report on confidential enquiries into maternal deaths in the United Kingdom, London, 2007, CEMACH.

Madams M: Maternal resuscitation; how to resuscitate mothers who die, *Br J Midwifery* 16(6):372–375, 2008.

Mitchell L: Cardiac arrest during pregnancy: maternal–fetal physiology and advanced cardiac life support for the obstetric patient, *Crit Care Nurse* 15(1):56–60, 1995.

Nolan J: The 1998 European Resuscitation Council guidelines for adult single rescuer basic life support, *Br Med J* 319(7148): 1870–1876, 1998.

Peattie PI, Walker S: *Understanding nursing care*, ed 4, Edinburgh, 1995, Churchill Livingstone.

Soar J, Spearpoint K: Resuscitation Council (UK) Guidelines, 2005: In *In-hospital resuscitation*, 2005. Online. Available: http://www.resus. org.uk/pages/inhresus.pdf, 6 April 2009.

Stringer M, Mack Brooks P, King K, et al: New guidelines for maternal and neonatal resuscitation, *J Obstet Gynecol Neonatal Nurs* 36(6): 624–635, 2007.

Principles of cardiopulmonary resuscitation: neonatal resuscitation

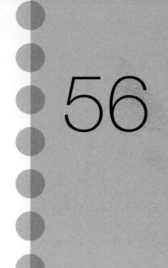

56

CHAPTER CONTENTS

Resuscitating the baby incorporates some of the fundamental principles used when resuscitating an adult but requires a different approach. However, the predisposing factors may be very different, often because the baby has not yet established respiration in the extrauterine environment. The aim of neonatal resuscitation is to initiate or sustain extrauterine life, limiting any cerebral damage.

This chapter focuses on recognition and action, suggested equipment and the midwife's role and responsibilities. The reader is encouraged to compare and contrast the care given when resuscitating an adult (see Chapter 55).

LEARNING OUTCOMES

Having read this chapter the reader should be able to:

- discuss in detail the role and responsibilities of the midwife prior to, during and following a neonatal resuscitation
- describe the signs that indicate that resuscitation is required
- describe the equipment and how it is used
- demonstrate/simulate a neonatal resuscitation technique, discussing how effective resuscitation is achieved.

Anticipation

The midwife may recognise the potential for neonatal compromise according to the known maternal or fetal risk factors. Such examples include:

- maternal disease, e.g. hypertension, diabetes mellitus
- maternal substance abuse
- previous poor obstetric or neonatal history, e.g. previous stillbirth, neonatal death
- known malpresentation, e.g. breech
- fetal abnormality
- prematurity
- prolonged rupture of membranes
- abnormalities of the fetal heartbeat indicative of fetal compromise

- fresh meconium within the amniotic fluid
- heavy maternal sedation
- precipitate delivery
- instrumental or operative delivery, especially under general anaesthetic
- obstetric emergency, e.g. prolapsed cord, antepartum haemorrhage, shoulder dystocia, eclampsia.

However, the need for neonatal resuscitation can occur without any warning, predisposing factors or obvious cause thus emphasising the importance for all midwives to be trained in and practise the skills of neonatal resuscitation. The presence of two midwives at delivery (wherever the venue) is a safeguard that allows one to care for the woman, and the other to begin resuscitation of the baby. However, the first element of resuscitation must be to call for appropriate assistance. The midwife must know how to do this, whether in hospital or in the community. In hospital it may be one emergency number to ring; in the community the paramedic service may be called using 999 (or if on a mobile with little/no signal 112) and the midwife must be familiar with their local arrangements.

A baby may require resuscitating at other times in the postnatal period; the fundamental principles of resuscitation apply in the same way. Examples include:

- occlusion of the airway, e.g. choking, feeding problems or mucus
- undetected congenital abnormality
- retained effects of respiratory depression after the effect of naloxone has subsided
- infection.

Pathophysiology of asphyxia

Asphyxia occurs when there is insufficient oxygen and excessive carbon dioxide and lactic acid in the blood. The consequence of this is a failure to breathe, which ultimately causes the baby's metabolism to shift from aerobic to anaerobic respiration. A metabolic acidosis is created. An anoxic baby may be in any one of four phases, depending on the level of intrauterine hypoxia:

1. hyperventilation
2. primary apnoea
3. gasping
4. terminal apnoea.

It is rarely possible to assess at birth which of these phases the baby is in. It is necessary to respond and then to assess the measures of progress.

Equipment

Resuscitation can be successfully completed with a minimal amount of equipment, in any environment, whether home or hospital. In the hospital environment it is likely that a standard resuscitaire with additional equipment will be available. At home a chest of drawers or table may be utilised, but care should be taken to avoid draughts.

Ideal requirements include:

- a flat surface
- towels and gloves (somewhere to wash hands if time permits)
- food-grade plastic wrapping (for preterm babies <30 weeks)
- a radiant heater
- a clock, with a second hand
- stethoscope
- oxygen/air source with flow regulation, reservoir and adjustable pressure relief valve (these should be checked prior to the delivery to ensure they are working correctly)
- T-tube or self-inflating resuscitation bag with valve and assorted size facemasks 00, 01
- Guedel airways sizes 0, 00, 000
- laryngoscopes (with spare bulbs and batteries)
- tracheal tubes, introducers and connectors
- suction apparatus with tubing and catheters
- drugs
- needles, syringes, scissors, tape, other extras, e.g. umbilical catheterisation pack.

Adaptation for the home includes a basic portable kit that can be utilised effectively. Maddy (1998) provides such an example, where suction, ventilation and oxygen apparatus for both the woman and baby are contained within one bag.

If resuscitation is anticipated the equipment should be prepared in advance of the delivery so that the baby can be delivered onto warmed towels, taken to a resuscitation area with a good heat and light source and where equipment is readily to hand. If resuscitation is unexpected this preparation occurs concurrently with the resuscitative measures used.

Principles of resuscitation

The principles are summed up as ABCD: airway, breathing, circulation, drugs. However, for the newly delivered wet, hypoxic baby, the principles begin with the need to dry thoroughly (except for premature babies <30 weeks gestation), remove the wet towel and cover the baby while assessing the colour, tone, breathing and heart rate of the baby, calling for appropriate help and noting the time (if a stopwatch is available, this should be started at the time of birth or at the beginning of the resuscitation period).

Drying the baby provides tactile stimulation and reduces further heat loss and hypoxia. It is important to discard the wet towel and wrap the baby in a warm dry towel. This measure should be undertaken immediately and as the baby is being transferred to the resuscitation area. Babies who are born prematurely (30 weeks and below) should be placed under a radiant heater without being dried and the head and body covered in food-grade plastic wrapping, leaving the face exposed. This has been found to be the most effective way for their body temperature to be maintained (Resuscitation Council UK 2005).

As this is being undertaken the midwife should assess the baby, taking into account the colour of the trunk, lips and tongue, muscle tone, respiratory pattern and heart rate. Blue hands and feet should never be mistaken for cyanosis in the newborn; assessment of cyanosis should be made by observing the baby centrally, even when the baby has pigmented skin. The mucous membranes (inside of the lips), tongue and trunk are alternative sites to assess. The heart rate is assessed by listening with a stethoscope and not by palpating the umbilical cord which can be unreliable. Mildly hypoxic babies usually respond well to drying; if the colour and tone are good, the baby is breathing regularly with a heart rate above 100 beats per minute, no further measures are required and the baby can be returned to his mother. However, if this is not the case, further resuscitation and assistance are required.

Airway

The airway must be open to facilitate air entry into the lungs. Loss of pharyngeal tone can occur in the floppy baby, causing the tongue to fall back and occlude the airway. To prevent this, the baby's head is placed in a neutral position, causing it neither to flex nor to extend. The prominent occiput can cause the neck to flex; to minimise this a folded towel approximately 2 cm in depth should be placed under the shoulders of the baby to bring the head and neck in alignment to keep the trachea straight (Fig. 56.1). Further support may be required in the floppy baby with the use of chin support or jaw thrust to maintain the upward and outward position of the chin. After each manoeuvre, the midwife should reassess the baby (colour, tone, breathing, heart rate) as the baby may begin to breathe spontaneously when the airway is open.

Chin support

The midwife should place a finger over the bony part of the tip of the chin, avoiding pressure on the soft tissues and hold the chin in position.

Jaw thrust

Where there is little or no tone, the midwife may need to place one or two fingers on either side of

Figure 56.1 • Neutral position

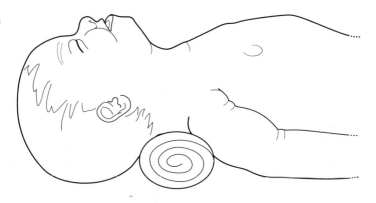

the lower jaw (at the angle of the jaw and avoiding soft tissues) to push the jaw outwards and forwards.

Tracheal suction

If the midwife is concerned that the airway is blocked, a direct visual assessment can be undertaken using a laryngoscope. A suction catheter should not be used unless the area is seen first and a blockage visualised, as inadvertent stimulation of the posterior pharynx and larynx with the suction catheter can result in severe vagal bradycardia, quickly exacerbating the situation. Although meconium can cause tracheal obstruction, routine suctioning is not recommended for babies born through meconium-stained liquor. Only someone experienced with intubation should undertake tracheal suction.

Use of oropharyngeal (Guedel) airway

This may be required when the baby has an abnormality of the face or mouth (e.g. cleft palate, micrognathia) or when there is difficulty maintaining the chin support/jaw thrust while undertaking other resuscitation manoeuvres. An appropriately sized airway (0, 00 or 000) inserted into the oropharynx will maintain the patency of the airway by pushing the tongue forwards, negating further manual assistance.

Airway size is assessed by holding the flange of the airway against the mid-point of the baby's lips, with the airway held horizontally so that the curved part of the airway curves around the baby's jaw; it should end at the angle of the jaw.

To insert the airway, hold the airway in the position it will sit within the oropharynx. Open the baby's mouth by depressing the chin and slide the airway over the baby's tongue, avoiding pushing the tongue backwards. The airway should slide easily into position. A laryngoscope can also be used to depress the tongue during airway insertion.

Breathing

When the airway is clear, breathing may follow spontaneously. If no effective breathing is seen, it is important to fill the lungs with air or oxygen as quickly as possible, usually via a facemask. Prior to the first breath, the baby's lungs are filled with fluid; physiologically the pressure required to inflate the lungs for the first time is higher than with subsequent breaths. Once the alveoli have been inflated, the presence of surfactant maintains the inflation. Inflation breaths are used to assist with removing the lung fluid; these are followed by ventilation breaths.

Practically this means that if mechanically ventilating the lungs the initial pressures should be 30 cmH$_2$O lasting 2–3 seconds for the first five inflation breaths. This is as effective as using a higher pressure for a shorter period and easier to achieve. The chest may not rise effectively until much of the fluid has been expelled from the lungs, usually within the fourth to fifth inflation breath.

If no chest movement is seen with the first set of inflation breaths, then the midwife should ensure that both the neutral position and the airway are correct, using methods described above, and repeat the five inflation breaths.

Facemask

The ideal facemask is circular with a deformable rim that will fit snugly around the baby's mouth and nose when even pressure is applied to form an airtight seal. The correct size should be used (00 or 01) and should not extend over the end of the chin or into the eye sockets (Fig. 56.2). Fingertips are used to support the jaw and seal off the mask (grasping under the chin will also occlude the airway). An airtight seal is essential to ensure adequate ventilation, and the head should be maintained in the neutral position. Care must be taken not to apply excessive

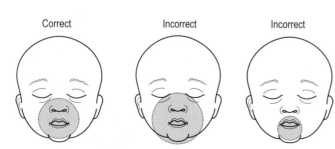

Correct	Incorrect	Incorrect
✔	✗	✗

Figure 56.2 • Correct positioning of the facemask (Adapted with kind permission from RCPCH, RCOG 1997)

pressure as this can result in facial bruising or mould the back of the head (Wood et al 2008).

The facemask can be attached to a T-piece connected to a supply of oxygen or air (with a pressure dial and pressure release valve to ensure correct pressures used) (Fig. 56.3) or attached to a self-inflating bag–valve–mask (BVM) system.

When using a T-piece to inflate the lungs, the open end is occluded by the resuscitator's thumb (the fingers are usually keeping the facemask in position) for 2–3 seconds then removed for the five inflation breaths and occluded and removed at a rate of 30 breaths per minute for the ventilation breaths.

If using a BVM, the blow-off valve should be tested before use by occluding the outlet and squeezing the bag. As the pressure rises, the blow-off valve makes a noise that confirms it is working and is safe for use. The principles of using BVM are similar to the T-piece in that a good seal is needed from the mask; the bag is squeezed slowly to produce a pressure of $30\,cmH_2O$ for 2–3 seconds (the valve will begin to blow when the correct pressure is reached). The bag is then released to refill and repeated until five inflation breaths have been given.

If the midwife has no equipment available, she can use mouth-to-mouth breathing. The baby's head should be in the neutral position and the airway patent. The baby's mouth and nose are sealed with the midwife's mouth and air from the midwife's cheeks is gently breathed into the lungs to provide inflation then ventilation breaths.

With effective ventilation the chest can be seen to rise. If this does not occur, the airway should be reassessed to ensure it is patent, and the position of the facemask/mouth should be reassessed to ensure there is an airtight seal, and the five inflation breaths repeated.

Following the five inflation breaths the colour, tone, respiratory effort and heart rate should be reassessed.

With effective ventilation the heart rate usually increases within 20–30 seconds as the baby responds to the resuscitation. If the heart rate increases and chest movement is achieved with the inflation breaths, the midwife should continue to provide ventilatory support via ventilation breaths at around 30 breaths per minute until the baby is able to breathe unaided. If spontaneous respiration does not occur, the presence of other complications should be considered and treated (e.g. effect of maternal opioid/drugs, neurological compromise) by the paediatrician. Assessment of the colour, tone, respiratory effort and heart rate should be undertaken following every 30 ventilation breaths. In practice the colour, tone and respiratory effort are usually assessed continually during the procedure and the manoeuvres adjusted according to the response shown by the baby to the resuscitation measures used.

If, during ventilatory support, chest movement reduces or the heart rate decreases, the midwife should reassess the airway to ensure it is still patent and the seal on the mask is still airtight. The eyeline of the midwife should be level with the baby's chest to visualise the chest movements more easily. The midwife's position should be adjusted to facilitate this.

If the heart rate has not increased quickly despite effective inflation and ventilation breaths, cardiac compression is necessary.

Circulation

Prior to commencing chest compression, the midwife should ensure that:

- the baby's head and jaw are in the correct position
- the mask is the correct size, with a good seal against the face
- the air/oxygen supply is working
- the inflation breaths have been given correctly.

Figure 56.3 • T-piece and mask

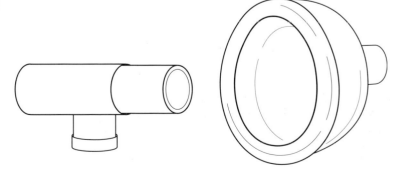

It is easier to undertake chest compressions with two people, but if help is not immediately available, the midwife should continue on her own.

The most effective method of compressing the chest is to hold the baby's chest with both hands, placing the fingers over the spine and the thumbs together on the sternum just below an imaginary line between the nipples (Fig. 56.4). It is important to avoid pressing on soft tissue or the ribs as this will result in ineffective chest compression and damage, which may exacerbate the situation. This two-handed method is thought to produce higher peak systolic and coronary pressure compared with the one-handed method (AHA & AAP 2006).

A less effective method of chest compression is to use the index and middle fingers positioned centrally on the sternum immediately beneath the imaginary line (Fig. 56.5). The other hand should be used to support the baby's back. This method is used where there is only one person undertaking the resuscitation and may be preferable to the two-handed technique when an umbilical catheter is being inserted as it provides better access to the umbilicus (AHA & AAP 2006).

The chest is compressed quickly and firmly to a depth of one-third of the anteroposterior diameter of the chest (1–2 cm). Time must be allowed for the chest to re-expand after each compression to enable the heart to refill.

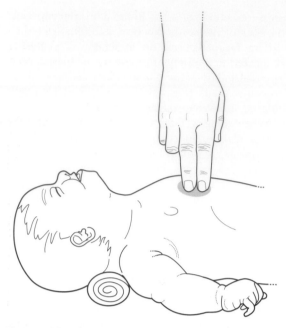

Figure 56.5 • One-handed chest compression

It is important that effective ventilation of the lungs continues and that the cardiac compression is synchronised with it. The synchronised rate is three compressions to one ventilation (3 : 1). In a 6-second period three cycles should be completed (a heart rate of approximately 90 beats per minute; bpm) but this may be difficult to sustain. Where two people work together, one of them should count aloud to maintain concentration.

The heart rate usually responds rapidly to effective ventilation and chest compressions. The midwife should recheck the heart rate every 30 seconds to determine if there is a response. Chest compressions should be stopped when the heart rate is responding but ventilation continued until the baby is breathing spontaneously.

Should the heart rate not respond, despite correct ventilation and compressions, drug therapy and transfer to a high-dependency unit may be required.

Drug therapy

Prescription and administration of drugs in this setting is the responsibility of the paediatrician who may administer them via an umbilical catheter. The midwife may assist in the checking and drawing up of such drugs, although many are pre-prepared. Drugs commonly required are sodium bicarbonate

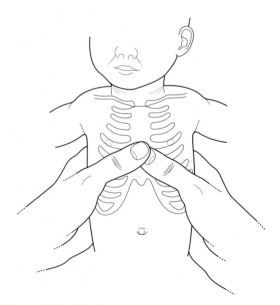

Figure 56.4 • Two-handed chest compression

4.2% (1–2 mmol/kg), adrenaline (epinephrine) 1 : 10 000 (10 µg/kg) (this can be administered via the tracheal tube) and dextrose 10% (250 mg/kg). If a volume expander is needed, a bolus dose of 10 mL/kg 0.9% saline may be given.

After the resuscitation

A successful resuscitation may mean that the baby will either remain with his parents or, if unwell, be transferred to neonatal intensive care. Body temperature should be maintained and feeding is essential due to the use of glucose during anaerobic respiration. The parents will need support and information to understand what has occurred and to appreciate whether any further dangers exist. The midwife will document all of the resuscitation details including the time the emergency call was made and when staff arrived, time of onset of respiration, nature of resuscitation, drugs administered and personnel present.

If the resuscitation is unsuccessful the paediatrician will make the decision to halt the resuscitation. Local protocols will vary, but it may be discontinued after 10 minutes without a heart rate but with full resuscitation support during that time (Resuscitation Council UK 2005). Considerable care of the parents will be required. The staff involved are also encouraged to gain support for themselves; the risk manager or supervisor of midwives may be instrumental in this.

PROCEDURE: neonatal resuscitation

- Move the baby to the resuscitation area. At the same time:
  - assess the colour, tone, respiratory effort and heart rate
  - send out an emergency call for appropriate personnel (if an anticipated problem the paediatrician should already be present)
  - set the clock and note the time
  - switch on the heater and light if not undertaken prior to delivery.
- Dry the baby thoroughly and remove the damp towel; wrap in a clean warm towel, with the chest exposed.
- Position the baby's head in the neutral position (see Fig. 56.1).
- Assess the colour, tone, respiration rate and heart rate (these are reassessed every 30 seconds):

  - if pink, with a heart rate >100 bpm and breathing spontaneously, keep the baby warm and return him to his parents
  - if breathing irregularly (shallow or slow), but a heart rate >100 bpm, provide tactile stimulation, keep the baby warm and the head in the neutral position. Continue to assess the colour, tone, respiratory effort and heart rate, returning the baby to his parents when breathing spontaneously, with good colour, tone and heart rate
  - if no response from the actions described above, or if there is no respiratory effort:
    - ensure a neutral position and an open airway, using chin support, jaw thrust or an oropharyngeal airway as necessary
    - inflate the lungs using a facemask and T-piece or BVM system, providing five effective inflation breaths and looking for chest movement. If no chest movement is seen, check head position and repeat inflation breaths
    - after effective inflation breaths assess the heart rate using a stethoscope to auscultate the heart beat. Count for 6 seconds then multiply by 10 to calculate the beats per minute. Where more than one person is involved in the resuscitation, the heart rate should be tapped out so that everyone is aware of the rate
    - continue ventilation breaths until spontaneous respiration occurs if the heart rate is more than 100 bpm. Reassess the colour, tone, respiratory effort and heart rate following every 30 ventilation breaths (continue the ventilation while counting the heart rate)
    - if the heart rate is decreasing or is below 60 bpm commence chest compression with ventilation at a rate of 3 : 1
    - reassess the heart rate every 30 seconds (while continuing ventilatory support) and stop chest compressions when the heart rate is above 60 bpm and increasing. Colour, tone and respiratory effort are assessed throughout the resuscitation. Ventilatory support is stopped when the baby is breathing adequately without assistance.

Resuscitation is summarised in Figure 56.6.

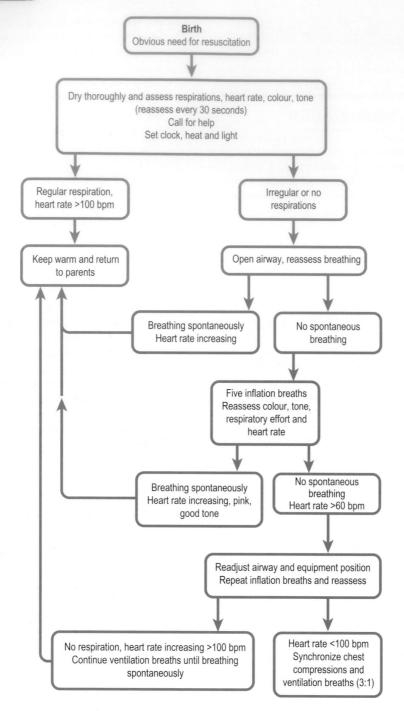

Figure 56.6 • Summary of neonatal resuscitation

ROLE AND RESPONSIBILITIES OF THE MIDWIFE

These can be summarised as:

- anticipation of potential problems and preparation of the environment and equipment
- recognition of the need to resuscitate
- competent resuscitation skills, including correct use of equipment and maintenance of the skill (regular updates and practice)
- recognition of the need to call for appropriate medical/newborn life support (NLS) trained assistance
- ability to support and assist the person called
- accurate contemporaneous record keeping
- information for, and support of, the parents during and following the event
- appropriate transfer of the care of the woman and baby
- familiarity with local resuscitation protocols.

Summary

- The midwife has a responsible role in the recognition and management of neonatal resuscitation. Equipment should be accessible and the midwife should be familiar with its use.
- Appropriate help should be sought quickly. Management includes drying the baby (>30 weeks) and assessing colour, tone, respiratory effort and heart rate. Manoeuvres to open the airway, ventilate the lungs and chest compression should be undertaken efficiently when required. Drug therapy may be required when the response is poor.

SELF-ASSESSMENT EXERCISES

The answers to the following questions may be found in the text:

1. How is the need to resuscitate a baby recognised?
2. Which predisposing conditions may alert the midwife to the need to prepare for resuscitation?
3. List the equipment required for neonatal resuscitation, indicating how each piece is used.
4. What measures can the midwife take to ensure the airway is open?
5. If a baby has a heart rate of 60 bpm, is pale and is gasping, what action should be taken?
6. List the responsibilities of the midwife:
   a. when anticipating the need to resuscitate
   b. during a neonatal resuscitation situation
   c. following a successful resuscitation
   d. following an unsuccessful resuscitation.
7. Demonstrate/simulate a neonatal resuscitation, giving verbal explanations for the actions taken.

References

AHA, AAP (American Heart Association, American Academy of Pediatrics) 2006: American Heart Association (AHA) Guidelines for Cardiopulmonary Resuscitation (CPR) and Emergency Cardiovascular Care (ECC) of Pediatric and Neonatal Patients: Neonatal Resuscitation Guidelines, *Pediatrics* 117:1029–1038, 2005.

Maddy B: The vital components of a resuscitation kit, *Br J Midwifery* 6(4):256–258, 1998

RCPCH, RCOG (Royal College of Paediatrics and Child Health, Royal College of Obstetricians and Gynaecologists): *Resuscitation of babies at birth*, London, 1997, BMJ Publishing Group.

Resuscitation Council (UK): *Resuscitation guidelines Newborn life support*, London, 2005, Resuscitation Council (UK).

Wood FE, Morley CJ, Dawson JA, et al: Improved techniques reduce face mask leak during simulated neonatal resuscitation: study 2, *Arch Dis Child Fetal Neonatal Ed* 93(3): F230–F234, 2008.

Abduction Movement away from the midline of the body

Adduction Movement towards the midline of the body

Agglutination Clumping together

Aortocaval occlusion Occlusion of the inferior vena cava and aorta by the pregnant uterus. Tends to occur if a heavily pregnant woman is asked to lie flat. Avoided by adopting a lateral position or using a wedge under the right hip. Also known as supine hypotension

Apical The apex of the heart

Apnoea Absence of respiration for >20 seconds

Bacteriuria The presence of bacteria in the urine

Bilirubinuria The presence of bilirubin in the urine

Biparietal diameter The distance between the parietal eminences, usually 9.5 cm in the term baby. This is the widest transverse diameter of the fetal skull to pass through the pelvic brim (during engagement) and to distend the perineum (during crowning)

Bishop's Score A scoring assessment used to assess the favourability (or ripeness) of the cervix prior to induction of labour. Considers the position, consistency, length and dilatation of the cervix and station of the presenting part within the pelvis. Each factor is awarded a score accordingly; the dose of Prostin may be adjusted according to the total score. A Bishop's Score of 6 or more considers the cervix to be favourable

Blanching Colour changes in the skin with fingertip pressure, turning the skin white. The colour should quickly return to normal as capillary refill occurs

Bradycardia A slow heart rate, <60 bpm for an adult, <80 for a baby

Constipation Infrequent or difficult defecation resulting from decreased motility of the intestines, which results in faeces remaining in the colon for prolonged periods. This extended time in the colon means that greater than usual amounts of water are absorbed, making the faeces hard and dry. Constipation can be caused by improper bowel habits, spasms of the colon, insufficient bulk in the diet, lack of exercise and emotions

Cyanosis Bluish appearance of skin and mucous membranes caused by reduced oxygenation

Cystocoele Bulging of the bladder into the upper part of the anterior vaginal wall

Denominator The leading part of the fetus, likely to meet the pelvic floor first. For a flexed vertex presentation it is the occiput, for the buttocks it is the sacrum

Diarrhoea Frequent defecation of liquid faeces caused by increased motility of the intestines. There is not enough time for absorption and it can lead to dehydration and electrolyte imbalance. Diarrhoea has several causes, e.g. infection, stress. Diarrhoea overflow may also occur in the presence of constipation

Diuresis Increased formation and excretion of urine

Dysuria Difficult or painful micturition

Erythema Redness

Erythema toxicum A blotchy red rash, sometimes with yellowish pinhead papules, which occurs usually between days 2 and 8 of age. Cause unknown, no treatment required

Extravasation Escape of fluid from the vessels into the surrounding tissues

Extubation Removal of the tube inserted during intubation

Fetal lie Relation of the long axis of the fetus to the long axis of the uterus. Where the two are parallel it is a longitudinal lie. Variations include transverse or oblique

Fetal pole An extremity or end, e.g. skull or buttocks (when in flexed position)

Fetal position The relation of the denominator on the fetus to a landmark on the fetal pelvis, e.g. occiput facing the left iliopectineal eminence equates to left occipitoanterior (LOA)

Fetal presentation The part of the fetus which is lying in the lower part of the uterus over the cervical os and would therefore 'present' first. Usually head or buttocks but could be face, brow, shoulder, hand, knee or foot

Fever A cause of hyperthermia, produced in response to the presence of pyrogens in the blood

Fistula An abnormal connection between two hollow organs or between a hollow organ and the body surface

Haematuria The presence of blood in the urine

Haemorrhoids Varicosities of the rectal vein. Can occur as a result of chronic repetitive straining to defecate, resulting in enlargement of the venous plexuses

Hydronephrosis A collection of urine in the pelvis of the kidney

Hyperthermia An increase in the core body temperature to >37.5°C. Also referred to as pyrexia: low-grade pyrexia is classified as a temperature up to 38°C, a moderate to high pyrexia is 38–40°C and hyperpyrexia is an excessively high temperature >40°C

Hyperventilation Increased rate and depth of respiration that results in excess carbon dioxide retention

Hypoglycaemia A lowered level of glucose in the blood

Hypothermia A decrease in the core body temperature to 35°C or below

Hypovolaemia A reduction in the circulating blood volume

Induration An area of localised oedema under the skin, often occurring with abnormal reactive hyperaemia

Intrathecal Within the meninges of the spinal cord

Intubation The introduction of a tube into part of the body, e.g. for anaesthesia – introduction of an endotracheal tube into the trachea

Laxative A medicine that helps loosen the contents of the bowel and encourages evacuation. Those with a mild action are referred to as aperients; those with a stronger action are called purgatives

Meatus Opening or passageway, commonly used when talking about the female urethral opening

Micrognathia A receding jaw

Milia Blocked sebaceous glands that appear as small white spots over the nose and cheeks

Nocturia Excessive urination at night

Observer bias Can occur when the previous findings are known and the observer subjectively alters their current findings, e.g. looking at a woman's previous blood pressure reading and expecting the current reading to be very similar

Occiput The back of the head

Oliguria Diminished capacity to form urine. In the baby, this is a urine output of less than 0.5 mL/kg/hour after 48 hours of age

Oxytocin A hormone released by the posterior lobe of the pituitary gland, responsible for contraction of the myometrium and epithelial cells within the breast

Parenterally Administered by any route other than through the mouth

Paronychia A staphylococcal infection of the nail bed, often associated with hangnails

Pharmacokinetics The way the body affects the drug, e.g. absorption, distribution, metabolism and excretion

Phimosis A condition in which the foreskin is retracted back from the glans penis and becomes obstructed, causing swelling and pain

Phlebitis Inflammation of a vein

Polydactyly Extra fingers or toes

Polyuria Voiding large amounts of urine

Postural hypotension Lowering of blood pressure occurring during a change of position from sitting to standing, or lying to upright. Frequently accompanied by dizziness and light-headedness, and sometimes syncope

Proteinuria The presence of protein in the urine

Pruritus Itching caused by localised irritation of the skin, nervous disorders, infection, e.g. fungal infection of the vulva, haemorrhoids, intestinal worms and some forms of jaundice

Rectocoele A prolapse of the lower posterior vaginal wall

Rigors Uncontrollable, involuntary episodes of intense shivering during which the temperature rises rapidly and then decreases after a short period. Often associated with the presence of bacteria or toxins within the blood, it may occur with severe cases of pyelonephritis in pregnancy

Shoulder dystocia Occurs when the normal mechanism of labour stops as the shoulders attempt to enter the pelvic brim but are unable to do so. Occurs with pelvic abnormalities reducing the pelvic diameters or increased bisacromial diameter (distance between the shoulders). This may be due to one (unilateral dystocia) or both (bilateral dystocia) shoulders becoming impacted at the brim or, with a large baby, delay occurs because of the tight fit

Sternal recession Occurs when the alveoli fail to remain inflated and the compliant chest wall begins to collapse around the stiff lungs. The sternum is seen to recess in, rather than expand out, with breathing movements

Stress incontinence As a result of reduced control of the internal and external sphincter, involuntary voiding of small amounts of urine occurs when the intra-abdominal pressure increases, e.g. during bouts of coughing, laughing or sneezing

Subinvolution The uterus is involuting at a slower rate than expected or remains at the same size for several days. This may be due to the presence of retained products of conception, blood clots within the uterus, uterine fibroids or infection. It predisposes to postpartum haemorrhage and is considered a deviation from the normal

Surfactant A phospholipid present in the lungs of the mature newborn that reduces surface tension in the alveoli permitting the lungs to expand and the alveoli to remain inflated

Syndactyly Webbing between the fingers or toes

Tachycardia A fast heart rate, >100 bpm for an adult, >160 bpm for a baby

Tachypnoea Abnormally rapid rate of breathing, >20 per minute

Terminal digit preference Occurs when a person recording blood pressure rounds the measurement to a digit of their preference, most commonly zero

Threshold avoidance Occurs when the blood pressure is recorded as being lower than the threshold for implementing treatment, when the actual measurement is at or above that level

Thrombophlebitis Inflammation of a vein with clot formation

Torticollis Congenital muscular torticollis occurs when the sternomastoid muscle is shortened or tightened on one side

Trisomy 21 A condition where there is an extra chromosome 21 present, resulting in three chromosome 21s in each cell. Also referred to as Down's syndrome

Urgency The need to micturate immediately

Urinary frequency Increased need to micturate, often voiding small amount of urine

Urinary retention The inability of the bladder to empty resulting in an accumulation of urine in the bladder

Urticaria A skin rash characterised by the recurrent appearance of an eruption of wheals (raised stripes of skin, similar to whiplash marks) which results in severe skin irritation

Index

N.B. page numbers in *italic* refer to figures or tables.